Bioethics in the Clinic

Recent and related titles in bioethics

Joseph S. Alper, Catherine Ard, Adrienne Asch, Jon Beckwith, Peter Conrad, and Lisa N. Geller, eds. *The Double-Edged Helix: Social Implications of Genetics in a Diverse Society*

Mark P. Aulisio, Robert M. Arnold, and Stuart J. Youngner, eds. *Ethics Consultation: From Theory to Practice*

Audrey R. Chapman and Mark S. Frankel, eds. *Designing Our Descendants: The Promises and Perils of Genetic Modifications*

Ezekiel J. Emanuel, Robert A. Crouch, John D. Arras, Jonathan D. Moreno, and Christine Grady, eds. *Ethical and Regulatory Aspects of Clinical Research: Readings and Commentary*

Jay Katz. *The Silent World of Doctor and Patient*

John D. Lantos. *The Lazarus Case: Life-and-Death Issues in Neonatal Intensive Care*

Thomas May. *Bioethics in a Liberal Society: The Political Framework of Bioethics Decision Making*

Stuart J. Youngner, Robert M. Arnold, and Renie Schapiro, eds. *The Definition of Death: Contemporary Controversies*

Thomas H. Murray, consulting editor in bioethics

Bioethics in the Clinic

Hippocratic Reflections

Grant R. Gillett, M.B., Ch.B., D.Phil.
Professor in Biomedical Ethics, Bioethics Research Centre,
University of Otago Medical School;
and Neurosurgeon, Dunedin Hospital, New Zealand

The Johns Hopkins University Press
Baltimore and London

© 2004 The Johns Hopkins University Press
All rights reserved. Published 2004
Printed in the United States of America on acid-free paper
9 8 7 6 5 4 3 2 1

The figure in Chapter 13 was drawn by Rudolph J. Zanella.

The Johns Hopkins University Press
2715 North Charles Street
Baltimore, Maryland 21218-4363
www.press.jhu.edu

Library of Congress Cataloging-in-Publication Data

Gillett, Grant, 1950–
   Bioethics in the clinic: Hippocratic reflections /
Grant R. Gillett.
      p. ; cm.
Includes bibliographical references and index.
   ISBN 0-8018-7843-8 (hardcover : alk. paper)
   1. Medical ethics. 2. Clinical medicine—Moral and ethical
aspects. 3. Bioethics. 4. Medicine—Philosophy.
   [DNLM: 1. Ethics, Clinical. 2. Bioethical Issues. 3. Philosophy,
Medical. WB 60 G479 2004] I. Title.
   R724.G549 2004
   174.2—dc22
                                2003015035

A catalog record for this book is available from the British Library.

To Rachel

Contents

Preface and Acknowledgments

The present work is personal and reflective. At one stage I was tempted to call it "Musings of an Overqualified Medical Misfit" or even "The Bioethical Detritus of an Intellectual Magpie," but I thought better of it. "Hippocratic Reflections" captures exactly what I wanted the book to be about.

First, it is clearly medical and historical in its tenor—ranging from the context in which my story as a doctor has been lived out to a variously informed reflection on that story and its happenings. It acknowledges a connection with the past.

It traces a continuity in thought and attitude with those who have gone before, something of which doctors are always aware.

It is grounded in a tradition and in practical experience, two foundations that can steady us in the dizzying maelstrom that is postexistentialist life and praxis.

It is reflective—a quality that many who know me may think I have little of, and indeed I do have constantly to curb my natural impulsivity and romanticism in order to make a go of it.

Be that as it may, these are my reflections on a life lived in the context of, but often straying from the path of, the Hippocratic ideal. I am indebted to many peers and masters for the ways in which they have stimulated and instructed me in my clinical and academic life so that I have become a little more able to reflect. Megabytes in my brain and on my disc mean that I can acknowledge only a select few of those generous (and often very astute) people.

A great influence on me and my attitudes to surgical practice was Philip Wrightson, a natural philosopher, a careful scientist, and a great lover of learning. I learned myself to be a practicing scientist largely from Don Webster, a physiological psychologist at a time when Skinnerianism was all the rage. His patience, regard, and care for me was generous to a fault and helped to set me on the right path. There are many clinicians whom I have admired and greatly appreciated working with over the years, and many of the anecdotes and remarks that appear in this book have been shared or inspired by them. A scrappy and incomplete list would include Gavin Glasgow, Bill Wallis, Graham Macdonald, Lindsay Symons, Alan Richardson, Alan Crockard, Gavin Kellaway, and Norman Grant. A very special acknowledgment must go to my colleague and friend Samir Bishara, my fellow surgeon for a number of years here in Dunedin, who provided an example of clinical dedication and generosity of spirit that one would have to go a long way to match.

The bioethics world has been unfailingly generous to me, but I must single out for special mention Tom and Cynthia Murray, who are more like *whanau* (Maori for family or kin) than anybody else with whom I have spent time anywhere in the world or at almost any time in my life. Other friends and colleagues have also been generous with their time, ideas, and constructive (and sometimes too gentle) criticisms. Carl Elliot, Dewey Ducharme (one of North America's last surviving dualists), Alastair Campbell, Alister Browne, Vincent Sweeney (who must count as one of the most generous hosts and truest friends that one could ever be so lucky as to encounter), Jim Thornton, Bill Fulford (whose energy and encouragement of others seems indefatigable), Peter Skegg (the most reasonable lawyer I have ever met), Philippa Foot, Dick Hare, Michael Lockwood, Stuart Youngner (whose port, cigars, and jokes are never to be forgotten), and Paul Mullen all spring to mind. I am, at present, very fortunate to be working in one of the most vibrant and stimulating bioethics communities that I have ever experienced, with a constant stream of young graduates and exciting visitors who make intellectual endeavor, whether in research or in teaching, more of a pleasure than a chore. It goes without saying that my colleagues in the Otago Centre are an unfailing source of lively conversation and healthy debate. Donald Evans, Neil Pickering, Jing Bao Nie, Lynley Anderson, Monika Clark-Grill, and Clare Gallop, all supported and organized by Vicki Lang, are a formidable team with which to work.

Some people are just special in a way that makes them a profound influence on your life—Nancy Johnson (Snow Queen) is one of these, and I know she has played that role in the lives of many.

Many philosophical colleagues have shown great patience with me and my surgical tendencies to want to bulldoze through the issues to the right answer and to be utterly convinced that I was correct. They include John and Hilary Spanos, Paul Snowdon, Alastair Hannay, Tim Bayne, Kathy Wilkes, Peter Strawson, Alan Musgrave, Andrew Moore, David Ward, Charles Pigden, Eric Matthews, Annette and Kurt Baier, Roger Crisp, and many more than are possible to name here. My students and colleagues in the philosophy department at Otago University have, in general, always provided me with a context in which critique and collegial support have been equally valued.

Over the last few years, I have also received great help and encouragement from friends and colleagues in the Australasian Bioethics Association, which is an innovative and affirmative community of scholars and peers in the bioethics world. The thinking that is fostered in the association is a never-ending source of inspiration and a spur to creative endeavor which I would warmly recommend to anybody thinking of visiting us here in the antipodes.

I must penultimately mention my many colleagues and peers on the staff of Dunedin Hospital who have listened, debated (mostly at lunch but sometimes in the operating theater), and forced me to clarify my ideas in a way that I hope makes them accessible to ordinary clinicians rather than just to bioethicists and philosophers. I am immensely grateful for their patience, interesting conversation, and clinical acumen.

There are also relationships that are so affirmative and enriching that one's "sense of life" is heightened, and their effects are pervasive. These relationships humanize us to the point where we become convinced that every human being, no matter what his or her failings, faults, and foibles might be, is of incomparable and irreplaceable worth (even such a flawed specimen as one knows oneself to be). This book is a culmination of all those influences and many more that I cannot begin to name. It is dedicated to my daughter Rachel, who, among the six of us in our family, is the one most interested in old and classical things. I believe that the Hippocratic writings are exactly the kind of thing that she finds unexpected value in and that delight her (thoroughly modern in other ways) soul.

Note to the reader: The various Hippocratic writings are quoted from the Penguin translation by Geoffrey Lloyd and acknowledged merely by an abbreviated title (The Oath, The Canon, The Science of Medicine, Airs, Waters, Places, Tradition in Medicine, The Sacred Disease, and so on) or by the initials HW.

Bioethics in the Clinic

Introduction

> For a man to be truly suited to the practice of medicine, he must be possessed of a natural disposition for it, the necessary instruction, favourable circumstances, education, industry and time. —THE CANON

I remember being gratified when, early in my philosophy studies, I realized that John Locke was a physician before he was a philosopher. My own career in philosophy crept up on me after I was firmly committed to medicine and had conceived a deep interest in neuroscience. A somewhat unlikely path led me to Oxford, the cultured and deceptively sedate-seeming den of the wild (or, more accurately, untamed) British philosopher, and there my interest developed into a pursuit with a goal and some purpose. The fertile fusion of Oxford philosophy and London neurosurgical practice led to thoughts about issues in medical ethics. Teaching the rudiments of bioethics to students in the health care professions while conducting my own clinical practice (conscious of glasshouses and stone throwing) has drawn me to the Hippocratic roots of medicine.

Hippocrates realized that medicine was uniquely placed to become a science because it necessarily involves observation, intervention, and theory. For a philosopher, medicine abuts metaphysical thinking about human beings against the moral challenges arising in the hurly-burly of clinical practice. Metaphysical and moral issues are vividly manifest in the human suffering that forms the daily bread of clinical life. What is so special about human life? What is the relationship between flesh and blood and the human soul? Is there a kind of life that is worse than death? Can the person die and yet the human organism remain, in some sense, alive? Can souls become sick? What justifies cutting into a living human body? These and other questions lurk in hospital wards, clinical offices, and operating theaters.

How does one cope with all this? Posed as an empirical rather than an ethical question, the answer is alarming. Our profession has an inordinately high rate of marital disruption, substance and alcohol abuse, and suicide. As an ethical question, it directs us toward the moral psychology of human beings in general and medical professionals in particular. An esprit de corps and institutional mechanisms help us to cope; there is also a culture of medicine, but at times certain elements of that culture seem themselves to be pathological. A kind of black humor inhabits the corridors of health care, and every doctor's mind is indelibly inscribed by medical aphorisms and musings.

Some are pensive: "How frail is human flesh and what hubris is required to address its ills."

Some are amusing: "To be an orthopedic surgeon, one needs to be as strong as an ox and at least twice as intelligent."

Some are wry: "A physician knows everything and does nothing; a surgeon knows nothing and does everything, but a pathologist both knows everything and does everything—just a day too late."

When I was a young doctor, I marveled at my superiors' compendious knowledge, their insight and wisdom, and their sanguine judgment. I aspired to those heights of assurance and adjusted my walk so that when I became qualified as a specialist, it had the right unhurried calm, impeccable timing, and suitable gravitas. There was even a time of such certainty when I found that the once-daunting peaks of philosophical scholarship were starting to look accessible, but that period was brief. Experience and reflection soon tempered my once-shining ideals. I like to think that in their place there is a considered judgment (albeit tentative on many issues) and a confidence in process rather than pronouncement on medical and moral issues. At this point of the journey of that most-to-be-envied of callings—the physician philosopher—it is far more often the case that the problem does not seem at all simple and that the response is one that everybody can live with rather than one that is known, beyond doubt, to be right.

Tristram Engelhardt has repeatedly drawn our attention to a divergence of moral values, principles, codes, or laws, claiming that these evince culturally diverse and irreconcilable conceptions of the good life and force us to accept a morality of permission; "there is no content-full, generally accepted, or even dominant account of the good life and of proper conduct." However he concedes that even committed adherents of one world view or moral code "can still understand those whom one acknowledges as moral strangers" (1997, 91). I want to explore the basis of this understanding.

According to the thin—permission-based—conception of morality, we must accept that human beings may differ fundamentally on what they value in life. This idea is taken to imply that communities should develop a process largely conforming to the liberal ideal of the social contract with maximal emphasis on individual freedom and minimal incursion of the needs and demands of one human being into the lives of others. Underlying this moral position is the view that two main axioms are definitive of human moral affairs:

1. We are autonomous individuals, each of whom has his or her own claim to the requisites of happiness.
2. We are all equally capable of arguing for our respective slices of the pie that provides us with those goods.

Principles and theories or codes of moral and politically acceptable conduct emerge as a product of philosophical attempts to codify our dealings with one another given that these axioms are self-evidently true. In fact, as Immanuel Kant noticed, this kind of position offers two possibilities for a fairly universal ethics (or moral theory).

First, an a posteriori universalism would argue as follows: "Look, these things that look so different actually serve similar values or evince the same principles." This is fine as far as it goes, but, as Kant argues in relation to general epistemology, such a stance merely reveals to us what tends to happen in the world as we find it. A certain kind of philosopher, impressed by the need for philosophy to be true to the real world as it is would say—"OK, but that *is* as good as it gets. The only thing you get a priori, in terms of knowledge is what we call *analytic truths*—propositions that are true by virtue of the meanings of the words comprising them—and, however you dress them up, moral truths (if there are any) are not like that. This kind of empiricist naturalism—naturalistic philosophers think we ought to ground philosophy on what the world is really like around here—might be persuaded by this line. It says nothing about what the world should be like.

Kant himself thought otherwise, arguing that we can identify truths that are synthetic or substantial and that tell us about the things that really concern us and yet can be debated a priori. This occurred in two areas: *epistemology,* where he argued on the basis of how things must be for there to be human life as we know it, and *ethics,* in which he argued that reason alone can reveal to us how human beings should conduct themselves.

I tend to agree with Kant and am going to offend many scholars in ethical theory by trying to argue (contra Engelhardt) that there are a priori moral truths that emerge from a plausible kind of naturalism.

Most moral philosophers claim that if there are moral truths, they are of one of two kinds: either they are sui generis (i.e., of their own unique kind in human experience) and normative (they tell us what we ought to do), or they are derived from reflecting on nature (and thus of a more familiar kind) and not genuinely normative but merely descriptive. In the first camp we find those who think we can discern moral truths that intrinsically commend certain ways of acting and thus have normative force (unlike typical statements of bare fact). The second camp sees moral thought as a kind of all-inclusive calculation of what complex of rules tends to make things go in a direction that most people favor. One then opts into that (statistically normal or politically dominant) order depending either on the extent to which one's own desires fall into line with those of others or on the desire to fit into an already formed human society with certain regulatory principles. The first position—intuitionism, despite its appeal, has always seemed somewhat arbitrary to those of us with a humanistic bent. In fact, the foundational moral truths for those who take such views are usually promulgated by those in a position of power. Thus, for instance, the intuitively obvious moral truth that each human being is an economic and psychological individual who ought to be treated so as to maximize his liberty has always been promulgated by relatively privileged white males.

What options, then, are open to an ethical naturalist apart from the hypothetical imperatives arising from desires to fit into some sociocultural setting? The question is usefully approached through a crucial ambiguity in Rawlsian theory. Does John Rawls give an account of humanity and morality that ought to have universal sway, or is the myth of the equally empowered community of all human beings just a good basis on which to proceed in moral reasoning? At certain points in his exposition Rawls veers close to an Aristotelianism of the first kind, and at others he seems to be arguing for a thin (neo-)Kantianism that approximates the second.

Rawls's discussion of reflective equilibrium implies that a crucial role is played by competent moral judges who can balance broad moral principles or values and more particular moral intuitions. Such a person is open-minded, reasonable in his approach to conflict and argumentation, adequately knowledgeable about the world and human affairs, aware of his own biases, and able to appreciate the values and interests of others (Rawls 1951). These qualities are directly reminiscent of the characteristics of phronesis or the practical wisdom required to live a virtuous life as a rational and social being. I argue that this is the key to a series of truths about human beings that are descriptive of human life and yet have normative force (or direct normative implications) for how we should live.

Like Kant, I argue that secure knowledge emerges from axioms that are non-negotiable and definitive of right thinking in a given area of human thought. If moral thinking concerns that which it is right or good for human beings to do with their lives, then it comprises statements about what one ought or ought not to do. I opt for a naturalistic version of the Kantian claim that moral truths are synthetic a priori truths reflectively evident to practically informed reason.

I claim that the naturalistic axioms on which we should found morality are as follows:

1. Human beings share a biological form or nature.
2. We are all members of an interactive community.
3. Different individuals have different perspectives on human situations.
4. Each perspective arises in a discourse that positions the subject in the human world and attaches value to the things that happen.
5. Much is to be gained by sharing the knowledge arising in different discourses.

These are all descriptive propositions (and therefore uncontentiously naturalistic), but an adaptive response to them (a response grounded in practical reason) generates moral or prescriptive theorems and corollaries that are plausibly definitive for human flourishing. These theorems fall into two groups, the first concerning the individual human being and his or her flourishing and the second concerning our interactions with one another.

Theorems:

a. A human being must belong somewhere or have a place to stand.
b. A human being is a unique individual.

Corollaries:

i.   We should appreciate the diverse knowledges that different individuals bring to any situation.
ii. We should attend to silences and discern why they are happening.
iii. We should be wary of moral "truth."
iv. We should give special attention to those who are experienced participants in a moral situation.

Theorems

The first two foundational theorems ground all the corollaries, and, because they arise from the general naturalistic axioms of human morality, they have fairly universal implications. The foundations are naturalistic in that they emerge from our conception of what a human life is and must be if the human being concerned is going to survive, grow, and develop into adulthood, but taken together they evidently generate the substantive normative corollaries that follow them.

A Place to Stand

Every human being belongs (even immaculate conception falls short of spontaneous origin), in that each has emerged from some womb or other (usually as a result of the conjoining of tissue from two human beings—cloning entails that there might be only one immediate forbear for some of us). If, once created, the human being is not nurtured through both intrauterine and early extrauterine existence, then that individual will not survive. Nurture consists of psychological support and care, so survival is conjoined with well-being. During development a human being enjoys relationships of a type that create the need to belong or share with others in significant ways throughout life. These relationships and the shaping that they bring about are therefore formative in human well-being (or its opposite), and there are discoverable constraints on that process in terms of psychological health. This fact is colorfully captured by the Maori phrase "a place to stand" and the concept of the people of the land—*tangata whenua* (where *whenua* is used to denote both the placenta and the tribal land). We are slowly learning that a sense of one's roots is essential for the health and well-being of any person and that its absence is a powerful source of discontent.

Belonging is, however, only one foundation for the human journey; the second is the room to develop as an individual.

Living One's Own Story

That each individual human being is unique (genetically and discursively) implies that every person is an irreplaceable resource for us all and should be valued as such. Of course, overriding values may occur from time to time, but placing value on the individual as an individual (acting with some independence from a platform of belonging) is plausibly the right way to go in the light of what kind of critters we are.

Corollaries: Our Relationships

The corollaries follow from the basic position, and they put substantial value on things that many people cherish (especially those who have turned to postmodernism as a reaction to white middle-class values). These valued things include moral responses such as learning from open discourse with others, a spirit of humility, listening to the voice of the oppressed, overcoming serious injustices that blight the development of individuals, sharing cultural and moral perspectives, deriding the exploitation of others and the concentration of economic or political power in the hands of an elite, and so on. All these beliefs about what we ought to do and be emerge as rational entailments of who we are and what makes us human. What is more, this set of beliefs and attitudes is particularly suited to medical ethics or bioethics, in which the power of the white middle-class male establishment can prejudice who will prevail in any meeting of so-called equals in a clinical setting. (The winners always tend to be either the doctors or the lawyers.) Thus, in the face of a claim that clinical ethics is bound to be hamstrung by diverse moral views, we say, "It ain't necessarily so!" We may well be able to find solutions to clinical dilemmas that all the parties can live with.

The quote from *Porgy and Bess* is particularly apt to the present discussion because appeals to the bible (whether that be *The Holy Bible, The Principles of Biomedical Ethics,* or anything with the word "foundations" in its title) come under intense scrutiny from a clinically informed and interactive approach to bioethics in which the skills of a good health care professional, and those skills that go to make up practical wisdom in general, are an essential ingredient.

For the sake of memorability (medical educators always use mnemonics), we could claim that ethical thought rests not only on axioms but also in fact on a formula.

$$E = MC^3$$

E = empathic understanding, M = moral tradition, C = consciousness—yours[1], mine[2], and mine of yours[3]. The aim of the formula is merely to reinforce the idea that the core idea of morality is intersubjectivity. A moral standard has intersubjective or even objective content such as that arising from a moral tradition (which might be no more than a family ethos or narrative context that creates expectations of how one ought to behave). The attitudes and intuitions that arise from living within that tradition equip one to meet moral challenges (for instance, whether to tell the truth about the result of a test or the decision as to whether or not to save somebody's life). I am influenced by my awareness of the complexities of the situation and the feelings evoked in me, the same kind of awareness on your side, and my awareness of your awareness and what you are experiencing. Only as I open myself to this tripartite consciousness (C^3) can I hope to evince the moral sensibility and *phronesis* that are self-transforming and conducive to eudaemonia in myself and my fellow human beings. Sometimes my ability to be conscious in this way is attenuated by cultural and positional distance.

We see this well illustrated in the discussion of "the case of the empty head," an issue arising in a New Zealand health care setting. (At this point, some readers might want to pursue the discussion in Appendix A, "On Metaethics," but it is mainly aimed at those who have philosophical scruples about the direction in which we are headed. It is not necessary to read if substantive bioethical issues or clinical ethics is your main interest.)

Part I / Foundations

CHAPTER ONE

The Case of the Empty Head

Cultures, Values, and Bioethics

> There are men who have turned the abuse of the arts and the sciences
> into an art in itself and, although they would not confess it themselves,
> their aim nevertheless is simply to display their own knowledge.
>
> —SCIENCE OF MEDICINE

How to Begin Doing Bioethics: A Case

Bioethics sometimes merely obfuscates what is already a difficult clinical decision by tabling a number of impressive-looking cards whose relevance to the situation is far from evident. Even worse, it can create a kind of expertise that disempowers both physician and patient. It should do neither. It should rather encourage and stimulate useful reflection on clinical practice so as to improve one's thinking about the human reality that is a clinical problem.

Many of us involved in bioethics have been hooked by a case that captures our interest and acts as an irritant to a mind comfortable in its own understanding of the world. Even after we have devised standard answers for dilemmas about informed consent, rescuing the at-risk (and possibly severely impaired) human being, abortion, euthanasia, and so on, we may still find that our ready solutions are inadequate the moment we begin to speak to members of different cultures and subcultures. That certain foundational ideas such as privacy and personal choice may seem curiously parochial raises the question: On what grounds can one say that certain values should guide us or that a certain practice is wrong outside the moral framework provided by a particular culture? This question has received various responses ranging from a fairly straightforward commitment to values based in medical conceptions of benefit and harm (Kopelman 1997) to a robust skepticism (Engelhardt 1997). Kopelman argues for certain unquestionable goods and harms related to international classifications of diseases. Engelhardt focuses on the different conceptions of the good life that are fostered in different moral communities and the different understandings of right and wrong that emerge from them.

Clearly there are serious disagreements about right and wrong, but there have been just as serious and sometimes cataclysmic disagreements about matters of fact even though a sense of convergence in beliefs is usually taken as a mark of progress and the acquisition of knowledge in scientific affairs. Similarly, one is sometimes struck by a sense of growing convergence in moral belief as "the global village" increasingly allows moral conversation between individuals and diverse groups of people. The tendency to convergence suggests that there is something about human intercourse that is likely to create an inclusive moral community and that the opinion prevalent in a given society or group at a given time is not the only source of moral authority. What is more, minority views have, in the past, been sufficiently persuasive to bring about moral reform of a majority, so it seems that there is a source of moral insight apart from the most popular or widespread view in a given society. This possibility gives us hope that we might achieve a rapprochement between diverse cultural groups sufficient for the emergence of a transcultural or universal ethics.

I do believe that we can converge on a transcultural or fairly universal basis for some key moral commitments, and I am encouraged by actual examples that evoke similar intuitions in competent moral judges from very different cultural contexts. Such is the case in a (minimally fictionalized) New Zealand example. (Similar stories have now emerged in many countries.)

The Case of the Empty Head

A young New Zealand Maori man of Tainui descent died from a severe head injury sustained in a road accident. He was, by law, subject to a coroner's postmortem examination. His body was returned to his relatives for the normal Maori mourning and burial rites. He was duly taken to the *marae,* or tribal meeting place, for a *tangi*. A central part of the tangi involves friends and relatives talking to the dead person, saying things that had not been said during his life, and farewelling him. This typically occurs over three to four days as the people involved gather, and all have their opportunity to say what has been unsaid or what is, in the light of his death, important. After this ceremony, he was buried. Subsequently, the relatives discovered that his body was returned without the brain, which was being held for delayed postmortem investigation. They were outraged.

If you are at all like me, and here I should say that in my neurosurgical and philosophical guises I am comfortable with the idea of brain death, then you intuitively understand the moral outrage of this young man's relatives. Notice the paradox. On the one hand, I believe that there is no difference in function between a dead brain and no brain at all. On the other, I feel the outrage of the family that the young man had an empty head at his *tangi*. My "rational" scientific self cannot understand the significance that my reactive self has found in this event. In fact, the gap between rational considerations and symbolic considerations has reached new heights recently with the discovery that in many places organs such as hearts have been retained by hospitals and medical research establishments and that individuals have been buried "heartless." Many folk recognize that, seen in one way, this means nothing in that the person's heart no longer has any useful function in a dead body. But in another way, a body without a heart or brain is hugely different in meaning from a body without a kidney or liver. This gap between the engaged reactive self, sensitive to symbolism and the human impact of events, and the "rational" abstracted self, I am now convinced, gives us an important response to arguments such as Engelhardt's that appeal to the wide differences between world views and varying conceptions of the good life.

Engelhardt argues that there are "as many secular accounts of morality, justice, fairness, as there are major religions" and concludes in favor of "different moral worlds" (1997, 91, 92). He contends that it is impossible to resolve substantial moral controversies by rational argument, which he equates, apparently, with the calculation of consequences on the basis of intuitively given and nonrational value commitments. He despairs of a substantive appeal to "human nature," "human sympathies," or "the character of rationality" (93) to address (in any rational spirit) the value diversity that he discerns or to arbitrate between competing conceptions of the good. Therefore he opts for the liberal notion of "authority . . . drawn from the consent of those who participate" (95) as the only rational basis on which to erect moral standards in a pluralist secular society. The claim for "permission as the source of moral authority" implies that we must regard moral narratives as inevitably bound to communities and cultures

(97) and that whole communities are not meaningfully corrigible in relation to their value commitments.

An argument for this claim, however, requires not only the existence of moral disagreement (examples of which are hard to find in Engelhardt's work) but also that basic concepts such as "caring" are the product of the moral narratives of particular communities; "it is only within such narratives and communities that one can, in fact, learn in a content-full fashion what it is to care or to have a good moral character" (1997, 97). But these arguments do not clinch the case.

The first reason for skepticism or moral relativism—apparent moral disagreement, even if well supported—is inconclusive because marked differences in practice at morally significant junctures in human life can arise from substantially similar value commitments. Praxis is a matter of habit (the well-worn inscriptions on a subjective body) and not totally amenable to reason, so the same deep-seated moral attitudes may be expressed very differently. For instance, Christians, Jews, Hindus, Tibetan Buddhists, and Parsis show their reverence for the dead in a variety of ways, some of which are regarded by members of other groups as being abhorrent and disrespectful (such as internment, mummification, donation for scientific dissection, cremation, dismemberment and feeding to vultures, or the towers of silence).

The second reason (the development of morality within specific traditions) is also insufficient because even if, in fact, one can develop a substantive morality only within a historical community and set of relationships, it is not necessarily true that the varying settings will produce incommensurable fundamental moral beliefs. It is possible that, as suggested in my introduction, even markedly different cultures and communities share certain universal moral attitudes or values informing those diverse practices. If different practices arising in different cultural settings may in fact result from deeply shared moral convictions and ways of dealing with the major life and health crises that face human beings, then there is real hope for rapprochement in bioethics, especially clinical bioethics.

Pellegrino and Kopelman are both quite ready to take a more direct route to the delineation of the values that should guide bioethics.

Orthodoxy and Imperialism

The orthodox medical model of human illness is committed to the idea that there is a right or best answer to each problem—the correct diagnosis, the best treatment, and so on. Thus in medical ethics there is a widespread attitude that there is a best possible answer about each case. This answer is usually formulated and outlined in rationally structured statements that express a belief, describe an action, or articulate a principle. This approach has characteristically led to methods of analysis that focus on a few principles based in some ethical paradigm (Beauchamp and Childress, 1989) or even, in some cases, a quasigeometrical "grid" (Seedhouse 1992). The preferred method is used to process the data from the case and to resolve the ethical questions involved. The principles most often relied on are *autonomy, beneficence, nonmaleficence,* and *justice,* and although they often conflict in actual cases, there is usually assumed to be a correct weighting that will yield the uniquely right solution to the problem.

Pellegrino argues for a link between medicine and its aims, and a substantial ethics based on "healing, helping, caring and health" (1997, 76). He and Thomasma ground the ethics of medicine in the ends that medicine seeks to attain (1988). Because of its vital link with the functions that make life go well, they echo the Hippocratics, regarding medicine as a very "natural science" and its practitioner as a *phronimos*—a person of practical wisdom, able to skillfully apply guiding principles to particular cases. Pellegrino understandably puts an emphasis on beneficence and the obligations of the doctor—"beneficence not mistakenly equated with paternalism, but beneficence-in-trust, beneficence which fuses respect for the person of the patient with the obligation not just to prevent or remove harm, but to do good" (1994, 363). I have a great deal of sympathy for this approach and its evident links to the legacy of Hippocrates but, for the minute, will pursue the idea that individuals from different cultures can respond deeply to each others' stories and develop moral empathy for them. I think this idea offers far more hope for cross-cultural initiatives in bioethics than the idea of coming up with abstract principles to which diverse groups might whole-heartedly subscribe.

Attempting to define such principles is difficult. For one thing, there are serious disagreements about weighty terms like *the sanctity of life*. For some thinkers, this means absolute commitment to saving life no matter what the quality, while others take it to imply reverence for what they consider to be truly human life. The first group regard the second as talking about quality rather than sanctity, but the second group deride the first for an unreasoned commitment to biological life rather than a holistic awareness of what makes human life truly human. *Autonomy* is similarly problematic. Does respect for autonomy indicate respect for any wish expressed by the person concerned or rather a commitment to comply with requests that meet some standard of reasonableness? If the latter, one must then ask, a la Engelhardt and MacIntyre (1988): "Whose rationality?"

We should also ask what counts as satisfying one of these principles. Does one respect autonomy by preserving an individual from his more foolish life choices so that he can take an otherwise precluded action when he regains his perfect mind? A friend of mine always avoids tetanus shots because he hates injections. Should we trick him into having one because if he gets tetanus he will need rescue at great cost, with uncertain probabilities of survival, huge risk to his ongoing well-being, and highly intrusive methods? Some would say that interventions in this spirit are paternalistic and, on that ground alone, are to be rejected.

And how ought one to weigh the relative importance of multiple principles in a real-life conflict? For instance, the principle of justice might suggest that one should not advance a particular patient before others on a waiting list, but the principle of beneficence might urge you to take serious note of her particular needs at that moment. How does one proceed? When we ask what a principle requires us to do in a given situation, we are (in some small way) negotiating the meaning of the principle itself because the meaning of any proposition partly depends on the conditions under which it would be judged to apply by a range of competent thinkers. (This is a common theme in hermeneutics and can be philosophically grounded in the work of Gadamer or Wittgenstein.)

Consider the following fairly basic questions: Is life itself always a benefit or may it sometimes be a harm? May there be conditions of survival that are worse than death? A Jewish ethicist may argue that where there is breath, there is infinitely valuable human life, which cannot be endangered by any of our actions. A Roman Catholic, Protestant, or secular ethicist may argue that there are certain states of living in which the value of the life has been destroyed (John Paul II, Thielicke 1970) and therefore may accept that brain death is death.

So far, this may seem like grist to the relativist and minimalist mill, and that Engelhardt is vindicated. What makes it seem inevitable that we should get stuck in moral disagreement is the idea that there are propositions about what should or must be done, couched in general terms, to which we would all agree if we shared a moral vision. Yet that is not the only possibility for a basis on which we might conduct our ethical lives.

If we could find some non-principle-based ground for moral discussion (for instance, what Nussbaum calls a "shared sense of life"), bioethics and its methods of deliberation would need rethinking. My hope is to find this ground in shared stories and the sense of life or worth that emerges from those stories, whatever their cultural setting. In fact, we are increasingly able to find in stories a sympathy and identification with characters whose community of engagement is vastly different from our own. Consider, for example, the appeal to white middle-class Westerners of books like *The God of Small Things* (Arundhati Roy), *The Sorrow of War* (Bao Ninh), and *Possessing the Secret of Joy* (Alice Walker). Sharing stories may not give us a method of solving ethical problems, but it may yield an inclusive set of foundations on which to discuss culturally diverse ethical discourse. This potential becomes clear if we look at the exclusive approaches to ethics that got our problem going in the first place.

There are two inherently exclusive approaches to ethics: *ethical imperialism* (as in the wide dissemination of the four principles of medical ethics) and *unprincipled relativism*. Both are kinds of hegemony that seek to take the dominant discursive position and silence other views, and both are highly abstract, tending to focus on moral rules or general principles rather than stories or particular situations.

In the first—or imperialist—view, we tell those holding other views that they have to change their way of doing things, what they believe in, or both. This kind of imperialism may succeed in ethics, as it has so evidently done in science and technology, through the spread of Western highly technologized medicine (and its intellectual hangers-on). In the second view, we concede that, whereas we might agree on "the facts," there is no principled basis for an agreement on our value commitments. Kopelman and others believe that a focus on medicine alone gives us a robust argument against divergent views. However, we are now beginning to realize that there are problems with this kind of fundamental secular orthodoxy because it carries with it an epistemic commitment to a theory of knowledge based on a sharp difference between facts and values and a moral commitment to what we might call the liberal ideal.

The sharp divide between facts and values is derived from the thesis that statements of fact are somehow direct reflections of observations, whereas statements of value, or morally relevant judgments, are not directly related to states of affairs. I argue that both statements of fact and statements with moral significance are closely related to shared human perceptions and that the latter are distinguished only because they concern aspects of situations in which people interact with each other. (The metaethical argument is summarized in Appendix A.)

The liberal credo is that people are free individuals with their own autonomy and rationally ordered preferences. The goods they seek are usually thought to be consumable and therefore gained competitively, creating problems of resource allocation. Satisfying the preferences of one individual depletes the resources available, and doing so can be based only on rational, individualistic considerations that command agreement, permission, or consent from the competing individuals. On the liberal account, individual preferences are legitimately constrained only when satisfying those preferences would cause harm to others. The corresponding theory of justice rests on the axioms I have rejected—autonomy and self-sufficiency in advocacy.

This view of individuals and their sociocultural relations does not fit well with many traditions outside the Western world. To exclude the insights of those traditions or neutralize them by squeezing them into the individualistic liberal framework is to take an exclusive or hegemonic approach to ethics. The intriguing possibility is that the alternative (and threatened) traditions and aspects of their spirituality may have something to offer "the free West" which it no longer has the resources to discern by itself.

It is also detrimental to ethical discourse to shrug our shoulders and accept social, political, or cultural relativism. "You have your beliefs and I have mine" or "You do things your way and we do them our way and they are different" ends the rational discussion of values within a community or human group. Indeed, that stance may represent a failure of imagination as to the human reality underlying moral thought and therefore obstruct philosophical inquiry in bioethics (or morality in general). For instance, the acceptance of the limited aspirations of peasants as an intrinsic part of a rural way of life may blunt our awareness of the frustration and discrimination that are part of such an attitude. To uncritically accept the irreducible relativity of values is to close the moral discussion in such a way as to exclude searching moral discourse about fundamental issues touching human life and death. It is also a potential betrayal of the abused, oppressed, and silenced minorities in some cultures to allow the moral regimes dictating their lives to persist with an abhorrent moral vision on the grounds that it is in accordance with the prevailing cultural values. Kopelman (1997), in fact, offers an initial counter to complacency and relativism when she argues that none of us really believe that our own or other cultures are so unified and harmonious that we should merely fit in with societal mores. We believe that moral dissent in human affairs is possible and worthwhile. History has repeatedly shown that individuals can discover the true importance of values that are systematically discounted in certain sociohistoricocultural settings, and we often admire such dissenters. Therefore, it behooves us to listen for and attend to the voices of protest in other cultures. If, for instance, it emerges that there is a widespread disempowerment and silencing of women in cultures that have rampant HIV infection or that perform female circumcision, then we cannot take dominant group pronouncements about cultural integrity as being the end of the debate. The combined voice of abusers is not a good place to ground reasoning about the morality of abuse. But if we are going to question the ethics dominant in a given cultural setting, where do we go to ground that questioning?

Inclusive Ethics and Moral Phenomenology

The current approach begins with the view that we all have in common and hold to be valuable certain types of human experience, such as the experience of being nurtured or the experience of having a friend. Certain other experiences are universally recognized as bad, such as rejection, callous disregard by others, and cruelty or vindictiveness. These experiences are signified or given meaning within a particular cultural context so that one might not recognize rejection when it comes from an unfamiliar cultural group. Yet this does not detract from the central point that rejection, when recognized, is *felt* as being bad no matter which culture you are living in or arise from. Such feelings are universal narrative moments of human subjectivity.

Different cultural significations (ways of giving meaning to situations) do give rise to diverse individual narratives (arising out of different cultural traditions) that illuminate moral situations in ways that the hearers of those narratives may not have anticipated, but we must be alert to the possibility that at bottom there is a kind of convergence of these "felt" values. Thus, we might be surprised by things we hear in others' narratives, but nevertheless we may come to comprehend why they tell their story the way they do. Consider the following case.

> Dr. Abelsen is talking with a Navajo patient who believes that words are thought to summon the spirits of the things that the words refer to. The doctor, wishing to get informed consent, speaks about the need for a splenectomy, which has a small but definite risk of death. Because the odds are overwhelmingly on the side of a good outcome, he wonders why his patient is reluctant to enter the conversation. He cannot make any progress until he is taken aside by a family member and informed that it is considered very bad to mention death or misfortune on

the occasion that a decision is being made because a shadow of death or misfortune then attaches itself to the acts that follow the decision.

If the doctor is sufficiently open minded, he might perhaps remark, "I have
never seen it that way" and learn from the experience. If he is a dyed-in-the-
wool exclusivist about medical knowledge and ethical procedure, however, he
will probably make some silencing and dismissive remark about old wives' tales
or superstition. This kind of remark can escape unwittingly from us before we
have time to reflect on the implications of the narrative we have heard for those
to whom we are talking. It is easy to treat what is significant to another with
implicit disdain. Once we realize the significance of the experience to the other,
we can then avoid the insensitivity, contempt, or rejection that we have inad-
vertently shown. Indeed, I would argue that if we engage with the other person
at the level of lived human experience, then what we should do becomes clear.

Being open to the meaning of situations for others and, as is inevitable when
we engage with narrative, inhabiting the subjectivity of another, even if only
briefly, are the fundamental moral dimensions for a view of ethics that aims to
take seriously the lived experience of moral situations rather than subordinat-
ing them to preformed and abstract metaphysical, epistemological, or ethical
assumptions. In fact, many of the most basic beliefs and abstract moral principles that divide cultures are "bracketed" (or set to one side) by a narrative or postmodern approach aiming to get in touch with the subjectivities of a discourse
on whose workings one is reflecting. That reflection questions the influences and
presuppositions of the discourse and is closely related to certain key themes in
postmodernism that, somewhat paradoxically, give us an alternative to a transcultural ethical impasse.

Phenomenology, Convergence, and Narrative

Where would we look for hope in seeking common ethical ground for diverse
views of life? It is instructive that members of different cultures tend to converge
on common intuitions such as the mystery of death, the special nature of the
mother-child relationship, and the need to belong. I believe that each of these
deeply implicates human beings as subjective bodies who are inscribed by certain profound experiences at key points in life. We are at heart (or in the roots of
our being) feeling and relating bodies who develop attributions of individual
selfhood as we enter into discourse and realize that each of us has a voice that

emanates from a given position in that discourse. The position I occupy is itself given by the body, and the body is the participant in the experience that it shares with others and through which, as I have noted, it becomes inscribed by that experience.

The body loses animation and subjectivity in death and therefore becomes other than human in any full-blooded sense of that word. At the beginning of life, the body experiences the nestling into, nurturing, and being held that bonds the child to its mother. The body moves in a familiar, comfortable, and unselfconscious way among those people who define the place where one belongs. In these experiences the body reacts to and resonates with the bodies of others; it is, we might say, inscribed by these experiences and the discourse that permeates them. Out of these patterns of relationship and inscribed subjectivity, each of us fashions a discursive narrative that becomes the lived self.

> I cannot feel comfortable in this place. There is no bustle, no mess, no people who fuss in irritating and yet strangely reassuring ways. Oh, I know that the nurses are very caring and competent, but I am out of place here and do not know how to make decisions or what I feel confident about any more.

> This is weird. Such a lot is happening. There are so many machines and so much information being displayed. Everybody is always rushing about so much and doing so many things. How can anybody find that place of calm, quiet certainty, and order in which good decisions can be made about me and my life? I do not feel safe here.

Both patients voice (each in her own way) the problem that many patients feel in understanding what goes on in a medical setting. The patient, on unfamiliar turf and trying to discern (as we all are all the time) what is OK to do around here, does not know how she should feel. Postmodern terminology asks "what kind of subjectivity is legitimated in this discursive milieu," but that just rephrases the subjective response. The discursive process allows us to form our narratives on the basis of bodily engagement and subjective response in a framework or context of legitimation. Legitimation determines what counts as reason, reflection, and right conduct in the construction of one's lived autobiography. MacIntyre (1984) argues that a tradition—nurturing my discursive self as meat, drink, and oxygen nurtured my bodily self—equips us with meaning, reason, and the techniques of reflection. These holistically connected discourses, subjectivities, reason, and values define moral situations.

The relativist stops the inquiry about morality and ethics at legitimation, but underneath is something more primitive (or bodily). We have a means of responding to others that has been inscribed on our bodies from before birth. We know when somebody likes us or is ignoring us because we are exquisitely and intuitively sensitive to these things. Any particular cultural narrative must draw on these foundations for the fundamental recognition of what is good or bad for beings like me. The actions of others toward me and the way I appear as an embodied being in their eyes is a primitive of my experience. Jean-Paul Sartre got this right when he noticed that the look of the other is a radical given whenever I encounter it (and no mere abstract conclusion from the other's behavior [1958, 268]). I cannot encompass what is seen by the look of the other, and I am aware that it can transfix me as an object for the other in a way that I never fully grasp. Jacques Lacan extended this into his discussion of the mirror phase of human development (1977). My learning to "resonate" with the other gives me an entrée into his subjectivity, and I can begin to appreciate my situation in interpersonal terms, but without it I have no hope. Establishing this link that is also a distinction (Carson refers to this as "the hyphen" in the doctor-patient relationship [2002]) is therefore much more basic than any principles as the foundations of ethics.

This relational basis for ethics deserves attention when health care professionals are told to maintain a "professional distance" in relationships with their patients. At its worst, this may leave the patient adrift at a time of vulnerability, uncertainty, and fear. Of course, we must conduct ourselves professionally, but we must also realize that we are confronted by persons who desperately need a companion at certain points in their life journeys. Discourse has forced us to consider culture; we must ask, therefore, whether culture can disrupt our relationships and obscure what is common between one human creature and others. Sometimes it does seem that lines of culture and ethnicity can obscure the fact that we are fellow creatures who share common affections (and afflictions) of the body and mind. But depending on how open I am to the other human being before me, regardless of the distances between us, differences in culture and discourse need not undermine the possibility of shared understandings of what morality demands. This is shown in at least two ways.

First, there is the moral reformer. Such a person works from within a culture, having been properly socialized to its norms, to change some moral stance taken by that culture. To succeed, the moral reformer must engage the consciences of others in their society. (The reason why they succeed is often due to political and economic factors that independently support their project of reform, but the tug of conscience is nevertheless an important factor in the change.) That possibility indicates sources for the imperatives of conscience that are somewhat independent of prevailing cultural norms. I believe these sources are found at the more immediately interpersonal level where empathic voices resonate in the experience of one's primary being in the world as a nurtured and relational body.

Second, conflicting subjectivities can be part of any person's experience. A given subjectivity arises and locates one within a given discourse and is, in part, the product of that discourse. Yet some discourses are discordant with others, and it is rare that any discourse, however influential in one's life, acts monolithically, given that we are all multiply located (and increasingly so). Therefore, one is not always insulated from the effects of discordant discourses. In the face of these intersecting voices and regimes of moral legitimation (however informal), most of us define and modify our self-conception through internal conflicts in subjectivity.

> Ben loved his involvement with his basketball friends, none of whom rated scholastic achievement very highly at all. He also wanted to enter medical school, in part to satisfy his own urge to help and heal and in part to repay his mother's investment of love and encouragement. The problem was that the image of the student studying hard for grades sufficient to earn entry to medical school did not sit well with the image of the neighborhood basketball court. After seeing the film *Good Will Hunting*, he found it somewhat easier to hold it all together.

When words and discourses conflict with each other in the shape they give to our personal narrative, something must guide or ground the subjectivity being produced. I have argued that we are subdiscursively grounded in the experiences that matter to us as relational and engaged bodily beings. I believe that these experiences have inherently to do with nurture, being cared for, receiving from and giving to others, feeling that one belongs, and those other intersubjective things that mean so much to each of us.

Grounding of Moral Claims in Phenomenology

To ground a moral claim or claims is to show some basis on which it should be upheld. This can happen in two ways:

1. The moral claim is grounded in a set of basic beliefs.
2. The moral ground is lived experience.

I have obviously favored the latter, but I have also espoused critical reflection in the form of an openness to the lived experience of the other, with a deconstructive bent. The deconstructive bent allows one to examine the genealogy of one's intuitions and their relation to one's own discursive position and commitments. Lived experience interrogates those commitments and intuitions. However, the project of favoring lived experience is, at a stroke, both postmodern and Aristotelian—an apparent paradox.

We ought also to notice that a basic moral claim can have two kinds of scope:

A. It can apply to beings sufficiently like me to accept it as I do.
B. It can apply to all human beings.

There are natural affinities between types of ground and scope statements. A claim grounded in an unassailable proposition such as "To take the life of another human being is wrong" is, prima facie, likely to have a scope of type A. The claim appeals to and can be debated by those who share with me certain basic beliefs and not others. An experiential ground is, however, inherently suited to all who share the experience. In both cases, the grounds can be questioned. In the former case, this questioning involves articulating arguments and reasons to maintain or reject some identifiable position. In the latter case, the questioning involves reflection on experience, one's dispositions and reactions, the meanings that informed those, and their sustainability in light of that experience. If the relevant experiences are such things as being born and nurtured, being accepted and cared for, belonging to some group of communicating individuals, being hurt, being excluded, and so on, then those experiences are universal to human beings, whatever their culture. Such experiences depend only on my bodily and discursive engagement with others, and participating in a situation of the relevant types causes me to feel a certain way as a result (for instance, if I see an infant being pounded against a wall). Thus, propositional grounds for moral judgment look unlikely to achieve universal scope, whereas an experiential basis seems much more likely to do so.

Experiential grounds are uncommon in moral theory except where there is careful attention paid to moral sense, moral perception, relationships, and praxis. Moral theorists of this type make appeals like "Can't you see that this is cruel?" or "Attend to your reaction, to what you feel, and what they tell you about the moral properties of this situation" or "Feel the vibes!" Such appeals depend, in ways that I try to enunciate, on a kind of narrative engagement in which the lived experience of others is sensed and incorporated into one's reflective practices.

Postmodern ethicists are skeptical about universal, rationally defensible moral beliefs and therefore focus instead on the context in which statements are made and things done. For this reason they are far better placed to embrace an experiential grounding for moral thinking (unless they make the mistake of detaching words and their significance from the real world contexts in which they function, as in certain varieties of structuralism, sociocultural nominalism, or other kinds of linguistic idealism). I prefer the form of life- or praxis-based approach to meaning found in the later Wittgenstein. Wittgenstein notices that words, though powerful instruments of mind making, are grounded in practice—shared experience. Moral theorists after Wittgenstein, like some postmodernists, should therefore attend closely to power, to the ways in which we operate on each other in discourse, and to the effects of those operations on the subjectivities to which our bodies give rise. In these actual dealings with each other, habits and reactions become inscribed on our bodies and shape our participation in human forms of life.

Power is part of the experiential grounding of an ethical claim, in that one can often detect when another person is acting in a controlling or dominating way without being able to articulate what is happening. Indeed, one's body will stiffen and exclude certain kinds of conversation without one being able to say why. The ability to articulate, discursively frame, and then reflect on the way one has been treated develops as we grow in our lived knowledge of one another and ourselves. If the individual occupies an oppressed position, then the individual can become very sensitive to subtle forms of domination and silencing. Yet the experience is two-edged in that it can both sensitize the individual and severely impair the creative development of the lived autobiography.

Silence is one response that arises from the combination of position and event. Silence becomes comprehensible to the extent that one has occupied the position producing it and felt the lack of accessible signifiers. Silence itself is therefore material on which one can base a moral response. It is common in clinical medicine, for instance, for patients to be disempowered and silenced by the lack of any discourse in which their subjectivity can be conveyed. There is no validation or legitimation for the narratives that should be told, and patients must indicate by silence, indirection, and disengagement that something of vital importance to them has been excluded from the conversation.

> Else wanted to say that she was sure it wasn't *nothing* that she felt, but what could she say? They had done all the tests, and the doctor was being so careful. It was just, well, how could the doctor know, behind her white coat, how insistent the pain was and how it came at the moments when Else least expected it or wasn't even thinking about it. Of course it was worrying, and of course it tended to play on her mind, but it wasn't produced by that. She should know; it was her body after all. This was different.

Discourse, I should here recall, is not merely speech and the language it uses but the whole context of signification in which doings, reactions, and feelings give bodily meaning to the words used and add reality and depth to the configured narrative. Ultimately, the narrative has ethical content because it impacts on the body and what the body must endure. In health care the bodies of professionals are also involved and can easily be overlooked because the bodies of patients (who are often only patients and not agents) are the targets of intervention. However, the bodies of health care professionals carry with them the inscriptions of the past and can significantly affect the way that the professional acts.

> The surgeon brushed past the family waiting somewhat anxiously outside the ward for news of their son. The nurse volunteered, "I really think that a word from you, professor, would mean an awful lot to them at the moment."
> "Isn't there a chaplain somewhere?" he snapped, "I don't do sensitivity."

In the triad of power, position, and subjectivity, we find the elements of discourse that Foucault was prepared to regard as universals in human experience, and we also find a basis on which diverse cultural narratives can be appreciated. (I shall return to the topic of silence.)

I ought to note that the experiential stance to moral thought is not necessarily irrational any more than are perceptual claims, such as, for instance, the statement "If you cannot see that this is yellow then you suffer a certain kind of blindness." In both the moral and perceptual cases, the grounding for the claim is provided by a certain kind of lived and appreciated experience rather than adherence to certain propositions, but claims of both types are able to be discussed and reflected on by individuals who have shared the relevant experiences. As those subjectivities are applied to situations remote from the original transactions where they have taken shape, more attenuated and complex discourse is involved. Thus negotiation, criticism, and the hearing of diverse narratives are able to open the mind to different significations or meanings of the more complex moral situations in which one finds oneself involved.

Sustained attention to our situated experience as beings in relation to one another within discourses where power, knowledge, and subjectivity are all interwoven results in a complex whole, in which one's identity and values can be understood only against the narrative of one's own life. We need to appreciate and draw on these insights into the nature of value to understand the healing traditions and ethical concepts that form the background to health care in different settings. This background provides and gives depth to the stories that patients bring to clinical situations so that an important part of the physician's art is understanding those stories and the part we play in them. What is more, there are times when we have to contribute the meanings that allow the patient to incorporate the story of their illness into their life narrative. "The stories that people tell have a way of taking care of them. If stories come to you, care for them. And learn to give them away where they are needed. Sometimes a person needs a story more then food to stay alive. That is why we put these stories in each other's memory. This is how people care for themselves" (Lopez 1990, 60).

I am often reminded of this as I talk to my patients, who must deal with problems as diverse as back pain and malignant brain tumors. The present approach to medical and ethical thinking enables one to appreciate the commonly felt human needs appearing in the culturally situated narratives informing the perspectives of caregiver, patient, and others involved. Such inclusive thinking encourages dialogue and an understanding of the whole picture encompassing the health care intervention rather than limiting our focus to biomedical facts and asserting the rightness of a particular formulation of the ethical issues

This orientation embodies a form of ethical particularism in which the multiple narrative constructions of a particular situated experience guide our moral responses.

> Christina was brain dead. The subarachnoid hemorrhage had plunged her into coma, and it was clear that she would rapidly stop breathing and her heart would stop if the cardiorespiratory support were not continued. Her twenty-eight-year-old daughter, Diana, had accepted the fact and realized that her mother was about to be taken off the ventilator and that Christina's wishes to be an organ donor should be carried out. Her thirty-two-year-old son had been contacted and

indicated that he could not believe his mother was dying. On discussing with Diana whether to continue her mother's cardiac support and delay the organ harvest, Diana mentioned that she had spoken to her brother, who had left home some three years previously and never spoken to Christina since but was now trying to fly back because, as he said to Diana, there are things I have to say to Mum before she dies.

Arguably, a decision about the timing of the organ harvest does not here depend on solely medical factors. Attending to the diversity of narratives that shed light on this situation gives rise to a new and richer tapestry of discourse about what is to be done. Such illumination informs our ability to communicate and think within and across cultures rather than over them. Such an approach imaginatively projects itself into the stories of those touched by a clinical situation, eschewing arbitration by competing metanarratives and allowing divergent narratives to cross-illuminate different features of the lived clinical reality.

This approach is Aristotelian in the sense that it is based in lived moral experience and the knowledge that emerges from it. An Aristotelian values the reflective conclusions reached by a conscientious moral judge as a result of engaging with and living through a number of morally challenging situations. Such a judge has what can truly be called *phronesis* in the sense of practical wisdom or informed moral knowledge of the conflicts in question. To the extent that the situations involve common human experiences, we would expect that the knowledge might be widely accessible, but if the issues are heavily shaped by specific cultural discourses, one would expect divergence in the practical conclusions reached.

I should lastly note that I am advocating not the mythical "view from nowhere" or universal point of view espoused by the epistemology and ethics of objectivity (Nagel 1986; Hare 1981) but rather a kind of intersubjectivity that is, necessarily, embodied and situated because embodiment is the medium of intersubjective experience.

Context, History, and Understanding

When looked at from the perspectival, or, more accurately, multiperspectival, stance that I have outlined, the case of the empty head is replete with moral lessons.

First, the medical representatives of the dominant culture failed to appreciate the reality of those who cared about and were identified with the young man. If they had ever opened themselves to feeling the things that Maori people feel or attempted to hear the narratives told in a Maori context, they would have grasped the wrongness of what they did and acted differently despite any rational justification for the actions they took.

Second, narratives occur in contexts that are not only synchronically discursive (presenting multiple simultaneous significations of a situation) but also diachronically discursive (historical). Maori people have made us in New Zealand aware of the importance of the history of dealings between peoples and cultures. Thus, the need for a biculturally informed health care ethics in New Zealand is tied to the history of European colonization.

The inseparability of history and ethics means that there are questions of safety for an individual from any colonized people: "Do I feel safe with you? Do you understand my situation?" These questions are not adequately addressed by interpersonal communication and empathy. Our movements, postures, attitudes, and conversation reflect our culture, so we cannot (either sub specie aeternitatis or interpersonally) shed responsibility for what our people have done to the peoples with whom we are in an ongoing encounter. Maori people have been, until recently, systematically silenced in New Zealand by denial of their language, dismissal of their discourse as primitive, failure to consult and honor their traditional sources of wisdom on key issues—the list could go on. It speaks volumes to bioethics in general that we have learned this from the Maori, whom the colonial insurgents officially respected as treaty partners, unlike many other indigenous peoples throughout the world, yet whose history is marked by the treatment of their culture as subhuman and the proliferation of stereotypes that one suspects are based as much in colonial guilt as in unsympathetic perceptions of a culturally alien "form of life."

In the case of the empty head, we see that there can be valid knowledge that does not need legitimation by our abstract and "rational" practices of signification according to the scientific reality in which we are immersed. We have imposed those arrogant abstractions in terms of some favored view of the facts, the right type of answers, the dominant discourse, or what counts as clear thinking "around here." Such thinking can silence the empathic weight that the body of the observer gives to the pain of the victim. We have seen this silencing in education, health care, policy formation, and the drafting of legislation so that it becomes yet another instance of systematic oppression rather than just a single tragic incident affecting a particular patient.

I have argued that postmodernism—with its problematization of the idea of power, position, the body, subjectivity, and narrative—is valuable in reflecting on these issues. A transcultural ethic can be based on such reflection combined with honesty in individual experience, openness to diverse narratives, participation in the ordeal of the other, and attitudes that are grounded in our common experiences of being human. This is quite distinct from a basis in universally agreed axiomatic propositions or rules. Such rules do not capture the bodily subjectivities, significations, and moral responses that are intrinsic to the varying narratives that arise within and in the meeting of different cultures. However, empathy, being nice, caring for people, at least as we sentimentally discuss it among the "civilized" and colonizing peoples of the world, will not turn this trick; much blood has been shed and too many lives, spirits, and identities fragmented and scattered into oblivion for that to be adequate. Transcultural ethics has to become truly open to rebuke and to real identification with the lived bodily experience of oppression and silence. That is both difficult to achieve and vital to the Western medical humanities if they are to meet the challenge of contemporary health care ethics.

Returning to the axioms:

1. Human beings share a biological form; therefore, we can appreciate each other's pain.
2. Each human being is unique; whenever one of us is lost or diminished, the world loses part of its human treasure.
3. We are all members of an interactive community that presents us with infinite opportunities for learning and growth.
4. There are multiple perspectives on every situation, and each one offers something to the others that would otherwise not be appreciated.
5. Each perspective is potentially empowering because our perceptions present to us opportunities.
6. The fundamental epistemic and practical virtue is communicative in that this virtue underpins our well-being as beings in relation.

I will carry these orienting axioms into my discussion of medicine and its origins.

CHAPTER TWO

Hippocrates' Children

> I will use my power to help the sick to the best of my ability and judgement; I will abstain from harming or wronging any man by it.
>
> —THE OATH

I remember walking through the doors into the National Hospital for Nervous and Mental Diseases in Queen Square, ready to begin another stint as a locum neurosurgeon, and being struck by the thought that all I brought to the job was the evanescent content of my head. That doctors carry the most essential tools of their trade in their heads is often obscured by the complex technological enterprise that is modern medicine. Surgeons have always had their tools, but devices and procedures are now rampant even though surgeons secretly believe that they are alone in being able to make a real difference to the course of human disease. In fact, knowledge has always been at the heart of medicine and its dramatic successes.

The search for knowledge about human beings and their world was, in Hippocrates' day, part of philosophy—or the love of wisdom, theory, history, and knowledge (Lloyd 1973). Only later did philosophy divide into those subjects we know as science, and medical science in particular, and the humanities, including philosophy (in its modern guise), history, political science, economics, and letters more generally. Even in Hippocrates' era there were loose distinctions, with the Socratic school at Athens best known for its pursuit of questions that we have come to see as being at the core of the humanities, and the school at Cos involved in the observation and documentation of the phenomena associated with human health and disease. It remained for Aristotle to combine the naturalistic methods of Hippocrates and the conceptual inquiries of Socrates.

We can, from the distance and perspective afforded to us by more than 2,000 years, see in Hippocrates an exemplar of the method that came to be definitive of the natural sciences and has lent the name "naturalistic" to certain approaches to philosophy. The Hippocratic method, as gleaned from the surviving writings of the school at Cos and the disciples who followed in the same tradition, consists of:

1. observation;
2. documentation;
3. a rejection of overarching theory;
4. an admixture of moral and scientific virtue.

Lloyd, the foremost translator of Hippocratic writings into English, notices "firstly, the detailed and meticulous clinical observations, and secondly the example he set of the doctor's devotion and concern for his patients, and his uprightness and discretion in dealing with them" (1978, 59).

It is useful to expand on these hallmarks of the Hippocratic teachings to understand the legacy that we inherit in an ethics for medicine in the twenty-first century.

The Scientific Core of Medicine

Why ought we be concerned about the doings of remote intellectual and professional forebears of some 2,400 years ago who knew very little about human health and disease and who were not schooled in the scientific method as we know it? Lloyd concludes that we should study them because of "the living ethical ideal that they represent," "the insight they provide into the origins and development of rational medicine in the West," and "the extraordinary influence they have had over medical thought" (Lloyd 1978, 9). I will therefore examine the contribution of Hippocratic thought to the ethos of scientific medicine as well as to the more familiar territory of ethics.

As Aristotle was developing a naturalistic approach to topics such as the soul, reason, and the proper ends of human life, the Hippocratics were formulating a naturalistic approach to human ills as part of a techne or rational discipline subject to some key guiding principles. Each disease was thought of as an imbalance or disturbance of the natural state of the body in a way that compromised the proper function of a human being. These ills were not attributed to divine action or supernatural influences, rather "each disease has a natural cause and nothing happens without a natural cause" (Airs, Waters, Places, 165). We can here see early signs of holistic thinking even though those who carried on the tradition tended toward methodism and the corresponding allopathic approach based on the doctrine of "Contraria contrariis curantor," (Temkin 1991, 13) or *to cure by opposing the cause acting contrary to the good of the body.*

According to this doctrine, the treatment of disease requires the doctor to oppose its cause with another material or physical cause such as a drug, change in environment, or dietary regime. This is the guiding precept of allopathic or conventional medicine, even though the idea of strengthening the patient's constitutional resources to combat the disease and restore the harmony of the body is making a comeback (which some of the big pharmaceutical companies are worried about). Holistic influences, in particular the holistic influence of psyche on soma, were recognized by Galen and other followers of Hippocrates but did not undermine the naturalism of the Hippocratic ethos because of Aristotle's view that the soul was the "temperament" or functional form of the operation of the brain (or, better, the soma). Galen saw no great mystery in psychosomatic illness because the psyche, as Aristotle had it, was a set of natural faculties. As informed scientific physicians, we can look back and marvel at the antiquated and somewhat strained pathophysiology based on the elements of earth, air, fire, and water, but we ought to reflect deeply on the firm foundations that were laid by the Greeks for contemporary medical science.

First, the Hippocratic writers were not only naturalists but also realists: they eschewed the idea of invisible forces that could not be observed and rejected the idea that our naming of things could alter the nature of those things (The Science of Medicine, 140). One of the dangers of postmodernism is to make this mistake—to think that naming or recognizing something makes it real. But this is to take an argument too far. It is true that the ways in which we think of things can influence our ability to detect and notice significant events and connections in the world around us, and it may be that the understanding of certain kinds of events is impossible without cognitive tools crafted for certain purposes. Yet the real causes of most things are not just ideas. The causes of human disease may be complex and hugely interactive with a number of holistic and discursive influences on a human individual, but, at the end of the day, our recognizing it to be so and saying that it is so do not make it so (except in certain decidedly discursive areas of life). Thus, we ought to beware of the nominalism that pervades postmodern thinking without denying the power of dominant discourses to influence clinical life at both macroethical and microethical levels (Komessaroff 1995).

Observation was also a forte of the Hippocratic school. Students were encouraged to visit Alexandria, where they would learn from the practitioners of dissection (and in some cases vivisection). This happened despite the fact that later Hippocratically inspired writers were to condemn vivisection and its violation of fundamental human values. It is worth noting that the supporters of vivisection justified the practice by using a utilitarian argument whereby the suffering of the condemned criminal was outweighed by the remedies that might be devised for the innocent (Lloyd 1973, 76). This is one of the earliest examples of the pernicious effect of utilitarian thinking in bioethics. The Hippocratic school, although it approved of dissection of the dead as a tool of medical science, itself recommended and taught methods that were justified in part by their consequences and in part by their compatibility with the art of medicine and a respect for human life.

The Hippocratic writers commend the need for careful and systematic observation of cases so that the practitioner's knowledge comes to exceed that of the layperson through his or her own practice and the development of methods for assessing it. Trial and error and the ability to learn from one's mistakes are an important part of this enterprise. "I warmly commend the physician who makes small mistakes; infallibility is rarely to be seen. Most doctors seem to me to be in the position of poor navigators. In calm weather they can conceal their mistakes but when overtaken by a mighty storm or violent gale it is evident to all that it is their ignorance and error which is the ruin of the ship" (Tradition, 75).

Is this the origin of the idea that the doctor is the captain of the ship in health care settings? The Hippocratic tradition makes it clear that the doctor is like the navigator in charge, who is responsible for the technical knowledge and skill required to conduct the voyage. But no Greek reading this would miss the point that the captain is answerable to the *owner* of the ship (i.e., the patient) for bringing the venture to a successful outcome (as defined by the owner). It is too easy to confuse the role of navigator with that of the person determining the end of a clinical regimen and therefore to substitute the perspective of the technician for that of the supremely interested party. The Hippocratics teach us that substantial benefit to the patient is not a topic for medical determination but should always be relativized to the situation of the patient. Indeed I have (in various writings) consistently defined substantial benefit as "an outcome which now or in the future the patient would regard as worthwhile," a conception that undercuts futile debates about physiological benefit, futility, purely medical indications for a given treatment, and the like.

The Hippocratics, as is evident from their attitude to medical error, understood their own lack of medical knowledge and did not seriously believe that medicine could be an exact science. However, this gave the physician no easy recourse to intellectual nihilism or laziness and complacency. "I contend that the science of medicine must not be rejected as nonexistent or ill investigated because it may sometimes fail in exactness. Even if it is not always accurate in every respect, the fact that it is able to approach close to a standard of infallibility as a result of reasoning, where before there was great ignorance, should command respect for the discoveries of medical science. Such discoveries are the product of good and true investigation, not chance happenings" (Tradition, 77).

This is a very sophisticated apologia for the pinch of salt required by a young and vital science unable, through achievements alone, to commend itself in the face of approaches to health and disease founded on less admirable tenets. The Hippocratic "science" resulted in significant advances in the understanding of human health and disease in which we find observation, careful reflection, and theory combined in a way that has characterized medical science ever since. Observations and theory from other sciences were welcomed, and the significance of the pulse, the idea of filtration and selective solution of metabolites in different body fluids, and many other concepts founds in later medical literature were debated in the light of evidence from actual cases and this wide body of knowledge.

Throughout the Hippocratic writings one discerns a vigorous and deeply committed search for the secrets that will help alleviate human suffering. We also find that this is not a one-way street in that a conception of the doctor's role develops alongside an appreciation of the important contribution of the patient. "Life is short, science is long; opportunity is elusive, experiment is dangerous, judgement is difficult. It is not enough for the physician to do what is necessary, but the patient and the attendants must do their part as well, and circumstances must be favourable" (Aphorisms, 206).

On this note I can usefully discuss the ethics that spring from Hippocratic roots.

The Ethical Core of Medicine

The Hippocratic Oath has traditionally been regarded as paternalistic and doctor centered. It focuses on physicians, but this does not entail that it is paternalistic, especially when seen in its own cultural context where physicians were journeymen, retained by heads of households like visiting tradesmen even though their education tended to rank them socially alongside those who retained them. In this context the physician was answerable to those he attended (or to those who stood in loco parentis as the interested employers of the patients concerned) and had no choice but to respect the wishes of the patient or householder. Only later in history did the institutionalization of medicine and the profession's own lack of knowledge combine to create the exclusive aura of superiority that some physicians still cling to.

The oath locates itself within the context of a belief in powers greater than those operating in the human world. This is of special interest in view of the pervasive naturalism of the Hippocratic corpus. It indicates, should we tend to overlook it, that our actions are not just transactions between cohabitants of the biosphere but are played out against a moral and spiritual landscape explored with great sophistication and depth by the Greek dramatists and epic writers. The Greek tragedies, in particular, showed human beings in touch with their own vulnerability and spirituality, dealing with life, death, and the drama of human relationships. Thus, we are reminded that the backdrop of the medical vocation is not the sterile canvas of the surgical specimen, the anatomy museum, the physiology laboratory, and the sanitized clinical record, it is the colorful and deeply complex tapestry formed by human life in all its fullness. The brain I operate on is not just a human brain, it is John's or Sue's or baby Joseph's, and what happens as a result of my gaze and my instruments invading it is of earth-shattering significance to the person concerned.

This philosophical reflection on the significance of events that one encounters in clinical life is characteristic of the reflective practitioner and can seem to make the physician priestlike or almost godlike (Temkin 1991, 26). One hopes that such godlikeness is linked to the more admirable members of the Greek pantheon rather than the petty, jealous, politically manipulative, or despotic Olympians. If the oath is followed, that should be the case: "I will use my power to help the sick to the best of my ability and judgment; I will abstain from harming or wronging any man by it" (The Oath, 67).

The idea of virtue and a respect for life is evinced in the promise not to give any poison or abortifacient where we see a deep commitment to the value of human life. However, such is the overriding commitment to compassion that one can imagine a very sympathetic Hippocratic voice thinking deeply about the kinds of debate that have surrounded abortion, unwelcome pregnancy, and the often desperate choices of women in the present era.

"I will be chaste and religious in my life and in my practice" (The Oath, 67). This remark must be seen in the context of the piety debated in the Socratic dialogue called the *Euthyphro*. The dialogue struggles to articulate an unambiguous ground for commitment to virtuous action and a proper sense of one's duty before God and humanity. Plato directs us toward a sense of goodness or human virtue coeval with the will that a worthy God would exhibit. This piety links the good of humanity and the will of God in such a way that the perennial wisdom of the dictum *love your neighbor as you love yourself* comes to mind, also linking two things that could be thought to be at odds with one another. We are now quite accustomed to the thought that there is none so vicious as he who hates himself, and the idea that in our shared humanity we stand in the presence of an imperative greater than any private concern encompasses right action both to others and to oneself.

When we turn to Aristotle on the question of what makes life go well, then the coincidence between self-love and love of the other becomes evident. We are happiest and most fulfilled when our interactions with others are rich and fulfilling. However, if one falsely identifies what makes life go well with possessions or goods for which we compete with others, then the scene is set for a significant misunderstanding of the good of self and of the good of others. In my discussion of moral theorems, I have noted the need for a place to stand and the room to develop one's own life story as a framework for ethics in which one seeks to enrich the lives of others rather than to compete with them.

"Whatever I see and hear, professionally or privately, which ought not to be divulged, I will keep secret and tell no one" (The Oath, 67). Here we have the moderate and careful statement about privacy found in the Hippocratic tradition. The doctor is enjoined to exercise judgment and discretion in the use of information from a patient, worlds apart from the draconian standards of medical confidentiality that have peppered the history of medical ethics. Confidentiality is not an absolute duty, but it is a mark of respect, and one needs to cultivate reflective practice so as not to abuse confidences whether through vice or incompetence (two sides of the same coin in the Greek moral lexicon). Notice that the undertaking is not narrowly defined with respect to any "clever-sticks" distinctions between practice contexts (public clinic or private office) or the mode of information gathering (voluntary disclosure or elicited responses to questions). The clause in the oath is all about astute clinical judgment as to what ought to be divulged, bearing in mind the role of the physician as a trusted and respected member of a community whose work inevitably brings him or her into contact with intimate details of the daily lives of patients, many of which should be kept confidential.

The practitioner or novice swears the oath traditionally on entry into the profession and links observance of the oath with good repute and prosperity. Thus, there is an implicit recognition of the central role of morality in a life that goes well—very much the Aristotelian orientation. Yet this cuts both ways. It indicates, if we are open enough to hear it, that the repute we have among our fellow citizens is a barometer that tells us not only about the standing of medicine in our community but also about the extent to which we are living according to the precepts we teach our young professionals. The linked ideas of respect, humility, trustworthiness, and beneficence are part of the medical ideal that is a powerful corrective to our worst tendencies.

Temkin identifies further practical and attitudinal mores that physicians are enjoined to embrace by the Hippocratic tradition:

1. they should be modest, gentle, and not obtrusive;
2. they should not be avaricious;
3. they should not only be public figures honored by their communities but also have their feet on the ground;
4. they should visit the sick;
5. they should have self-control and restraint;
6. they should be excellent craftsmen and not showmen. (1991, 23–27)

There is, nevertheless, supposed to be an element of detachment and an objective assessment of efficacy that should moderate our more empathic reactions: "a surgeon should be full of pity but not too easily moved to hurry or cut less than required" (Temkin 1991, 33).

Of particular interest is the idea that doctors should not be overly motivated by money and, if necessary, should be prepared to treat the sick without a fee being paid at all (Lloyd 1978, 15). These precepts decry the thought that good medicine for those in need should be vulnerable to the distortions produced by commercialization. The Hippocratic practitioner is supposed to respond to need and not the ability to pay, thus setting medicine apart from those arts in which individuals deliver their services only to those who can pay for them. Although the idea of a state-funded health service was completely foreign in ancient Greece, this idea of justice in which services are provided with regard to need should give us pause when we contemplate the problems for medical science and the impartial assessment and application of putative remedies arising from the capture of the medical profession by commercial interests. The prominent role of major pharmaceutical companies (as recently seen in academic appointments and the funding of biomedical research) comes uncomfortably close to the type of injustice here envisaged.

The Hippocratic corpus envisages knowledgeable professionals, who consult their colleagues, are free from envy and avarice, and form an honorable company dedicated to relieving suffering and a respect for persons. They have, from time to time, to make decisions involving considerable risk of harm, and sometimes they proceed urgently in the face of uncertainty under the necessity imposed by mortal danger. These are the realities of clinical practice, which cannot be regulated as if it were based on the certainties beloved of scientists and accountants, and which relies on the sound intuitions and wise judgments that are the stuff of virtuous conduct informed by extensive clinical experience.

Internal or External Morality

Pellegrino and others pursuing the Hippocratic tradition have noticed that medicine is a distinct subculture into which one enters after a period of acculturation and that it generates its own moral understandings. They follow Alasdair MacIntyre (1981) in arguing that such a subculture has its own internal morality, here grounded in goods and excellencies intrinsic to the complex human form of life that encompasses clinical medicine and its associated institutions and practices (Pellegrino 1982; Ladd 1983). The emphasis on the informed intuitions of practitioners who are experienced and wise in the techne of medicine is close to the ideal I have outlined as the ethical core of medicine. Therefore my exposition of the Hippocratic writings can profitably engage with the debate surrounding the idea of an internal morality (Veatch and Miller, 2001).

Pellegrino (well aware of the Aristotelian—indeed, Thomist—resonances of this idea) uses the internal morality of medicine to discriminate between ends that are properly in accordance with it and ends that are not, where the root values have to do with the health or well-being (in some objective sense) of the patient. He argues that a number of activities in which the profession has become involved are not consistent with that end but serve more questionable or even vicious ends such as the beauty myth, military or judicial purposes, or personal gratification (however misguided).

One is immediately aware of the dangers of such a view despite its excellent dialectic pedigree. Veatch attempted to capture these dangers in his attack on the idea that "one need not look beyond medicine itself to know its morality" (2001, 627).

He has three objections:

1. there are many diverse medical roles, and therefore no unified goal or *telos* to medicine in the way that is required for such a view;
2. medicine itself has multiple ends, all of which are ambiguous and sometimes conflicting;
3. the purposes that any craft or vocation pursues takes on value only from the culture in which it is embedded.

Nevertheless, these are all problematic.

Diverse Medical Roles

There are indeed a number of Hippocratic professions—medicine, nursing, pharmacy, physiotherapy, psychotherapy, psychology, homeopathy, occupational therapy, and speech therapy, to name but a few. But the different individuals work together in teams, and each person's role is subservient to the one aim of improving the well-being of the patient. We are, according to Aristotle, all making contributions to eudaemonia (or a harmony of the "demons"— forces that give life its energy and vitality) by addressing things that detract from it or distort it. This "harmony of the lively forces" contributes to health that is a sine qua non of a good life. It is a misconstrual of what we are aiming at in this cooperative enterprise to argue that our different roles preclude a common telos, although *phronesis* in the varieties of techne that we have individually mastered may have very different forms (but that is not unusual even within medicine itself).

Diverse Ends

Veatch's argument here rests on changing medical views of the use of life-saving technologies and shifting or diverse cultural beliefs about such things as "brain death" and "cardiac death." Unbridled relativism seems to give way to a pragmatic naturalism in these areas that would have been instantly recognizable to Aristotle or Hippocrates. A moment's reflection makes it clear that shifts in our allegiance to such ideals as saving life wherever possible is not so problematic as Veatch makes it seem. There was a time when we first discovered how to rescue "hopeless cases" and did so indiscriminately. Having mastered these skills, however, we have found that the results were not always in accordance with our intuitions about life and its worth when some patients were "rescued" to what most people felt was a life worse than death. Thus, our conceptions changed, and the idea that futility and beneficence were definable in purely pathophysiological terms was abandoned in favor of something like substantial benefit or "an outcome that now or in the future the patient would regard as worthwhile" (Campbell, Gillett, and Jones 2001, 12). Only those who are wedded to flat-footed standards of clinical duty (defined in terms of mandatory interventions) fail to see this change as consistent with the coherence and integrity of the Hippocratic tradition. Thus, the supposed confusion of medical ends seems itself to rest on a confusion about the telos of medicine.

An External Framework of Value

I have argued that the Hippocratic practitioner works within an ethos that has a deep regard for certain very general or natural facts about human beings and their flourishing. Within the collective narrative that forms a common basis on which to construct livable life stories, there are infinite unique paths that any human being can take. Despite this diversity, certain universal and shared features of the human condition (I have argued) are close to the heart of what concerns Hippocratic professionals. Thus, a kind of understanding of human life and the proper response to human needs, injuries, afflictions, and vulnerabilities is a product of the Hippocratic vocation. That is important because Hippocratic practitioners individually and collectively have great powers to harm their fellow human beings and therefore must bear a proportional burden of responsibility. I would argue that this yields an internal morality and that at crucial points in our lives when, as professionals, we face potent moral challenges, it is vital that we are steeped in it.

This last point should alert us to the dangers of elitism and Gnosticism, ever-present temptations to those who find themselves set apart by any calling no matter how intrinsically virtuous it may appear to be. Doctors are fed the message that they are highly valued, are set apart from the common run of humankind, and have an essential and important part to play in the affairs of their fellow mortals. This is heady stuff and can be quite intoxicating for the bright young things who find their way through all the obstacles and enter our select order. Some of these are already misfits before we get them, and things do not get any better in the pathological milieu of veneration and abuse in which they can find themselves immersed. They can become unbalanced and blinded to the common intuitions of humankind, and we should always be wary of a concept that seems to reinforce the specialness of doctors—such as that of internal morality. Armed with empathy, pragmatism, and humility, we can avoid the dangers, but it is a path alongside which the madness sometimes seen in our intensive care units lies in wait for some of the brightest and the best.

Charlotte Paul, a New Zealand epidemiologist and contributor to numerous societal and academic debates in bioethics, picks up this debate about internal versus external morality and applies it to the constraints and statutory mechanisms that have evolved in the regulation of medical professionals and medicine as a whole (2000).

New Zealand was rocked by an ethical scandal in 1988, when a judicial inquiry headed by Judge Sylvia Cartwright (the Cartwright inquiry) revealed that National Women's Hospital, our major obstetrics and gynecology teaching hospital, had conducted an extensive "clinical trial" of cervical cancer management without obtaining consent from the women concerned. The hypothesis was that cervical carcinoma in situ did not typically progress to invasive cancer of the cervix and could be observed rather than excised, avoiding the need for hysterectomy. For nearly twenty years this policy was followed and the results published although there was no properly constructed clinical trial or systematic safeguards to deal with possible sources of bias in the data (Cartwright 1988; Paul 1988). When this trial and its defects were exposed, there began a period of sweeping ethical transformation in New Zealand health care.

Paul examines the resulting "external" constraints, comparing them with the existing "internal Morality," "those values, norms and rules that are intrinsic to the practice of medicine," in dealing with the ethical failures of health care professionals (2000, 499). She contrasts internal morality with external morality (as represented in socially, politically, and legally generated regulations) and notices that various groups in society delivered diverse verdicts on internal and external morality. Some thought that internal morality was adequate but had failed due to circumstances in the actual situation; others believed that internal morality was itself likely to promote such unethical conduct because of the intrinsic character of the medical profession. Paul, an often critical voice in New Zealand medicine, then delivers her own verdict on the consequences of the Cartwright inquiry: "The operation of internal morality was ignored in the making of policy after the Cartwright inquiry. The external controls, designed as if they had the whole task of regulating the moral conduct of doctors, have been clumsy and unsatisfactory, as could have been expected" (502). For instance, she reviews the role of consent and patient autonomy and concludes that it is "the tradition and context of medical care that makes a difference to consent" (502).

I return to the topic of consent in due course, but for the moment it is vital to notice the importance of respect and the recognition of the patient's close interest in his or her well-being that we find in the Hippocratic writings.

In her criticism of the imposition of external morality, Paul remarks that "Complex regulations can disempower those forced to observe them" and that such disempowerment can work against the interests of patients and undermine the trustworthiness of the profession. Her final comments are telling: "Distaste for the self-serving nature of some professional activity should not blind us to instances where internal morality has worked in the interests of patients. Instead we need to examine how it works, how it can be adapted to new circumstances, and how it is connected to external morality" (2000, 502).

The Hippocratic corpus outlines an approach to medicine founded on the best interests of those whose bodies we address in our clinical practice. We are encouraged to be open to the data that arise in clinical life and to learn from it so as to grow in the art of medicine. In this learning, reflective correction of our techniques and rational self appraisal are of central importance and ultimately give rise to a humane science fit to confront illness and suffering in all its guises. A conception of the virtuous practitioner is central in this vocation. This conception circumvents much of the debate about an internal morality for medicine and brings us face-to-face with the sociopolitical context that surrounds and in part conditions our clinical practice.

The Virtuous Practitioner

Hippocratic practitioners clearly need to cultivate certain virtues. They need to be trustworthy and committed to discovering and respecting the patient's real interests. They must appreciate widely different life stories and the role of illness in those stories. They must then incorporate their clinical learning into practicing the art of medicine, systematically incorporating scientific and therapeutic developments. This requires their empathy and humility, and a right use of their powers as healers so that they can participate in liberating their patients from affliction. They must have a number of traits: imagination, self-criticism, generosity of spirit, loyalty, justice and patience, even irony. And in all of this they must cultivate their own growth as people so that they become more complete in their ability to help those who turn to them. None of these things is fit for legal regulation, and they lie at the core of both internal morality and the ethical provision of clinical care. Given that most of us are only travelers on the path of virtue, to have such ideals is fine provided we do not make the mistake of thinking that because we travel virtuously we have arrived in some way that elevates us above our fellows.

In this spirit I can examine the science of medicine.

CHAPTER THREE

What Is Medical Truth?

Medicine has for long possessed the qualities necessary to make a science. These are a starting point and a known method according to which many valuable discoveries have been made over a long period of time.

—TRADITION IN MEDICINE

From Praxis to Science

I have noted that the medical science of Hippocratic times was founded on certain principles. It was naturalistic and made use of the science of its day; it relied on observations rather than hypotheses about the nature of humanity and the universe, and it was fueled by a concern for the sick. It developed as a practice based on knowledge rather than opinion, fostering "industrious toil and the passage of time" such that it grew like a seed in well-tended soil (Lloyd 1978, 67–68). The knowledge contained in the Hippocratic corpus, as we have seen, was light on theory and virtually unaided by technology. Its seed was the teaching of those who had treated the sick, along with what could be gleaned from dissection and more general natural science. The soil in which medical knowledge grew was the character or person of the student.

The Hippocratic disciple was "initiated into the mysteries of science" pragmatically (Tradition in Medicine, 68). As a person one was enjoined to be attentive to the observations of the past and to employ a method of discovery using careful and sustained observation coupled with judicious intervention (71). This combination of observation and intervention made medicine the ideal model for the scientific investigation of nature (83), and one became a master only by submitting oneself to the discipline of undertaking such studies. Implicit in the corpus is a deep suspicion of high-flown theories based on insufficient observations. The Hippocratic writings also recorded their disapproval of the unholy alliance between medicine and money (which often went along with quackery in their day) but is more typical of orthodoxy today.

The pragmatic approach proper to a techne requires both contemplation and technical skill and emphasizes the subtle interaction between praxis and knowledge. Hippocratic knowledge is painstakingly gained and carefully accumulated from reflection on case material.

Medicine has not always been so judicious in its procedures and attitudes. In place of the relevant scientific knowledge, it has sometimes made do with ungrounded opinion and artful conjecture based on empirical rules of thumb. At other times, political and financial interests have unduly affected its development. There have also been times when certain theories and procedures of data gathering have excluded certain observations from its corpus of knowledge.

In nineteenth-century Hungary, this hegemonic tendency affected Ignaz Semmelweiss, who suffered as a physician, an academic, and a person when he introduced the theory of infection into the understanding of "childbed fever," or pelvic inflammation and septicemia, and targeted unsound sanitation in obstetrics. Semmelweis's inferences seemed intolerable because they implied that doctors themselves might cause their patients' sickness and death. This reversal of the image of the doctor—from healer and helper to death-bringer—so upset the mythology of medical practice (and was true in nineteenth-century medicine) that it was unthinkable in that discourse. He was silenced by the abuse of medical power and privilege in a way similar to the events that shaped the cervical cancer scandal in New Zealand (Cartwright 1988). In both cases, the problems occurred in large university hospitals responsible for the advancement of medicine as an enlightened and virtuous discipline with a prima facie allegiance not only to academic standards but also to excellence in clinical practice.

In contemporary medicine we see a continuation of the Hippocratic method but with a vastly expanded technological repertoire and against a more mature scientific framework. Medicine's catalogue of astounding achievements includes, for instance, the virtual eradication of mortal bacterial infections (such as that which Semmelweiss identified), the identification and treatment of many cancers and other neoplastic conditions, the correction and stabilization of previously untreatable hormonal diseases, and the development of preventive measures for viral and other diseases that have killed in epidemic numbers.

This success story is not, however, universal. Many of the diseases now challenging us do not fit neatly into our existing theoretical accounts, rooted as they are in an empirical science that has embraced Hippocrates' naturalism to the point of hegemony. Contemporary biomedical science treats the body as a machine that can be understood through physiology, biochemistry, and pathology. This model, derived from Descartes, leaves the soul as a disconnected "ghost in the machine," so psychiatry, in the minds of many doctors and patients, treats illnesses that are "all in the head" or "not real." But many doctors and medical researchers are intolerant of any theories that question this model and flirt with something more holistic. We are similarly intolerant of methods that stray from those aimed at discovering the pathological conditions that are thought to cause certain diseases.

We have come so far by extending Hippocratic pragmatism and naturalism into positivistic biomedical science, that it is easy to understand the tendency to extrapolate from our successes to date. Yet perhaps we have nearly exhausted the problems amenable to classical reductive scientific explanation, and a scientific revolution is creeping up on us. We can pursue that suspicion by reflecting on the effect of positivism on the Hippocratic tradition.

Positivism and Medicine

The positivistic tradition is founded on the idea that we establish by observation the truth or falsity of hypotheses or theories in the form of propositions (or sets of propositions) that represent the world as it actually is. Newton-Smith summarizes this view as follows: "The scientific community sees itself as the very paradigm of institutionalized rationality. It is taken to be in the possession of something, the scientific method, which generates a 'logic of justification.' That is, it provides a technique for the objective appraisal of scientific theories" (1981, 1).

The objectivity of science goes hand in hand with scientific realism: the idea that representation and reality are distinct and can be compared in such a way as to demonstrate the truth or falsity of the theories involved. In this view, science reveals the nature of the world and the processes going on within it, and allows us to discover the facts about human health and disease. It comes as a surprise to many medical scientists that there are significant shifts in scientific theory: "viewed *sub specie aeternitatis* scientists (even physical scientists) are a fickle lot. The history of science is a tale of multifarious shiftings of allegiance from theory to theory" (Newton-Smith 1981, 3).

Popper is himself somewhat modest about the knowledge claims of science: "The old scientific ideal of *episteme*—of absolutely certain, demonstrable knowledge—has proved to be an idol. The demand for scientific objectivity makes it inevitable that every statement must remain tentative for ever. It may indeed be corroborated, but every corroboration is relative to other statements that, again, are tentative. Only in our subjective experiences of conviction, in our subjective faith, can we be 'absolutely certain'" (1959, 280).

Despite Popper's modesty, most practicing scientists think that they have grasped part of an interconnected "totality of truths equally open to all scientific inquirers who may share their techniques and experiences" (Hacking 1996, 44). However, the pragmatist philosophers of science challenge this theoretical and pictorial unity, arguing that "it is not high level theory that has stopped the innumerable branches of science from flying off in all directions, but a widely shared family of experimental practices and instrumentation" (1996, 69).

Crombie for instance, criticizes the putative unity of science as a theoretical endeavor and makes a post-Wittgensteinian suggestion about scientific reasoning and "normal science" (1988). He remarks that different sciences focus on a diverse range of theoretical and practical activities that are interconnected and resemble each other in various ways reminiscent of the conceptual affiliations between games that Wittgenstein famously characterized as "family resemblances." Following Crombie, Hacking identifies seven "styles of scientific reasoning" that illustrate this diversity: (a) postulation; (b) experiment and measurement; (c) hypothetical modeling; (d) taxonomic ordering; (e) statistical analysis; and (f) historical or genetic explanation; to which Hacking adds (g) laboratory science (1996, 65). A similar diversity can be identified in medicine (Wartofsky 1997).

Postulates and axioms are evident in basic theoretical commitments such as the idea that structure underpins function. Structure is investigated by increasingly sophisticated methods, including electron microscopy and nuclear magnetic resonance scanning. We conjecture that the macroscopic and microscopic structures we encounter have analogues at even lower levels, thus revealing the causal connectedness of human function and dysfunction. We are now beginning to examine these most general axioms and postulates in exploring the top-down determination of structure by context (in embryology, for instance).

Experimental exploration and measurement are interwoven with the investigation of structure and function and conceptions of the data that should be of interest to contemporary medical science. This conceptual work reflects the axiomatic foundations of biomedicine.

Hypothetical modeling is another activity conducted in "reflective equilibrium" (cognitive not moral) with other techniques defining medicine. It is more detailed than the axiomatic thinking basic to biomedicine and generates models such as that of "immune surveillance," neoplastic transformation, the genesis of atherosclerosis, and the axes of psychiatric diagnosis.

Medical taxonomy is founded on the philosophical idea of natural kinds. The idea comes from the work of Putnam (1973) and Kripke (1980), who argued that there are general terms that designate things naturally occurring in the actual world, such as gold, tigers, water, neutrinos, and white blood cells. These terms "carve nature at its joints" and underpin realist metaphysics (for medicine, the metaphysics of disease). An object or type of thing really does belong to such a category if it appears in the best current scientific knowledge in the relevant area. The linguistic community defers to the scientific experts, and therefore the category becomes de facto a product of orthodox scientific theory in the area in question. Science, in this view, reveals to us the real structure of the actual world and therefore identifies enduring categories in nature. A radical and serious challenge to the scientific theory governing the phenomena in question therefore has metaphysical implications. Such a shift can affect even basic questions about when a certain scientific kind or phenomenon (such as oxygen) was discovered and by whom (Hudson 2001).

There is a vigorous debate about whether diseases are natural kinds (in the sense defined) and represent objectively specifiable dysfunctions of the organism they affect (Boorse 1975). I and others have argued that defining diseases by reference only to aberrations in the natural or normal biological function of the human organism is problematic. Classifying something as a disease involves not just describing but evaluating a pattern of changes in an organism (Fulford 1989; Megone 1998; Gillett 1999a). But the basic premise of biomedical science is that something like the objective metaphysical claim about human disease and dysfunction is true and ought—*sans phrase*—to underpin the taxonomy of biomedicine.

Statistical analysis is a method of finding noncoincidental correlations between phenomena, and statistical association is a way of linking taxonomic categories—such as elevated blood pressure and atherosclerosis. These statistical associations may be supported by showing that drugs with known effects on certain biochemical processes have a statistically demonstrable influence on the course of disease. The conjunction of methods is often used to unravel a pathophysiological story about disease.

Historical or genetic explanation of the occurrence of a pathological abnormality in light of what we already know about bodily structure and function is also used to understand diseases and their therapy. This kind of explanation links to our conceptions of natural kinds and laws of nature, and our commitment to the causal connectedness of natural phenomena informs the models and taxonomies central to the web of belief that is contemporary biomedicine.

Laboratory science is a growing part of medical science as the quintessential means of isolating and investigating the processes and events that lie behind (clinical) phenomena.

This colloquy of theory and methodology yields a classical model according to which there is a preferred description (or representation) of every disease, composed out of the cognitive materials provided by the paradigm (or network of theory, technology, and practices) that is contemporary clinical biomedicine. The enterprise is Hippocratic in that it is pragmatic, causal and naturalistic, based on observation, and grounded in a scientific model of human function, and the problems it solves have what we could call a "classical structure."

One such classical problem is subarachnoid hemorrhage due to a berry aneurysm on one of the cerebral arteries. A berry aneurysm is an out-pouching of a cerebral artery caused by a deficiency in the arterial wall. We believe that increasing blood pressure during life causes the aneurysm to stretch and then split. The aneurysm ruptures, causing a hemorrhage around and sometimes into the brain, which can be fatal (on either the first or a subsequent occasion). We detect the hemorrhage on a CT scan and find the aneurysm by imaging the cerebral blood vessels. Then we try to obliterate the aneurysm and prevent recurrent hemorrhages. A neurosurgeon does this by exposing the blood vessels inside the skull and following them to the point where the aneurysm is shown to be. A small spring-loaded clip is used to obliterate the "neck" of the aneurysm, where it arises from a cerebral blood vessel.

This problem and its resolution is a testimony to the practice of meticulous postmortem examination of people who have died from strokes, the development of imaging techniques to reveal structures inside the head, theoretical modeling of a pathological process in the light of relevant observations, and the development of surgical techniques and supporting therapies (analgesic, anti-septic, anesthetic, and pharmacological). Despite its technical complexity this is a comparatively simple conceptual exercise aimed at a simple anatomical anomaly and the problems arising when one tries to correct it. Other problems are not so easy.

For instance, why do some individuals develop essential hypertension (raised blood pressure predisposing, among other things, to brain hemorrhage, stroke, or heart disease)? Why do people develop allergies? Why does cancer become arrested in some patients and advance rapidly in others when the same allo-pathic treatment is used? These questions are not well addressed by contempo-rary biomedical science, and yet the scientific approach of positivist biomedi-cine remains dominant both in treatment and in funded research into the conditions (including these) that present themselves for medical attention.

Science and the Fall

Science in general and the science of medicine in particular is now being challenged by alternative approaches to healing and, independent of these, a philosophy of science that, through thinkers like Kuhn, Rorty, and Foucault, is critical of all claims to objective truth.

Kuhn (1962) introduced the idea that science is not merely the gradual accu-mulation of truth to provide a unified structure of knowledge that encompasses natural phenomena; rather, it is marked by revolutions in which old paradigms are attacked, ravaged, and discarded, or else abandoned through creeping dis-affection as new paradigms take their place. He noted that the reasons for para-digm shift do not always lie within the cognitive content of science and may not reflect debates within "the logical structure of scientific knowledge" (94). Paradigm shifts not conducted strictly according to scientific principles (108). In fact, Kuhn argues that the competing paradigms often do not compete on the same playing field according to the same rules and may require a revaluation of scientific standards. "When paradigms enter, as they must, into a debate about paradigm choice, their role is necessarily circular . . . each paradigm will be shown to satisfy more or less the criteria that it dictates for itself and to fall short of those dictated by its opponent" (93, 109).

New paradigms accept different base theories and methods of investigation and validate their data in different ways, thereby reconstituting the science they comprise (Kuhn 1962, 108). A fairly localized example of this process might be the switch in medical theory that reconceptualized Graves disease of the thyroid gland as an autoimmune rather than hormonal problem. The original theory was that some change in the hormonal system and the regulatory and cell-based factors governing thyroid hormone secretion produced a function-driven enlargement of the gland. This idea was displaced by the discovery of an antibody, specific for thyroid tissue, which attacked the gland producing an excess of thyroid hormone and swelling of the gland. This challenge to existing theory is no more than a local change in biomedical theory and shakes no foundations. A similar change in theory was the discovery that Burkitt lymphoma (previously classified as a neoplasia or cancer) was caused by infection with a certain virus stimulating the cells to embark on a course of disproportionate growth and reproduction. Before this discovery, infective diseases and neoplasia had occupied different groups in our pathological classifications, but as a result of the discovery new theories were developed to allow us to investigate the possibility that viral infection may play a causal role in cancer. Thus, an answer previously marked wrong in any medical examination (i.e., that some cancers are caused by infection) became right; what was untrue became true. However, at a basic level, the role of DNA as part of the original genetic explanation of neoplasia and then as part of the mechanism proposed for viral action defused the need for a fundamental revision of medical theory.

Somewhat more radically, we have now reconceptualized the processes leading to the changes in cells that occur during embryological development. It appears that these are not unidirectionally driven from bottom up by DNA codes but, at least in part, are due to contextual influences arising from their structural setting in the embryo or fetus.

Even more radically, we have to reconsider the reductive basis of biomedicine when we face the challenge of holistic therapy and the idea that the psychosomatic organism considered as a whole may influence even detailed molecular and pathophysiological processes contributing to the orthodox profile of disease as delivered by the diverse technologies of clinical science.

Similar points are made vigorously, if slightly immodestly, by Foucault when he comments on Kuhn's characterization of scientific revolutions:

> this extent and rapidity are only the sign of something else: a modification in the rules of formation of statements which are accepted as scientifically true. This is not a change of content (refutation of old errors, recovery of old truths), nor is it a

change of theoretical form (renewal of paradigm, modification of systematic ensembles). It is a question of what governs statements, and the way in which they govern each other so as to constitute a set of propositions which are scientifically acceptable, and hence capable of being verified or falsified by scientific procedures. In short, there is a problem of the regime, the politics of the scientific statement. (Foucault 1984, 54)

Foucault is not speaking about competing representations of reality but rather "a regime of knowledge" that governs the rules of formation of statements, rules that, although unstated, determine what will count as scientifically respectable according to legitimated concepts of observation, demonstration, confirmation of theory, validation of hypotheses, and so on. There is no direct comparison of representational pictures here; the relevant rules are enforced through the complex of mechanisms constituting "the regime"—editorial policies, research grants, invitations to conference speakers, academic appointments, and so on.

Foucault therefore asks searching questions about "the governance of statements" and the constraints on the corpus of knowledge. He argues that such things are sensitive to relations of power, both economic and political, for instance, the power we wish to exert over human health, sexuality, and social behavior. The concerns he raises figure prominently in the kinds of discourse that determine our thoughts about the social role of individuals and their reproductive activity because the "deviant" and the insane are prime targets for medicopolitical control. Foucault highlights the sociocultural and political aspects of medicine and their intersection with its scientific endeavors. These aspects contribute to the regime of truth that produces the surgical technology and pharmaceuticals fuelling the clinical and research industry that is central in contemporary biomedicine.

Foucault's analysis is sufficiently radical to call into question the very nature of biomedical science and its distinction from dogma or opinion based on financial interest, expediency, and professional power networks. Clinical science does, however, have a pragmatic response to this worry, and it recalls the Hippocratic remarks about medicine as a paradigmatic science.

Language Games, Diverse Practices, and Clinical Medicine

Wittgenstein's account of language, thought, and knowledge grounds meaning and truth in practices through which we interact with those things around us. The meaning of any term is given by its use within the relevant human practice (1953, 43); truth is a function of meaning, and the use of terms in accordance with the rules operating in the relevant practice is the closest we can get to truth for any statement. Thus, if I say to a trainee surgeon "That is the carotid artery" when surgical dissection has in fact exposed the carotid artery, then my statement is true. If others were to contradict me, they would be saying something false. I could also say, "This is the supply line to the engine-house of thought" and be speaking the truth, although making a specific point different from the simple anatomical statement. No doubt, there would be some way of characterizing this structure according to traditional healing systems that would perhaps emphasize its place in a connected network of bodily functions.

Wittgenstein likens words to tools and their meanings to the functions of tools, a perspective yielding a conception of truth firmly based in praxis or human activity. In this conception we could liken the use of words from different discourses to the use of tools from different activities, so that judgments about whether the words did the job well (or yielded knowledge) would be like asking of, for instance, a hammer or a whisk whether it did its job well. We might then conclude that a hammer was a good tool in the work shed but not for cooking and vice versa for the whisk. Thus, in Wittgenstein's terms, the aptness of a meaning to convey the truth about a situation is like the aptness of a tool to perform a certain job. For instance, a mistake similar to that involved in complaining that a whisk is unsuited to carpentry occurs if we complain that words used about persons, their decisions, and their relationships with others do not fit the biomedical context (Clark-Grill 2000). It is possible that a mistake of a similar kind might be involved in asking statistical or biomedically framed questions of certain holistic healing systems (but more of that anon). To look for some common intertranslatable language for these different discourses would be like looking for whatever it is that all implements have in common, which, as Wittgenstein noted, is a futile exercise. "Imagine someone's saying 'All tools serve to modify something. Thus the hammer modifies the position of the nail, the saw the shape of the board, and so on'—And what is modified by the rule, the glue-pot, the nails?" (Wittgenstein 1953, 14).

The fact that different meanings are used to capture different facets of situations implies that they do not stand in a straightforward opposition to one another. We all inhabit the same world, and we use sets of tools whose function we understand to the extent we participate in the relevant discourses. Our participation is practical, and therefore a pragmatic approach to knowledge and truth is plausibly the one most suited to clinical medicine (Toulmin 1997). That different discourses have different associated purposes or activities undercuts the claim that a unitary standard of truth applies to all statements about health and illness (Davidson 1996). Wartofsky, picking up this point, suggests that in this impasse we are condemned to a diversity of knowledges in clinical science. "The medical object is not given, it is constructed in the course of the activity of medicine, and in this sense it is a historically constructed object, the product or artifact of the relevant history of medicine. And so, too, is the practitioner or medical specialist, who comes to be that concrete individual by engaging in that practice" (1997, 63–64).

Wartofsky is careful to distance himself from the claim that the functions identified and investigated by biomedical science are nothing but constructions of medical practices, and he affirms the realist position that they have an objective (or knowledge-independent) existence but argues that our ways of thinking do depend on the therapeutic and theoretical concerns of biomedicine. Pellegrino endorses this essentially realist conception, arguing that medicine must have a metaphysics in common to all of its "disciplines of the most general kind" (1997, 82), and yet he wants to respect what we could call a sense of the clinic and the kind of inquiry that is clinical medicine. Pellegrino's hope is that medicine can, through reflection on its nature as praxis, "enhance our grasp of the universal" (81) while reinforcing the realities specific to its own sphere of activity. But how does this affect the discourses of bioethics?

Here we can find some guidance by examining a Hippocratic discipline with longstanding and thorny problems about its proper object—psychotherapy. Lacan, the most renowned postmodern exponent of Freudian psychoanalysis, addresses these concerns of psychotherapy in his discussion of the scientific status of psychoanalysis (1979). He notes that a basic minimum for any science is that it should have a definite object, although the object "changes, and in a very strange way, as a science develops" (1979, 8). His case for this claim concerns modern and classical physics, but our present topic is the metaphysics of disease.

We tend to classify a state as a disease state only if the patient complains of a problem; so, for instance, a low eosinophil level is not be regarded as a disease. However, such is the imperialism of scientific pathology and pathophysiology in medicine that many things of which patients complain, such as headaches arising from cervical spondylosis or "chronic fatigue syndrome," do not have the status of recognized diseases because we have no adequate account of their pathogenesis and pathophysiology. Other things, however, are regarded as diseases, to be investigated and possibly corrected, on the grounds that they represent deviations from certain norms (such as anemia, obesity, osteoporosis, or hamartomas). The norms themselves are, therefore, to some extent an artifact of the diagnostic sciences and biomeasurement. (For instance, obesity depends on identifying a person's body mass index.) Lacan examines briefly the ability to generate such formulae associated with the objects of scientific inquiry and concludes that "a false science, just like a true science, may be expressed in formulae" (10). He uses the example of alchemy, but other "false sciences" like phrenology, tarot, and palmistry also spring to mind. Thus, measurement, precision, and formulae do not provide grounds on which to distinguish true medical science from pseudoscience. Nevertheless, such grounds are needed for a robust concept of truth, rather than legitimation (according to shifting relationships of power) as the goal of medical knowledge and inquiry.

The Return to Praxis—To What Works

Lacan suggests that we retrace our conceptual steps in the evolution of science and reexamine the idea of a praxis (in much the way that Toulmin, Pellegrino, and Wartofsky have advocated). Any praxis occurs within and defines a field of activity in which its practitioners work. Its concepts allow one to locate (conceptually), interact with, and manipulate or operate on the objects that play key roles in the phenomena constituting that field. Lacan then "gobsmacks" us by suggesting that the development allowing a praxis to become a true science hinges on one thing—"the purity of the soul of the operator."

This is startling because it puts a seemingly moral property, "purity of soul" (whatever that means), at the pivotal point of a decision that seems to be concerned with a matter of fact—whether a discipline is a true science. A moment's reflection soon discloses that this may not be as wacky as, at first, it seems. We are, after all, considering an evaluative decision: whether something is or is not good enough to be called a science. Thus, it is not prima facie unreasonable to think in terms of evaluation of the engineers of our knowledge structures. The worry is that a powerful regime might exercise a suasive and normative influence on science that did not coincide with the science in question "tracking" (or correcting itself in the light of) the actual phenomena it purported to be about. Hacking's "self-authentication" as the normative component of science enhances that worry (1996, 67).

Lacan and Hacking take seriously Foucault's claims regarding legitimation and power as exercised by scientific regimes, but they also suggest that the theoretical commitments of any regime are, in some sense, corrigible. This possibility is related to the role and implications of moral dissent in overturning widely shared moral views (such as the claim that slaves are not really human and therefore can be treated in ways that one would not treat "real human beings"). A decision about the status of a branch of science or a scientific paradigm might, in a similar way, have evaluative content and yet be open to the intricate relations between truth, power, and knowledge. It seems an open question as to whether the judgments of a given regime of truth and the discourse legitimated by it are corrigible. We might find that the pragmatism advocated by Hacking, Pellegrino, and Toulmin gives us a way to avoid the closed circle of power, legitimation, and truth that is taken by many to be the inevitable conclusion of Foucault's analysis. We get out by applying the tools provided by an epistemic regime to the actual sufferings of human beings (which have always been insistent and unavoidable in the Hippocratic ethos) and seeing whether they help us.

A second, related argument also bears on Lacan's claim: some of the qualities indispensable to good scientific inquiry do have a distinctly moral flavor. These include honesty, curiosity, openness to argument, a desire to get to the real data and scrutinize them critically and reflectively, willingness to be humble in the face of conflicting opinions or theories, a passion for truth no matter who is the first to discover it, a readiness to acknowledge and acclaim the achievements of others, and so on. Therefore, there is a moral quality to genuine clinical science, and it is reinforced by compassion and a properly professional attitude to investigating the phenomena that cause human suffering.

We can add Foucault's acknowledgment that not all sciences are on an equal footing in their vulnerability to "external power." He argues that sciences such as theoretical physics and organic chemistry are relatively immune to such influences. What is it that makes a science more likely to approximate truth as a traditional Popperian realist (or representationalist) would understand it and less likely to be subject to power relations shaping its discourses of validation? Medicine is difficult to evaluate when viewed in this light.

On the one hand, it is practical and has palpable results, so the cycle of conceptualization, intervention, monitoring of results, and refinement of theory can be kept in touch with real world events at the coalface that is the clinic. Toulmin (invoking a Wittgensteinian concept) speaks of a medical *lebenswelt* (life-world) comprising *lebensformen* (forms of life) or "different substantive enterprises that have survived the pragmatic tests to which they were subjected in the evolution of those enterprises" (1997, 53)—a conception close to the Hippocratic foundations of medical science. This gives us a reality check on medical truth.

On the other hand, there is a discursive regime conditioning contemporary biomedical science, the outlines of which I have already sketched. This regime exclusively fosters certain kinds of theory (reductive and ultimately biomolecular) and a relatively mechanistic conception of human function subject to statistical scrutiny. It has invisible but palpable control of the medical research industry and over many facets of clinical life, including the legal constraints on best practice—which tend to track technology rather than clear evidence of efficacy. Given the interests converging at the point where medicine meets power, the political process, and economics, we might worry that medicine itself is more prone than other branches of science to ideological and axiomatic distortion. Even the focus on evidence might be a convenient and effective means by which orthodoxy cements its hold on the profession and thereby on the human population it serves.

If we accept that a naïve, or even modestly critical, realist view of scientific knowledge is unsustainable, wherever the regime of truth can be shown to have significant political, economic, and cultural determinants, how can we justify the view that we should ground our medical interventions on proven pathophysiological knowledge (emerging from the orthodox paradigm) rather than opinion? Where and when can we ground medical orthodoxy so as to hold fast to what is good and sketch guidelines for those areas where orthodoxy is not confident? What should our attitude be to those areas where alternative techniques seem to have anecdotal success and call into question the regime of truth that rules medicine?

Orthodoxy and Insecurity

Foucault's challenge to the conventional notion of truth and his focus on the role of power in determining what is accepted as valid knowledge are disturbing to those who espouse the Hippocratic vision. But some concrete examples give us reason to believe that the scientific ground of medicine cannot totally be swept away by these doubts about human knowledge. For instance, in studying the anatomy of the neck, one cannot question that the carotid artery is lateral to the thyroid gland and strap muscles. We are equally certain of other things: spinal cord compression causes loss of function in the limbs distal to the area affected, spontaneous subarachnoid hemorrhage can be prevented by clipping berry aneurysms on cerebral blood vessels, meningitis can be treated with penicillin, and so on. We can therefore add to Foucault's favored exemplars of nondubious science (theoretical physics and organic chemistry) the disciplines of anatomy, laboratory physiology and biochemistry, and some aspects of clinical medicine, pathology, and clinical epidemiology. Thus, in some areas of medical knowledge where we are close to an effective set of interventions and a framework that is neutral between contested areas of therapeutics (such as anatomy and histopathology), we are in no doubt about what counts as truth.

However, we do not have to look far in our clinical sciences for claims that are much more subject to scientific fashions. We might claim, for instance, that drugs in homeopathic doses have no effect on human physiology according to well-established pharmacological experiments. Yet perhaps in a complex and holistic system, even a minute adjustment of certain parameters might, as is found in chaos theory, have profound effects on events that transpire thereafter. Or, to invoke political claims made by Foucault and others, we might dispute that the essential causes of mental disorder are ultimately to be elucidated by close attention to neurobiology and neurochemistry. Can we, in the face of such possibilities, erect any boundary (even if it is fuzzy, shifting, and difficult to define) between those aspects of medical knowledge that are vulnerable to post-Kuhnian and Foucauldian critiques and those that are not?

The Return of the Techne: Reflective Practice

I have hinted that we might find what we need (as Pellegrino claims) in the Aristotelian idea of a techne—an art informed by technical knowledge and reflection showing a dynamic interplay between praxis and conceptualization. This approach (as Toulmin showed) has clear conceptual links to Wittgenstein's analysis of meaning and truth arising within language games and forms of life and evades, to some extent, the challenge directed at traditional epistemology.

Traditional epistemology posits a relation between two independent terms: the world and the thinker. The two relate through the ideas of the thinker. Thus, we have the traditional epistemic problem: If the thinker knows about the world only through (theoretically informed) ideas (and observations), how does she know what things are really like objectively? Traditional idealists and many postmodern writers conclude that ideas, language, or discourses are internal and self-regulating such that different discourses result in hermetically sealed constructions of reality. Truth then becomes located to a particular discourse. The idea of truth is then multiple, and there is no pressure to adjust or moderate a statement by apparently contradictory claims with their roots within different discourses. Not so with a lebenswelt and its lebensformen. Medicine can tolerate and even welcome to some extent the opportunities for cross-fertilization inherent in such a multiplicity of truths but is not totally elastic. We need epistemic norms robust enough to furnish some constraints on what counts as legitimate methodology and theory in clinical practice because what we do affects people.

The pragmatists direct our attention toward the purposes and interests served by knowledge structures in order to evaluate their usefulness for the domain in question. A clinical description should serve to identify features that guide our Hippocratic efforts to understand and alleviate human suffering. Take the following example.

> Emma, a woman of eighty-three, was admitted with a brain hemorrhage. She recovered from the initial shock of the hemorrhage and seemed to be improving, but some three days later she began to "deteriorate." I was called to review her case to see whether surgery was now required. On my way to her bed, the nurse looking after her said that the previous evening she had called her family to her and said her good-byes to all of them. Once I had heard this, it was clear that further scans, tests, and other measures located within the pathophysiological model of events were no longer to the point.

One should not conclude from this story that Emma did not die as a result of her brain hemorrhage, but one should notice that it was a change in her as a subjective human being and not in her hemorrhage that led to her death. This shift in attitude has radical implications for the axioms that ground biomedical science and our appreciation of health and disease.

The understanding of a clinical situation in human terms is a different understanding from that yielded by medical science and its tests. Holistic understanding is, no doubt, different again. The understanding that disputes the genetic programming model of embryonic development is different again. Clinicians inhabit a number of discourses and must become adept in several of them if they are to understand what is happening to their patients. The human and biomedical discourses alone form two very different maps that picture the same terrain, and they approach that terrain from such different sets of concerns (and therefore perspectives) that they may not be intertranslatable. There are alternative conceptualizations of the situation of the eighty-three-year-old woman, and we make an evaluative selection in diagnosing her "deterioration." To grasp the situation, we have to understand, at least in some small part, her narrative because her response is part of a moral reality that has to do with the place of her condition in the totality of her life. Her body must be seen as a subjective body such that the "soul trajectory" has determined the course of her physical trajectory in a way that is obvious when we hear the nurse's report. The closed framework of "scientific" or biomedical knowledge is not sufficient for the case. This concession, as in general epistemology, does not undermine a substantial conception of truth (as related to purpose-driven cognitive maps of a domain of praxis); it merely permits alternative conceptualizations where the phenomena concerned are complex and may be produced by the interaction of multiple factors.

Truth is a function of a given cognitive map (and therefore lebenswelt). Because it is advantageous not to have a series of isolated and impressionistic maps of any domain of activity, human thinkers tend to make connections between intersecting (and sometimes irreconcilable) concepts and constructions. Some thoughts, such as the thought that the eighty-three-year-old woman wanted most of all to live, even when seen in this tolerant light, come out as just plain false. Others, such as the thought that she saw her admission and stroke as the point at which her life would end, come out as true. Each thought is assessed in an appropriate way; the idea that the hematoma had extended and was killing her comes out as false because the relevant tests show it not to be so (not because her death can be explained otherwise). Each true thought fits well into its own conceptual or cognitive map of the situation and to some extent validates the use of that map at that time. We hope that at least some of the true thoughts we have in such a clinical situation (in this case, the one at the human level) allow us to move with assurance and propriety in our actions toward the patient. On that ground, the thought about the meaning of this event in the whole context of her life as a human being is good, it has what truth-bearing and adequately action-guiding thoughts ought to have. It has, we could say, both epistemic and practical value because these, for a pragmatist, coincide.

Wittgenstein points us toward the mastery of an area of praxis (and its accompanying discourse) as the basis of knowledge. Truth emerges from a mastery of the rules operating in an area of discourse and a willingness to be open to the corrections and informal constraints on truth claims that arise in the relevant praxis.

Therefore, moral virtue and epistemic virtue are intertwined. It takes a certain kind of person to achieve the relevant openness to experience (Nussbaum 1990), and it takes a certain kind of cognitive skill to conceptualize what experience reveals. Any praxis involves whole people, subjective bodies, and their intersecting trajectories. Appreciating that this is reality is central to clinical practice. Medical knowledge does more than assess theories on the basis of a supposed relation between theory and data. Clinicians engage with patients; they try out ways of conceptualizing what is going on until they discover regularities that are worth conceptualizing and working with so as to achieve mastery or competence in their practice. The result is Hippocratic knowledge, the multifaceted set of skills that can effectively and reliably deliver our patients from suffering.

Truth, Virtue, and the Techne

These vague moves toward a post-Kuhnian epistemology for medical science take us back toward the epistemic and practical values endorsed by Hippocrates. I have used the term *epistemic virtue* and linked epistemic and moral virtue, in a way that Plato and Aristotle both could be taken to suggest, as different facets of the same jewel. But is this position robust in the face of a postmodern critique of clinical practice and its scientific products?

Foucault argues that power and relations of power control the legitimation of statements within any given discourse. This applies a fortiori in medical discourse where a set of power relations confer an exalted status on the conceptualizations and validated judgments of doctors as distinct from others. Doctors decide "what is really going on," "the good of the patient," "good evidence for this or that," "a reasonable therapeutic option," and so on. The story of the patient can be left out of this set of discursive constructions, and, even more radically, the privileged discourse excludes the patient's opinion about whether the medical story actually fits his illness. If postmodernism teaches us any lessons, they would include the idea that the thoughts or discursive constructions of situations that most deserve our endorsement are those that do not serve oppressive power imbalances. This implies a moral constraint on genuine clinical knowledge. True knowledge, despite reflecting a discursive arrangement put in place by a power group (such as clinicians in medicine), should not obliterate or otherwise negate the perspectives (or subjectivities) of others involved in the relevant situations. For this reason, a patient should not be the focus solely of that type of knowledge leading to a limited range of biomedical interventions. Clinical knowledge should be able to be owned equally by the sufferer and the agent who hopes to alleviate that suffering. Thus, considerations like respect, participation, mutual concern, understanding, and so on have key roles.

It emerges that the proper evaluative aspects of clinical practice, the moral commitments of good doctors, and the sharing of information and power are inseparable from genuine clinical knowledge. A Platonic conception of *the good* as the ultimate constraint on human thought (one shared but not made so explicit by Aristotle) implies that goodness is a sine qua non for true knowledge, and it looks as if clinicians would be well advised to take that conception to heart. Lacan's remark about the purity of the soul of the operator is therefore vindicated (for medicine at least) in that clinical practice is an area in which the relation between the good and knowledge emerges more clearly and closely than in any other area of scientific endeavor. What is more, the penetration of our knowledge by the good allows us to speak of a set of scientific and professional norms for medicine that coincide with the internal morality that emerges from its Hippocratic ethos.

Hippocrates thought that clinical science is the exemplar of science in general because it methodically and sensitively charts the accumulated wisdom that comes from observing and intervening in real and pressing natural phenomena. The inseparability of praxis from science in medicine can be used to understand the nature of reason in general. Reason, on this pragmatic account, has much more to do with acting well than with building theoretical structures that cater to a shifting elite who dominate our ideas through a regime of truth. True reason cannot be separated from the openness to experience and care for human suffering with which the Hippocratic writers attempted to infuse it.

Postmodern Illness and Virtue

The intrusion of postmodern thinking into medical ethics reinforces the direction that the present inquiry is taking. Charles Taylor, Ian Hacking, and Art Frank have each explored medicine through the lens of the postmodern perception "that illness is no longer a purely biological state—no longer a brute fact of nature—but rather something in part created or interpenetrated by culture" (Morris 1998, 71). The idea that disease is a "biocultural" phenomenon (to pick up Morris's term) provokes a rethinking of the image of medical truth as a representation of kinds of dysfunction understandable in the limited terms of biomedical science. The fluidity and uncertainty that results are captured in an assessment of disease theory and medical nosology after the impact of postmodernism. "Social forces, in effect, always reconfigure the contexts of human life. Truth, within this poststructuralist vision, is plural and contingent: it is truth (with a lowercase *t*) situated within history, limited by the outlook of specific disciplines, shaped by the interests of dominant groups, perplexed by the inherent indeterminacy of language, caught up in a flow of social power: uncertain, temporary, ironic" (73–74).

What social forces reconfigure is, notably, truth, and not the virtues required by the current account to discern and respond to the multiple truths found in the narratives of patients. In the poststructuralist context (one that has gone beyond the structure of signs, texts, and political functions that might otherwise make a human life no more than a cipher for a conglomeration of fragmented moments of signification), we look for the appropriated story. In the story, the teller presents/presences him or herself to us so that the narrative is inherently relational (Frank 1996, 144). The story is told under certain constraints; the patient does not control the way his or her body appears in the story, and the very fact that the subjective body has fallen under the medical gaze indicates that it is not doing that which it normally does. We need to appreciate the alienation that has crept into the subjective body to understand the patient's dis-ease, that which is not allowing a harmony of subjective bodily function. Now such dis-ease/harmony might arise from within or from a mismatch between the subjective body and its environment. To appreciate it, we must be ready, as Hippocratic practitioners:

1. to recognize the narrative coherence of the patient's story;
2. to identify the multiplicity of tellings, listenings, and interpretations that characterize that story;
3. to notice and explore the contradictions in this multiplicity; and
4. to deepen the appreciation of the participants in the health care event.

Brody (1987) coins the remark "My story is broken, can you help me fix it?" as the key to the clinical encounter, and we should notice that, just as it is for any good orthopedic surgeon, our first task is to identify the fracture and, from an appreciation of the normal anatomy (or narrative structure), assist the patient to mend the story.

An openness to individual meaning and the diversity of narratives within different cultures and subcultures that our healing work may involve, in the light of a commitment to preserving what is valued by the human being before us, is bound to enhance our ability to remain open-minded in the face of normal clinical science (or the existing paradigm, as Kuhn would have it) and its discursive regime.

There is, therefore, a significant convergence between, on the one hand, the epistemic and moral virtues of the Hippocratic tradition (marked by compassion, empathy, and pragmatism) and, on the other hand, the conception of clinical science that emerges from the postmodern critique. This convergence allows us to move ahead in specifying some of the hallmarks of virtuous practice for the Hippocratic professional in a postmodern era.

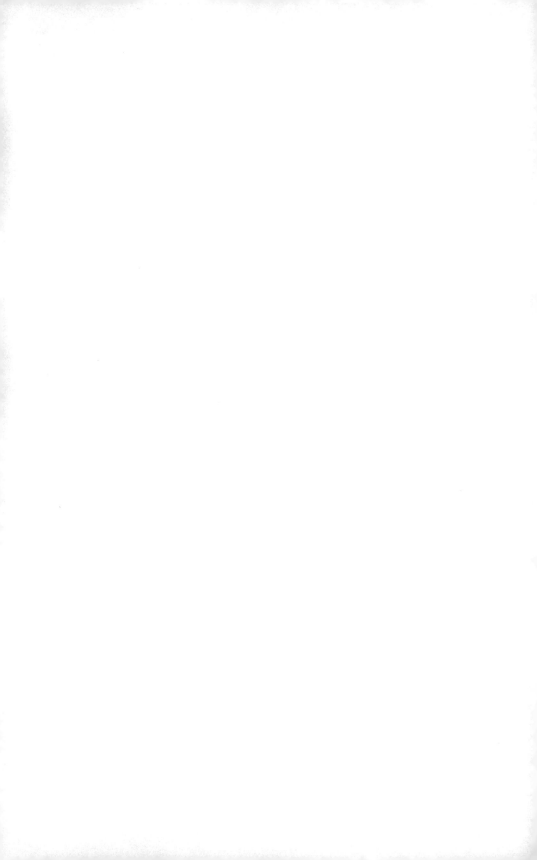

Part II / Clinical Practice

CHAPTER FOUR

Getting over Informed Consent

Although it were no easy matter for common people to discover for themselves the nature of their own diseases and the causes they get worse or better, yet it is easy for them to follow when another makes the discoveries and explains the events to them. —TRADITION IN MEDICINE

Informed consent is supposed to be a byword for patient-centered clinical practice, but it is time for it to grow toward a more effective understanding of medical decision making that allows patients to participate in and therefore take ownership of those parts of their life narratives that must be spent in medical treatment. In fact, informed consent is one of the three topics on which I am most commonly asked to lecture by medical audiences (end-of-life decisions and surgical innovation being the others). I well recall plunging just such an audience into stunned silence when, while the autonomy brigade was in full cry in New Zealand medicine, I announced that I did not believe in informed consent. This chapter explains why I made that remark.

Informed Consent and Being Lost

The proper attitude to informed consent begins by recognizing that the patient is on a journey and has strayed from his or her chosen path of life into the wasteland of illness and disease. Here the patient meets a strange context— the clinical world—which runs according to its own rules—many of them unwritten—and has its own hierarchy. (I will call this world *Clinicum*.) Clinicum definitely has doctors as the elite, even though statutory seniority might seem to attach to administrators. Yet the doctor, while walking the discursive mountaintops of the land of Clinicum, is also the primary point of contact between the medical system and the patient, and here the requirements are different from those necessary to succeed in a hierarchy (although the kind of success conventionally sought is, I suspect, a "boojum").

The doctor is the patient's guide to this strange landscape and its apparently alien inhabitants who move to the beat of a different drum from the real world—of friendship, sports, the coffee shop, courtship, and messing about. Of course, the alien-ness is a mask as is obvious once one has a *kosher* place in the clinic or, for a patient, when one of the "aliens"(naturalized inhabitants) makes contact. Nevertheless, illusion or not, the need for someone to be a trusted guide is great for every patient. The doctor is ideally placed to fill this role because the other inhabitants of Clinicum often, consciously and subconsciously, model their behavior on that of the doctor. A distant and aloof doctor has a somewhat sacrosanct presence, but a friendly and reassuring doctor who anticipates the patient's fears and uncertainties, and crosses the divide that is professional distance (in one of its many guises) creates an inclusive atmosphere. The Hippocratics recognized this problem. "Physicians come to a case in full health of body and mind. They compare the present symptoms of the patient with similar cases they have seen in the past, so that they can say how cures were affected then. But consider the view of the patients. They do not know what they are suffering from, nor why they are suffering from it, nor what will succeed their present symptoms. Nor have they experience of the course of similar cases. Their present pains are increased by fears for the future" (Science of Medicine, 142).

When we look through the eyes of the patient (imaginatively or through our own ill health), we realize immediately that the patient needs a map of the land that he or she has strayed into. Doctors, nurses, and other Hippocratic professionals who have been here before and have some idea of what the journey is likely to involve therefore need to provide that map, and the patient must also be encouraged to think about it so as to be part of the team that can bring the journey to a successful conclusion. That end is not served by informed consent as commonly practiced and is much better served by regarding the patient as a partner in the problem-solving exercise that is health care. "Partnership means that patients and doctors must change, sharing responsibilities as well as information and decision making. It takes two to tango" (*British Medical Journal*, 1999).

The doctor must be convinced that partnership is the right way to go, or it will not work. If it does work, though, the doctor will find that the narrative of managing illness is improved just as much as the narrative of living through, or bearing up under the burden of, that illness. I learned this in a very telling way.

> I used to be convinced of the doctrine of informed consent way back when I saw as though in a glass darkly. In the name of informed consent, I would engage my patients in earnest discussion about their illness and my proposed cure for it. The problem was usually of the form: "How can I get them to consent to the operations I think they should have?" Clinics were on Thursday afternoons, and they were often very crowded and very stressful. I used to work hard for my patients and feel responsible for their health care outcomes. I explained, drew diagrams, used metaphors, talked about odds in creative ways, and "wore myself to a frazzle." The Thursday afternoon tension headache was a regular feature of my life.
>
> One day my patient asked to see his X-rays. I thought "Why not?" and pointed out the problem in his spine that needed an operation. I did the same with the next patient. This worked so well that it became a regular habit. What is more, I found that patients would ask reasonable questions about options, and together we sometimes opted for a course of management that I thought less than optimal. It turned out that I was not always right in my convictions about best management (as is the case with many distinguished clinical experts in the light of objective evidence). After a few weeks, I began to notice that my headaches were less frequent and less severe. I lost less time off work, and as a result the tension was turned down even further. I would sometimes come back to my office and remark to my secretary, "I have such wonderful patients."

In the mode of the reflective practitioner, I ought now to ask why this was so.

In the Name of Autonomy, Beneficence, Nonmaleficence, and Justice, So Help Me God

Beauchamp and Childress (1989), and others who worship the fourfold godhead of bioethics led by autonomy, have outlined the nature of informed consent, in which we all, at least at some stage, have believed.

Informed consent is based on the idea that every individual of sound mind has the right to make decisions about his or her own body and what will be done to it. We then ask what standard of information is required to allow an individual to make an informed decision of this kind. The goalposts also move depending on key court decisions. However, the difference between *spontaneous* and *responsive* disclosure is sometimes not reflected in ethical or legal discussions of these decisions and the resulting standards.

Spontaneous disclosure concerns information given either in spoken, written, or video form; it should tell the patient what the problem is, what is likely to happen, what interventions are possible and what they aim to achieve, and it should convey the risks of any planned intervention. The crucial legal test (one that is instructive for ethicists) is *material risk*. A material risk is a risk that would be taken into account by a reasonable person in making the decision in question. In effect, this means that serious but low-probability risks, such as quadriplegia or incontinence, as well as more probable but less serious risks, such as wound infection or bone-graft pain, should be mentioned. The reference to a reasonable patient rather than this particular patient implies what is often called an *objective patient standard* as distinct from a *subjective patient standard.*

Responsive disclosure comprises information given in response to the patient's requests and so on. Both subjective and objective standards assume that the patient's questions must be answered honestly and with the accuracy to be expected of a qualified specialist in the area. Thus, the standard for responsive information is fairly clear in the Sidaway decision and others (*Sidaway v. Board of Governors,* 1985; Skegg 1988). The subjective patient standard focuses on the level of disclosure dictated by a particular patient's concerns (*Rogers v. Whitaker,* 1992). In the *Rogers v. Whitaker* case, an eye surgeon did not disclose the risk of blindness in the contralateral eye (estimated as 1 in 14,000) even though his patient clearly had a major concern about her vision in that eye. Although most professionals would have realized from her remarks that she had this concern, the surgeon concerned did not mention the risk of sympathetic ophthalmia. The patient became blind, and she sued him. The court ruled that the surgeon should have realized that the risk of contralateral blindness was of material concern to this patient despite its very low probability and that therefore it should have been mentioned. The decision dramatically underscores the need for the doctor to buy into the patient's story and appreciate the patient's dilemma, just as the Hippocratic writings indicate.

The aim of informed consent is to enable the patient to make a reasoned decision about his or her treatment. If the surgeon puts herself in the patient's shoes, then it becomes obvious that the patient needs to know what is wrong, what is proposed, what will happen if it is not done, the likely benefits of the proposed intervention, the chances of success, and the material risks. Information to the patient should cover all these points with a clear indication of the options open. It is the patient's choice as to what will happen, although the doctor, if we take note of the Hippocratic remarks, is best placed to make a recommendation. Note that this is a recommendation and not a prescription, and patients should be aware that such decisions are theirs alone to make.

The patient should not feel coerced to make any particular decision. Coercion can take many forms apart from direct pressure by surgeons to go along with their recommendations. Some patients feel coerced by the fact that they have waited for a long time for their treatment, and they worry that hesitancy or time taken to think about things will move them to the bottom of the waiting list. Other patients feel that they have to make a decision immediately in the surgeon's consulting room or clinic. Yet others feel uncertain but worry that the surgeon will be offended if they want to discuss it with someone else or seek a second opinion. The surgeon should therefore make the patient feel comfortable about taking as long as is needed to make an informed and careful decision, while giving a clear and realistic indication of any risks associated with delay of treatment. It is often helpful to send the patient a copy of the letter to the referring doctor so that the patient can see exactly what is being proposed and be as clear as possible about the decision that has to be made.

Necessity is a concept that covers treatment that must proceed even though consent is not possible. In some situations where the patient's wishes cannot be ascertained, the doctor ought to do those things that clearly would be done were the best interests of the patient the sole consideration. In such a case, however, the onus is on the surgeon to show that there was no alternative but to proceed given the facts available and that what was done seemed necessary to safeguard the well-being of the patient. Legitimate questions then arise about the soundness of the surgeon's clinical judgement and the attempts made to ascertain the true wishes of the patient. The patient's best interests would be judged according to something like the standard I have laid out elsewhere—*an outcome that now or in the future the patient would think was worthwhile.*

Therapeutic privilege refers to the discretion of a clinician to judge that disclosure of a certain sort would harm the patient and ought, therefore, to be withheld. But the doctor needs to make a careful and informed judgment about that harm because there is virtually no defense if the patient later says, "But I would want to have known, even though I would have found it hard to cope with." I believe that the doctor has a responsibility not only to "spill the beans" but also to try to equip the patient to deal with the spillage. Thus the preferred option is always to develop skills allowing the patient to receive even the worst of news, perhaps because, along with that news, the patient is assured that the doctor will be present to help. The guideline is therefore that one should use therapeutic privilege only in the most difficult cases where disclosure is almost certain to harm the patient.

Clinical research and innovative treatment are also bound by these same principles. It is mandatory that the surgeon disclose that certain interventions are part of a research trial, are unproven, or are innovative and depart from standard clinical practice. Generally, clinicians (with advice from patient groups) can write a fairly comprehensive information sheet about the research or innovation so that patients can understand it.

Clinicians following the partnership model such that "both parties . . . share information and make decisions jointly" (Coulter 1999) will find that, even when partnership is not really possible, their style of clinical management is influenced by the experience.

But how do we decide whether doctors do well or do badly, given that patients sometimes do not accurately recall what they have been told (Byrne, Napier, and Cushcieri, 1988)?

The Track Record: Characteristics of Integrity

When reviewing a consent process, we have to ask about the quality of the information given, the extent to which the patient was satisfied, felt pressured, falsely reassured, or persuaded to do what he did not want to do, and so on. What is more, the judgments required are retrospective, and the facts are often obscure or poorly recorded, so we can have little confidence in what was said, how it was said, or the extent to which a partnership was created. We are not, however, completely bereft of guidance because we often have access to some information about the physician's clinical practice.

The clinical history of a particular physician can give us, at best, a conclusion of the type: If it was Doctor X, and the facts are less than clear, then he probably acted something like this. But it remains to justify this kind of appeal when a particular set of events is our concern. Justification emerges from Peter Winch's discussion of the story of Billy Budd: "Billy Budd, a fore-topman of angelic character, is impressed into service on the *Indomitable* from the merchantman *Rights of Man* on the high seas. He is persecuted by a satanic master-at-arms of the *Indomitable,* Claggart, in a campaign that culminates in Claggart's falsely accusing Billy before [Captain] Vere, of inciting the crew to mutiny. In the stress of this situation, Budd is afflicted by a speech-impediment which prevents him from answering the charge. Frustrated, he strikes Claggart, who falls, strikes his head and dies" (Winch 1972, 155).

Captain Vere is in an unenviable situation. He must maintain order after the recent mutinies at Spithead and the Nore, and he feels that British naval discipline is hanging by a thread. Naval law dictated that Billy Budd should hang for striking a superior officer, but one's sense of natural justice prompts the thought that he had been so strongly provoked that a lesser penalty would be warranted. Vere, at the drumhead court-martial that he summons to try the case, is visibly moved by Budd's plight, and yet he recommends the death penalty, arguing that a more severe law than our common humanity should prevail. Winch, reflecting on Vere's judgment, considers that his actual decision, in and of itself, is evidence that counts for its own rightness despite our inclinations to opt for clemency in the light of the facts. Winch argues that the reactions and opinions of a good moral judge in a morally challenging situation ought to be taken into account in making a retrospective moral decision. But how can he argue in this apparently circular manner?

Winch notes that the virtuous person, faced with a moral challenge, is uniquely placed because he or she actually participates in the problematic situation. The many diverse and unnamed factors that should influence a properly weighted moral judgment bear directly on the participants but are only indistinctly present to a distanced spectator.

Given this fact, Winch asks certain questions of the agent whose decision is in question.

1. Did he or she appreciate the moral conflict involved?
2. Did he or she act with endorsable moral sensitivities and dispositions?
3. Did he or she act sincerely aiming to do what was right?

If the answer to these questions is *yes,* then it is likely that the agent did what was right in that situation, all things considered. Such an orientation seems entirely apt for those situations in which we wonder about the emphasis put on certain features of a clinical decision—its likelihood of success or failure, the extent to which the patient is coping, the dangers of the proposed intervention, the prognosis without it, and so on. In such cases, we rely on doctors to be trust-worthy guides—to discuss the clinical problem in such a way that it is easy for patients to decide and commit to what is in their own best interests.

This is not a blanket endorsement of "good doctors." If one is judged as having done the right thing according to this test, not only would the doctor have to have a good track record of dealing with patients, but also we would need convincing that the doctor appreciated the uncertainties and challenges of the intervention proposed, and that the situation in question was one in which the doctor actually did do his or her best (an unimpaired performance without conflict of interest). Because detailed evidence on all these points is unlikely to be available, this is an area of ongoing disputes. Therefore, in the interest of justice and effective patient care, safe procedures are needed to try to ensure generally good practice (to which I shall return below).

In my own case, the issue is summed up in the saying, "This is like catching the bus to Mornington." Let me explain.

> Mornington is an inner-city hill suburb in the town where I live and is served by a commuter bus. The bus service is reliable and has few accidents (although they do happen occasionally). Now, I regularly perform an operation called "anterior cervical diskectomy" in which a prolapsed intervertebral disc is removed to re-lieve pressure on the spinal cord or nerve roots in the neck. This operation has, in certain hands, a fearsome reputation. If there are complications, they can be very serious and include paralysis from the neck down, troublesome and deep-seated infection of the discs or bones in the neck, and so on. But I have been doing this operation three or four times a month for nearly twenty years, and that has never happened. So, to put the risks in perspective, I tell my patients about those risks and then remark, "But honestly I do not lose any sleep over this. In my hands it is no more risky than catching the bus to Mornington." Innumerable patients when their consent is later checked by a nurse or resident, spontaneously come out with this line and, if not, those checking the consent sometimes ask, "Did he mention the bus to Mornington?"

This, in an informal way that can be systematized and improved, is the kind of safeguard needed to make sure that patients and those monitoring informed consent are aware what is going on. But it does not always work. One elderly lady, having been admitted for an elective procedure on her lumbar spine, said to the nursing staff in the operating room, "Oh, yes, Dr. Gillett told me all about it. He said I would end up in a wheelchair but that I needed the operation anyway." Needless to say, I hadn't (said that), she did (need the operation), and she didn't (end up in a wheelchair); indeed, she was a lot more mobile after the operation than before.

Why are some doctors so good at communicating with patients and others have great difficulty? I was once told (by an ethicist), when I said that our job as ethicists in medical schools was to train medical students in the virtues, that what I proposed was impossible. I do not agree. Aristotelians maintain that young people, full of ideals and absolutes as they are, become virtuous only as a result of experience and training, and that once set on the right course, they will see the value of, and tend to develop into, good human beings. I have already remarked that this is done by directing the attention of the novice to features of a situation that are morally important, by encouraging imagination and empathy, by inculcating right habits and dispositions, and by engaging in reflective discussion of experiences. Being a trusted guide in a health journey requires all these things. They come about through a certain kind of conversation between doctor and patient which Ron Carson summarizes beautifully in his reflections on the metaphor provided by the hyphen in the doctor-patient relationship. "The hyphenated space in the doctor-patient relationship is a liminal place of ethical encounter, alternating voices and actions—back and forth, address and response—seeking mutually satisfactory meaning by means of which an illness that has threatened to fray or sever the storyline of a life can be woven into the fabric of that life. The hyphen points to the prospect of overcoming silence with meaningful conversation" (2002, 180).

Carson also speaks of the joining together in a common enterprise and the setting apart from one another that the hyphen between doctor and patient so graphically represents. The doctor must bring to this relationship the clinical and discursive skills that are required for it to work. Only by making it work, by forging a team involving the patient, can doctors improve this process for patients and for themselves.

The Hyphenated Relationship and Empowerment

The liminality (or thresholdlikeness) of the hyphen consists in the ambiguity of location in the doctor-patient relationship. It occurs in the real world but also within the world of Clinicum. It is a relationship of respectful unequals in which one partner necessarily wields more power; it is also an agent-patient relationship in which any healing must, in part, be the work of the patient. In some medical curricula, attention is paid to helping medical students come to recognize the great influence they wield when they deal with patients. What is less common is explicit acknowledgment of the power dynamics in the physician-patient relationship in relation to informed consent. Even if the patient believes their consent to be valid, he or she may not have been sufficiently empowered to make decisions that reflect their life narratives.

Usually, the physician knows much more about the medical condition of the patient than anybody else, and therefore the patient naturally looks to the physician for the most complete information about what is going on. For this to work, the patient must trust the physician, but in the normal situation there is a message conveyed by the fact that the patient does not get to see the physician's investigations or notes. The implicit message is that the information belongs on the powerful side of the medical relationship and should be controlled by the doctor or the system.

> Bill, a bluff ex-farmer, had become a shopkeeper in a rural town. He had hemifacial spasm—a condition that screws up the side of the face so that the patient is often taken to be winking at people to whom he is talking (much to his and their embarrassment). This condition causes frequent misunderstandings, particularly for a shopkeeper, and he wanted to be rid of it. The operation is a microvascular decompression of the seventh cranial nerve (which innervates the muscles of the face). It carries a 25 percent risk of ipsilateral deafness. In the event, Bill did not completely lose his tic but he did lose the hearing in his left ear. The issue came up at a clinical meeting where his case was being discussed by a group of neurosurgeons and neurologists. One of the neurologists asked how Bill had felt when he realized he was not free of his tic but he had become deaf in one ear. Bill said, "Well, I accepted that because Mr. Gillett warned me about it before the operation and what's more he used words that were a bloody-sight easier to understand than this stuff you jokers have been spouting for the last half hour."

" 'Nuff said." There is more to the dynamic here than the fact that the doctors knew more than Bill. Bill had clearly felt that he knew enough to make a reasoned decision, even though the neurosurgeon was more educated and seemed a busy and important man. I doubt whether he was told all the possible complications to posterior fossa microsurgery, but he would have known enough to know the major risks he was facing. In fact, the problems are manifold. The neurosurgeon need not be unfriendly, and yet, explaining a surgical procedure, he may speak in such a manner that makes it hard for any patient to interrupt. He may convey the idea that the patient's operation is merely one among many of his duties so that the agenda for any clinical encounter is severely constrained. In fact, after giving Bill the information that he thought sufficient, if he did not ask whether Bill had any questions or would like more information, Bill himself may not have felt able to create an agenda of his own and therefore his concerns may not have been addressed. In actual fact, it is evident that they were and that the interview was conducted so that Bill could understand and think about the risks. Often that does not happen, and that single factor seems to be the most important reason why doctors get sued (Warren 1980; Studdert et al., 2000). Often, one feels that, despite the clinician thinking that a clinical encounter has been comprehensive and informative, the interview was all on the doctor's terms and at the edge of a world that patients feel to be quite beyond them and into which they should not presume to trespass.

This problem can be overcome only by a change of attitude such that clinicians come to see themselves as merely part of patients' lives. They enter at the points where patients have strayed into the badlands and may be very unsure and insecure about what is going on. If physicians become trusted guides, they can make patients more confident in their own ability to take part in the problem-solving task. My showing my patients their X-rays and conveying the attitude that they could appreciate the problem opened my own eyes. It showed the patients that we can approach the clinical problem with open eyes and open minds, and it conveyed to me how simple and yet profound the idea of patient participation is. This simple measure, which clinicians increasingly are taking up, achieves several things:

1. It tells patients that the information is accessible and that they can take an intelligent interest in it.
2. It allows patients to see the difficulties and uncertainties involved in medical diagnosis and treatment.
3. It tends to dissipate rather than increase the stress on patients, just as one feels less stressed the more one understands where one is on a trying journey.
4. It gives the patient permission to inquire about their tests and their treatment; they have, as it were, been invited across the gap dividing them from their own medical information.

5. The patients find, often to their surprise, that they can understand what is going on and, as a result, feel able to claim some ownership of the decisions being made.
6. Ownership and responsibility go hand in hand; therefore, the patients' sharing the burden of decision making relieves some of that burden on the clinician.

Think of the difference between playing a hand of cards close to one's chest and laying it down to play in a cooperative manner for the purposes of instructing a novice. If we adopt the open-handed attitude in clinical situations, it is possible for patients to be more active and learn more about their treatment options. This empowerment enables patients not just to consent (in a way that is informed and voluntary) but to assume some control over a medicalized part of their autobiographies. Empowerment of that kind gives reality to the hyphen as the mark of a problem-solving alliance. Yet the hyphen must be embraced by the clinician, and the rules for this "language game" are laid down on the playing fields of Clinicum by body language, conversation, dress, deportment, and the techniques of engagement. According to the reformed attitude, decisions cannot be made absent the patient, recommendations have to be formulated as clearly and considerately as possible, uncertainties have to be shared, and we have to be open to the possibility that the outcome or process may not be exactly as the clinician initially plans. Only so can the participation of the patient become a reality in clinical life. The advantages of such an approach are legion. They include patients becoming educated observers of their own illnesses and their management, and, therefore, co-travelers on the path of therapy.

The neurosurgical treatment recommended for the sufferer of a brain tumor—call her Rosalind—brings the issues into clear focus. Will she take the risks and side effects associated with surgery—possible paralysis of a limb or, depending on its location, loss of speech—or will she refuse an operation, given that it cannot cure her? Empowerment enables patients to decide on the best option for them, all things considered, whether their problem is a malignant brain tumor or a chronic pain problem.

Any course of treatment involves conflicting considerations. There are some diseases where, in Hippocratic terms, "a man is attacked by a disease more powerful than the instruments of medicine," and in such cases experienced clinicians often realize that they can only harm by using their medical skills. Other cases are less clear-cut, and in these our resources, if used intelligently, can produce a good outcome. We can communicate these uncertainties in such a way that the patient realizes that the problem is taxing and difficult and that a good outcome cannot be guaranteed. Most patients can appreciate such difficulties, but often they are offered no more than a glimpse into a complex and kaleidoscopic situation glossed by false medical assurances that we have it all under control. It is no wonder, therefore, that they become disillusioned and even cynical when our confident assertions prove empty and worthless. Statues with feet of clay should not accept the status of gods.

In the closed-hand model, consent functions as a relatively forced choice made under a set of constraints and contingencies largely unknown to the patient, according to a time scale fixed by somebody else's narrative and on turf controlled by the medical establishment. The realities undermine in practice any abstract value of autonomy, and it is understandable that the ideals of communication and decision making endorsed by such a model do not achieve patient empowerment in practice. Real empowerment actually enables patients, through free, responsive, and rational cooperation with a clinician, to devise a management plan that leads to the outcome most congenial to their own perceptions and values. Only so can patients take some responsibility for their own health care; it does not happen by loading them with a great deal of complex information, giving little in the way of help to understand that information, and leaving them "free" (or autonomous) to choose this or that possible (or fanciful) escape from their dilemma.

A Narrative Approach and Empowerment

Narrative ethics (and its postmodern awareness of power, subjectivity, legitimation, and silence) are ideally suited to serve the ends for which informed consent was designed. But going beyond informed consent, narrative ethics are alert to and take account of the power differentials that distort moral relationships and silence the voices of those traditionally disempowered by an institution and its discourses (Gillett 1997). We must now consider the silences that abound in clinical encounters and the points at which patients cannot grasp what they found unsatisfactory about their care. The language of autonomy, beneficence, nonmaleficence, and justice does not throw these points into sharp relief, and it paradoxically leaves patients feeling "all at sea" or "out of control" in a way that they need not. A narrative appreciation of the patient's predicament addresses disempowerment and silence without aligning the physician and patient on opposite sides in claims about rights and duties. Postmodern theorists offer us an appreciation of the problems of naming those aspects of discourses in which certain people are condemned to powerlessness. Deconstructing such situations often shows that there may be no intention to marginalize the patient by those who hold the power and that, in fact, the powerful players may not even realize what is going on.

If, as Murray suggests, narratives put us in touch with "stories and images of good, fulfilling, meaningful lives" (1997, 54), then the stories encountered in clinical practice, particularly when we hear the multiple voices telling them, show us complex moral dilemmas in a way that moral principles and duties may fail to do. Such insights reveal the plights of the marginalized and powerless (which, to some extent, includes all our patients) because they tend to capture the lived experience of the person who is vulnerable, who can enunciate only a truncated or attenuated narrative. Postmodern and narrative ethics enable us to say, with the songwriter, "I've looked at life from both sides now" and to have some hope of telling and hearing truth as it shows itself to each point of view.

The empowerment of patients forces doctors and particularly specialists, to relinquish their godlike, even if gracious and kind, control of clinical management. By so doing doctors, and indeed health care professionals in general, are released to take part in a much more cooperative and ultimately satisfying adventure. That new adventure still has its sticky patches, and some characters in any narrative are just "ornery" or "awkward," but, by and large, empowerment and the relative equalization of roles in health care is more healthy both for those who are cared for and for those who care.

To return to my headaches, the answer now seems as plain as day. After adopting the open-handed view in a visible and inescapable way, I was no longer inflicting on my patients my answer to their ills and thereby taking on the karma of the success or otherwise of their treatments. I was sharing the load of responsibility, sharing the ownership and control of clinical decisions in which I took part, and learning to work *with* subjective bodies rather than just work *on* them. In this way, my relationship to the people who were those subjective bodies underwent a radical transformation. Their sufferings, hopes, and even their silences became a little more accessible to me.

And so, on into the silences.

CHAPTER FIVE

Listening to the Silences

The authors . . . have omitted a great deal of what the physician should
learn from his patient without his telling him; details of which vary from
case to case but the interpretation of which may be of vital importance.

—REGIMEN

In this passage the Hippocratic writers chide other medical teachers for failing
to take note of what the physician can learn from an appreciation that goes
beyond the "history." The same sensitivity is, however, also worth exercising in
listening to that story.

I recently lectured a class of medical students about the mind, as part of their
brain and behavior course. The session was at nine on a Monday morning, and
they knew that the content would not be examined, which made any turnout
seem quite impressive. During the lecture, I wrote the word *misty* on the board
and asked them what it meant. It was a winter's morning in Dunedin, so there
was an obvious explanation. In fact, the word was meant as the title of the Errol
Garner jazz classic that, on the same occasion one year previously, had a special
significance for me. The incident captures the essence of the mind-brain relationship; a brain scientist might have told me a great deal about the neurocog-
nitive circuitry that was active, but to explain what *misty* meant to me reaches
beyond my own brain into my relationships, my autobiography, and the symbolism of my culture.

To appreciate what things mean to me is to catch a glimpse of my conscious world or lived autobiography. The descriptions or significations needed to do that are not available in the terminology of biomedical science as taught in medical schools (although some of the wider aspects of human life and the concepts that articulate them are creeping into the curricula). These wider terms are the key to the silences that pervade clinical encounters. To understand these silences is to begin to appreciate the patient's world and the journey that the patient is on, which, as I have tried to show, is essential if one wants to be a trustworthy guide for the patient in the world of the clinic. So, moving on from informed consent, we must learn to attend to the gaps in the patient's story. These may hold the key to the "brokenness" of that story and therefore may be central to resolving the problem that is the illness.

Locating the Silences

Two kinds of silence are endemic to human suffering. The first is found where there are gaps in a person's psychological life, and the second is imposed by the medical setting and its legitimated discourses.

Silences have many origins, only some of which have consciously grasped reasons, and many of which in a clinical situation are not of this type at all. I could invoke the idea of unconscious thoughts, but it is better to call them unspoken so as not to assume a tendentious theoretical framework. Silences arise from several sources: sometimes there are words that *are not spoken;* sometimes there are words that *cannot be spoken;* and sometimes there are *no words to speak.* Any of the three might represent a "gap" in the patient's story or might reflect the constraints of the discourse permitted in the clinic: "Granted, most professions have their own lingo that excludes outsiders, but none is more intimidating than the medical profession" (Jaffe 2000).

Katherine Montgomery Hunter underscores this point when she notices the special nature of medical discourse. "At its source in a medical center, medicine is practised by means of a series of narrative accounts of illness told in a relatively self-enclosed dialect and according to strict rules that define the genre" (1991, 8).

The same point is made by Foucault in relation to the discourse of medicine and to the medical gaze. Medical discourse often alienates patients from their own bodies and their suffering, and conveys the idea that what is going on is best understood in terms that patients have no familiarity with or confidence in. This can also alienate health care professionals from any fellow feeling with patients. If that happens, an instinctive or intuitive understanding of the patient's situation is excluded from the clinical encounter. That empathy can also be excluded where the patient and the doctor are separated by the patient's disability. Any of these varieties of silence might, at any stage in the illness, confound the clinician as well as the person who is suffering.

Words that *are not spoken* express thoughts that cannot be shared. Perhaps the person feels ashamed of them or senses that they would not be well received. Everybody has areas of life about which they would rather keep silent, and when the audience is from an "upstanding" middle-class group, there may be certain things that are off limits. For instance, many patients who are abused are ashamed to tell. The shame may be due to what they perceive to be their role in the abuse, to their family environment, or to being somebody to whom such things have happened. What is more, the abuse arises organically in the midst of a complex life story replete with values, commitments, and relationships, and the abused person may value that life context as his or her only place of belonging. Patients may therefore be scared that reporting abuse or involving the professionals will cause the loss of their only place to stand. Intensely personal reasons for silence, such as these, interact in a complex way with the social structures and norms that typically prevail in a Western middle class–dominated society, of which the doctor is a representative.

A more localized and clinical reason for silence occurs when patients are reluctant to tell doctors that, for instance, they have used alternative therapy or that they still have a drink when they get home from work. They fear that they will be cast aside by the doctor whom they need to look after them. The doctor is also confronted by a complex array of formal and informal professional role expectations that range from an injunction to facilitate the patient's care by cooperation with other health professionals to an enjoinder to maintain standards of professional practice that can be very judgmental of anything unusual or unscientific. The doctor's resulting embarrassment, intolerance, or discomfort is usually readily apparent to the patient and, understandably, creates a barrier between them.

Words that *cannot be spoken* express thoughts that cannot even be framed. The patient may be suffering in a way he or she cannot really articulate. "I don't know, I just don't feel like doing anything, what's the point?" might evince depression or just a no-win situation. The patient may have had a horrendous childhood, have had little or no chance to develop life skills, lack any realistic opportunities to "get a life," and suffer chronic physical ailments, perhaps due to poor nutrition, untreated transient infections, and fatigue. The case record may note "depression" (Rx Prozac, amitryptiline) or "Does not want to go to work," and obscure rather than illuminate the patient's suffering. Such a mismatch between the clinical text defining the medicalized patient and the lived autobiography of a real person, produces a kind of silence that need not but often does arise in the clinic. "Reinterpreted as a diagnosis, however preliminary, the transformed and medicalized narrative may be alien to the patient; strange, depersonalized, unlived and unliveable, incomprehensible or terrifyingly clear" (Hunter 1991, 13).

The discourse of medicine helps produce this kind of silence by excluding from its legitimate accounts of illness complaints that may be real to the patient. The ennui and strength-sapping effect of chronic pain such as cervicogenic headache can make every minor achievement (getting a drink of water, for instance) a major battle. This battle, draining the subjective body of its life, is hidden by the phrase "axial pain," which, for instance, attracts the lowest weighting on our (New Zealand) booking system for elective spinal surgery. Yet it is typical of the morbidity caused by cervical spinal problems. Imaginative engagement with a subjective body that feels "like that" brings a different dimension to one's assessment of the patient.

There are *no words to speak* about some of our afflictions. Some events cannot be captured by clinical discourse or indeed any discourse. I want to focus on two further ways in which experience can be excluded from articulation and therefore from our conscious understanding (and self-understanding). Both are, for want of a better word, *psychic*—they concern the interface between the subjective body and the resources we have to make narrative sense of our lives.

The first source of exclusion is best approached through Lacan's concept of *tuche* or trauma (1979, 129). This is an encounter with the real world—a point at which one is affected or touched by life. Some encounters give rise to ill-defined malaise. Lacan observes that any event, interpersonal or otherwise, affects us in ways that are captured by words and in ways that go beyond those words. The latter effects are inarticulate, inarticulable, but, despite their inchoate nature, they impact on the psyche and alter us psychologically such that emotional work may have to be done to allow the person concerned to reconstruct a livable autobiography. Their impact is similar to that of poetry, which resonates with a person's psyche in ways that go beyond the meanings of the words themselves—Wittgenstein remarks that "a poet's words can pierce us" (1967, 155). This "piercing" is not a thing that one can adequately describe.

The second source of exclusion is evident in the insight that descriptions are selective and focus on some aspects of experience at the expense of others. A simple example is the case where I notice that my friend is not in the coffee shop where I was to meet him and ignore everything else about it. Now, consider the problem of "fit" between the traditional forensic category of provocation and marital-abuse situations. The blame attached to inflicting grievous harm on another person is mitigated by provocation, conceived as something immediately prior to the injury and causing loss of self-control. However, this conception of provocation is strained if a woman waits until her husband is asleep and sets fire to the bed; she does not act "in the heat of the moment" (please forgive the pun). However, the "heat of the moment" provocation that applies to male actions, does not cover the helpless and desperate situation leading to such behavior, even though the assault may be just as understandable and perhaps excusable. (The fact that it occurs in the same bed that was the site of some aspects of the abuse may also be important.) In such a situation, the net effect of those moments of the life story culminating in her action may be to undermine rational or conscious control of the woman's action, even though the loss of control is more protracted and the act itself may be both conscious and deliberate.

Any of these types of silence may both be important in clinical practice.

Personal Silences

Some aspects of one's lived autobiography are opaque, uncomfortable, or inexplicable (even all three). Some of this extraconscious material results from the many ways that the body follows (or even forms) its own patterns of adaptation. Examples of the use of extraconscious techniques and skills are the football striker who consistently scores crucial goals and the clinician who facilitates the development of trust in a patient. In the one case, we see a smooth and polished athletic performance, and in the other a skilled interpersonal engagement with qualities that cannot easily be fabricated and result in the patient having confidence in the doctor. In both cases—the sporting or the clinical—conscious attempts to produce the required results might just get in the way.

However, some of the moments of lived autobiography cannot be silenced in any sustainable way and clamor to be explored and dealt with. These aspects of one's being, despite being poorly articulated, are often significant at an emotional and personal level. As such, they must be treated through the use of a full range of reflective and integrative techniques (perhaps originating in discourse).

Only if the relevant subjective forces can be melded can one bring harmony to one's function as a psychosomatic being.

Freud spoke of the dynamic Unconscious (Ucs), directing our attention to an area of the psyche which was not transparent to the subject but exercised a profound psychic influence on the individual's ability to construct a livable life story (1940). For Freud, the content of the Ucs resulted from childhood traumata. The details are not important, but some extremely plausible themes emerge that should inform clinicians as Hippocratic practitioners. He recognized the importance of the primary family group as the source of many deeply affecting events in the formative years of the psyche. He sought the unconscious and its "memories" of traumata where gaps in the coherent narrative of a life cried out for explanation and illumination.

If we imaginatively reenter Freud's world, early twentieth-century post-Darwinian Europe, we find ourselves immersed in an intellectual climate where the brain as an associationist network is inscribed by experiences to create inscriptions, only some of which form conscious memories. The inscriptions are physical and connected to the "keyboard" on which the nervous system plays out an ongoing fugue (or variations on a medley of themes). The subjective body responds to the score written in our nervous systems, and our words (particularly our scientific and clinical words with their sharp edges and clear certainties) struggle to keep up with the tonal and melodic riches that it produces. Yet the score makes a kind of sense so that an astute clinician learns to work with it and assist the body to function in harmony at every level. Thus, the patient's narrative requires an ethics of the body, replete with its harmonies and silences, and here lies the key to the well-being of patients, their authenticity, and that elusive quality to our interventions that will count as beneficence.

These themes are developed by Lacan, whose complex writings help us understand the silences resulting from what Freud called the unconscious. In sketching his views, however, we ought to recall that he has been widely criticized for his profoundly androcentric view of the psyche. Yet if we proceed with caution, given that medicine itself and the bioethics of recent years is a preserve stalked by decisions and principles, his insights may be not only a la mode but also a step in the right direction.

Lacan's mirror phase ties the human being into the world of discourse as a potent shaping context (1977). In this phase the child first becomes aware that an image of himself appears in a mirror as a single surveyable thing and that therefore he appears to others as a unified object and is referred to as such. The relevant signifiers identify me as a discursive individual and provide the materials that I use to give narrative shape to my life. But these signifiers are used by others who inhabit an ordered world where "the name of the father" rules. Lacan uses this phrase to indicate the authority and legitimacy of the order that prevails in the world through language.

The individual experiences the world through the medium of discourse as well as in a more direct and bodily way. Lacan's *tuche* (or encounter with the real world) is similar to the trauma (for Freud), in that it occurs within a context of discourse and therefore has a significance to the individual but is not totally encompassed by signification.

The significance attached to any moment in life is outstripped by reality in two ways. First, there are layers of significance implicit within words as used by others but not evident to the psychological individual (especially during childhood). Second, there are aspects of an encounter that are not captured by signifiers but may still affect the individual (as I have noted). These latter aspects of a given encounter that escape discursive capture by the subject can result in the subject becoming affected by "unspeakable" problems. Those problems are therefore indicated by silences in a way that is shown by actual clinical examples.

The Silences of Anorexia

Some of the more important of these themes emerge from an outline of the problems we have in understanding and treating anorexia nervosa, which I have discussed in some detail elsewhere (Gillett 1999a). This problem continues, despite some recent trends, overwhelmingly to be a disorder of young women. The most plausible syntheses identify several factors in its genesis:

1. the need to cope with the woman's role vis-à-vis food and family;
2. the danger of food to one's appearance and acceptability to others;
3. the societal pressure toward sexual attractiveness as a moral demand on women;
4. the view of one's body and oneself as a commodity competing in a market;
5. the onset of the signs of mature sexual identity;
6. the mixed moral messages to young women about their sexuality;
7. the need for independence and authenticity in forming one's self;

8. the conflicts between relationships and career that are typically greater for women than men;
9. the need for each person to construct their own livable autobiography;
10. the possibility that dieting can trigger a biological disorder of eating.

An important feature emerging from this complex of factors is that the young woman concerned feels that she is losing control of her life and that she cannot reconcile the conflicting demands on her and construct a livable self-narrative so as to preserve what she values. She tries to control those aspects of herself which can be controlled and thus mark out a clear domain of self-determination. Her efforts result in her keeping her childlike body, and she creates the illusion that she can postpone or reverse the onset of womanhood. This, as Orbach notes, is a dramatic solution to a tangled and intractable problem that strikes deep at the heart of the story that is the young woman's life because it calls attention to "deeply painful but salient aspects of women's existence which are often obscured" (1993, 125, 4).

Bordo (1985) speaks of "the crystallization of culture," exploring the joint roles of discourse and context in configuring the psyche or subjective body of a young woman. In anorexia, the young woman creates tracts of silence to exclude people from whole areas of her life. Anorexia grows within these "no-go zones" where others cannot address or engage with it in any meaningful way. Those problems are also largely inaccessible to therapy, at least in conventional terms. It is plausible to synthesize these accounts by suggesting that the silence of anorexia arises from the complex factors responsible for it and the attempt to retain a zone of control in which the young woman's life is not being intruded on by the knowledge and requirements of others.

Among other things, that the silence is protective and is itself inextricably tied to anorexia's multiple causes suggests that simple measures such as force-feeding ignore the psychic tangles that need resolution. Force-feeding may, of course, be forced on the therapist as a desperate measure to save the patient's life, but ultimately that life can be saved only by the young woman accepting herself as capable of living with the issues that she needs to resolve and constructing a narrative that allows her to do so.

It follows, even from this brief sketch, that the silences of anorexia can be intensified by the attempts of orthodox biomedical science to be reductive about the disorder and suggest that there is a singular biological lesion or disorder at its heart. In fact, the alienating effect of turning it into yet another instance where the patient has not just actually but also conceptually lost control of her own body may be considerable. Theories that reinforce the whole idea that the problem is susceptible to an individualistic explanation and approaches that neglect the context in which the disorder develops are intrinsically likely to be counterproductive. The young woman concerned has, ex hypothesi, a brokenness in her life story (possibly exacerbated by a lesion in her neurophysiology) and it (unlike the lesion) cannot be treated biochemically; it can be approached only by exploring the silences that trap her in the pattern of self-harm to which she has committed herself.

In this case, we find a colloquy of silences central to the patient's narrative which the discourse of the clinic struggles to deal with. But the silences of anorexia merely reflect the silences imposed by orthodox medicine and its scientific basis. This discursive regime, I have argued, trades on the exclusion of individual, relational, political, cultural, and holistic factors that are not amenable to a biological focus on the organism and its internal function. There are other voices, which not only do not fit neatly into biomedical discourse but also ask us to redefine the norms of disease and health to remove the narrow biomedical assumptions from them.

The Silences Imposed by Medicine

The authority of biomedicine, as have discussed, has grown from its roots in the Hippocratic tradition and has been fueled by the therapeutic ethos of medicine, the political role of the medical profession, and the self-professed foundation of clinical medicine in the scientific method. These are powerful sources of legitimacy. Nevertheless, there are tensions in the discourse of contemporary health care.

The most dominant influence, if not the most venerable, is positivist science allied to "the principle of contraries." The theory favors causal manipulation of physiological variables by allopathic interventions validated in ways that eliminate subjective patient factors. The model theorizes the body as a complex physiological machine so that its own "wisdom" can neither be conceptualized nor listened to. I have suggested that the theory is problematic and that we need a different orientation to explore the silences of the clinical encounter. Therefore, I am tempted by the obvious resonance between homeopathic theory (and some other holistic approaches to health) and the Aristotelian model of a good life.

In these alternative conceptions, a healthy state is that which has managed to achieve a balance of a number of factors, none of which should be fostered to the exclusion of others and all of which play a vital part in human function. In Aristotelian approaches to human well-being, there is an obvious and indispensable role for mentors who are sensitive to the story, needs, and personality of the developing individual and have themselves an appreciation of what makes life go well. In homeopathic theory the therapeutic role is played by a practitioner who is experienced at spotting patterns of illness and discerning the points at which the illness maps on to the pharmacopoeia that is deployed. The practitioner thinks of the body as showing a certain kind of imbalance with a need to mount a corrective response to that imbalance. The attraction of such a holistic theory is that it respects and works with the unique and integrated human being concerned rather than overpowering the disease by an externally introduced agent.

As such, whatever one thinks about homeopathy or other types of holistic medicine, and despite that they run counter to the metatheory behind the current evidence-based orthodoxy (Cochrane 1972), the metatheory coheres well with only some of our clinical intuitions. These tensions within the orthodox camp run deep.

There is, or should be, a certain humility in orthodox medicine considering the vast array of ailments that we do not understand: myalgic encephalomyelitis, addiction, rheumatoid arthritis, most varieties of cancer, multiple sclerosis, back pain, allergic rhinitis, and so on. Most of us recognize that these things are multifactorial, and we plug away with orthodox theory to help us identify important independent variables. If that is the wrong metatheory, then partnership with holistic understandings of the subjective body might be, in some areas, a more fruitful avenue to explore.

A shift toward holism and the ethical considerations arising from the silences I have identified, both, in their own way, direct our attention to the innerness and intricacy of the subjective body which may be seriously disrupted by the clinical gaze and its technological armamentarium. (I shall return to holism below.)

Recognizing the Contents of Silence

Recall that the silences arose in two general ways: either because of factors within patients of which they may be unaware but which have an ongoing effect on their health, or because of things of which patients are aware but for which they cannot find words within approved clinical discourse.

The ethical challenge posed by the need for partnership and negotiation in clinical care is especially relevant because mutual respect and openness of mind are the ruling values in discourse of that type. The stories of illness told by clinicians are, as we have seen, medical stories replete with the metatheory proper to external rescue or intervention overcoming the source of badness (disease, silencing forces, moral condemnation) in the patient. But I have argued that silences indicate badness so intertwined with goodness that the job of picking them apart can be done only with real sensitivity to the "inside" of things, as experienced by the patient (consciously and unconsciously) and as (perhaps intuitively albeit incompletely) understood by the patient. If that is true, silence itself, or a sensitivity to what is unsaid and puzzling, is our guide to what needs caring attention.

Further insights arise in the clinical setting of old age care.

Istvan is a patient in an aged care facility in Hungary. In the midst of the conformity to rules that prevails in the institution, he insists on one concession. At the end of every day, he changes from his working clothes to have his dinner. This sometimes delays him and also delays the second course of dinner. The doctor in charge has tried to stop Istvan from doing this because the institution must be run in an orderly and structured way for the good of all. The result was to make Istvan somewhat irascible and uncooperative. He also became taciturn when left to himself and unmotivated to participate as he usually did in occupational therapy and ward recreation. The issue is raised at the weekly meeting, and the staff wonder whether Istvan should be started on antidepressants. But one of the nurses at the meeting had listened to Istvan's story.

As a younger man, Istvan was in a Nazi concentration camp. After the war he would often recollect that time. "We were made to eat like a bunch of pigs at a trough, wearing whatever dirty things we had worn all day." After the war he had insisted on changing every night before dinner and would often say, "It is so nice to sit down properly as a family and eat dinner together."

What does Istvan's story tell us? Are the requirements to have an orderly dinner time in the institution enough to override Istvan's wishes? Does Istvan's recent irritability, anhedonia, and psychomotor retardation indicate clinical depression? How could we make that judgment without knowing Istvan's story? Perhaps there are many patients for whom a pinch of narrative understanding would temper the need for a chemical corrective, but they are not as independent or determined as Istvan and therefore their compliance condemns them to more conventional remedies.

The need for empathic and imaginative listening is a constant theme of those who are impaired in their ability to communicate with us and to live an unassisted life. The narrative "filling in" induced by attention to silences in the patient's story may be particularly important in areas where we are questioned about the parental role of a community vis-à-vis its "differently abled" members.

Disability, Being Cared for, and a Life of Your Own

Those who live with quite a different range of abilities and challenges from those that most of us enjoy are often frustrated by attempts of able-bodied members of society to control their lives. This shows up in a number of areas, but the problems are thrown into sharp focus in the area of sexuality.

Young people are reckoned to have growing autonomy in the area of their sexual lives. Thus, even though sexual contact with a child by an older person is considered to be exploitative, we recognize that it is different when children or young people of a similar age negotiate a mutual sexual encounter on their own terms. We could call this a similar age proviso on sexual behavior. All in all, until the age of sixteen (or thereabouts), it seems appropriate to speak of exploitation and abuse in certain relationships although the similar age proviso might be a reason not to do so.

It is normally expected that vulnerable individuals should be supervised and protected by their parents. So the identification of the person (or body) *in loco parentis* is important in discussing these issues when we move beyond the normal confines of a family and look more broadly at the diverse living situations of people of mixed abilities.

We need also to consider the peer support and guidance that is an important part of most young people's sexual learning (though for some this is quite damaging). Peer support can be provided either within the family or outside of it, and confidential and intimate relationships of this kind with peers form a context in which the details and uncertainties of sexuality can be shared. Given that sexual relationships are often confusing on both sides, a heavy parental and moralistic hand in such matters can only make many aspects of the sexuality of the young and immature strained and stressful. This is conducive neither to personal growth nor to the development of responsibility.

The problems of sexual learning are often compounded in those with "disabilities." However, the silences of sexuality and disability can be a cloak for inhuman and degrading practices of the worst sort, and therefore some kind of balance needs to be struck between an atmosphere of tolerance and an atmosphere of protection and parentalism. To strike such a balance, for most vulnerable young people, is not a theoretical or rational exercise but requires practicality, wit, and sympathetic company so that solutions to a variety of situations can be negotiated within the proper spirit of *whanau* (loving/familylike context) and safety (a context of security, growth, and the nurture of oneself as a whole being).

Many of the able-bodied community find it both shocking and somewhat distasteful that disability and sexuality should be linked at all. This aversion is unrealistic and unhelpful for two reasons. First, sex is enjoyable, and second, it can be damaging.

We ought to recognize that young people with intellectual disabilities may have relatively few areas of their lives in which they achieve genuine satisfactions and pleasing relationships. Sexual activity may be an area in which some particular disabled persons can experience genuine emotional satisfaction and build pleasurable relationships. However, it remains to balance these positive experiential factors with the ethical safeguards needed to compensate for the dangers and uncertainties that arise for anybody but do so particularly where silences abound.

Protection and Autonomy

We normally expect parents to provide a certain amount of protection for children in sexual matters while those children go through the extended process of developing their own autonomy. This is a difficult role because we realize that a young person's sexual and reproductive choices may not be those of the parents, and yet we also realize that a sink-or-swim attitude is irresponsible. In the past we arguably have overemphasized parental responsibilities and rights to control sexual behavior in the young, but there are two arguments supporting parental supervision and influence that have nothing to do with Victorian and authoritarian attitudes.

The vulnerability of the immature argues that young people may put themselves in positions that they do not fully understand, without realizing the consequences of those choices or the difficult interpersonal consequences that could arise. The result is that they find themselves in situations with which they cannot cope. The problem is worsened when their knowledge about what is at stake in a particular choice (or course of events) is incomplete. This may involve biological facts but more often concerns interpersonal knowledge about the effects of one person's actions on others. Any young person, and particularly those who are intellectually disabled, may find the area of personal relationships quite perplexing but choices about sexual behavior and sexuality fall squarely within it.

These difficulties are aggravated by inexperience (that often goes along with disability). Life knowledge and life skills developed in relevant experiences are used to solve novel problems in personal relationships. Relatively naive young people lack these skills and are likely to find themselves in situations where they do not feel comfortable but they do not know what to do.

The lack of relevant life skills is probably a more useful idea in relation to sexual questions than the idea of incompetence as it appears in the informed consent and psychiatric ethics literature, and it is far more in keeping with the partnership and narrative themes of this book. However, if we were to think in terms of competence, consent, and choices, then we must realize that human reproduction and the possible implications of sexual contact may not be understood by intellectually disabled young people. That lack of knowledge would mean that they were unable to safeguard their own best interests in this area. Therefore, a degree of sensitive "parentalism" is usually appropriate when young people are facing such problems, and there are other considerations that tend to the same conclusion.

Young people with intellectual disability often show a degree of impulsivity commensurate with their general level of maturity (or immaturity). Therefore, they may put themselves in situations where their long-term interests are seriously compromised because they are unable to cope with the mess they find themselves in. Caregivers or advisors can act well in such an impasse only if they appreciate the unfolding life story and the things that may seriously disrupt or damage the young person and others in the context of that life story.

Sexual choices are often further complicated by an imbalance of power in which an older or more savvy acquaintance is able to influence a young intellectually disabled person. I shall deal with this in more detail under the topic of exploitation, but a simple story makes the issues vivid.

> Teresa lives in supported housing with a group of other young people under the
> supervision of an onsite "buddy." She begins seeing a man, somewhat older than

she, who she quite often invites in for "morning tea." Teresa is quite proud of her ability to make a cup of tea or coffee for her special friends from within the complex (and others) and of the nice biscuits she buys from the supermarket. The supervisor or "buddy" notices that Teresa's new friend often stays for some time and raises the topic with Teresa. She becomes very coy, giggles a bit, and then gets aggressive: "Anyway, why can't I have a boyfriend like other girls?" Inquiries reveal that Teresa's boyfriend is known to the disabled services and that he has been sexually predatory on other young women like Teresa. In at least one case a pregnancy resulted, at which point he stopped making contact.

It is clear that young intellectually disabled people, while needing encouragement to develop autonomy and the life skills that go into that, also need some protection because of their inherent vulnerability in the face of sexual challenges and choices. This protection should surely approximate that afforded by normal parental care, and the judgments required are, if anything, more demanding than those required of the parents of ordinary teenagers who are usually surrounded by peers and siblings with a more developed set of social skills.

Responsibility for consequences is also important. Challenges such as pregnancy, possible parenthood, and serious disease involve a level of self-care that may not ordinarily be required in the sexual encounters of adolescence. Often, the parents or host institution of a young person will assume a disproportionate load as a result of these consequences because the individual's disability may preclude him or her from taking on the burdens that are involved. This may have a profound impact on the lives of parents, but an institution also has an interest in avoiding some of the more serious and costly (in every way) effects of unwise choices. Thus, there is a good reason why certain safety-net features should be in place to mitigate the effects of unwise sexual choices if such choices are going to be possible and permitted.

Neither of these arguments supports a complete prohibition of sexual activity among intellectually disabled young people in institutions. They rather suggest that responsibility does not end with the giving of permission for sexual activity to occur and that the young person concerned should be able to share his or her story and participate in relationships with others who can offer the kind of support and contribution that any young person would normally look to from whanau and peers. Inarticulacy does not negate that story. In fact, it requires us to attend more closely so as to fill in the blanks with empathy, imagination, and a sense of where the teller of the story is wanting to go.

The Similar Age Proviso and Exploitation

If an underage person is involved sexually with a mature adult, we are suspicious that the imbalance in age and experience has disadvantaged the younger person. Therefore, we afford legal protection to them even though we accept their sexual choices when we are relatively sure that they involve equals.

However, if both parties are relatively inexperienced and lack the relevant life skills, then they may find themselves in a position they could not envisage, can only imperfectly grasp, and would not have chosen if, per impossibile, they had understood the implications of their actions. This argument tends to offset to some extent a permissive attitude to more or less consenting sexual choices between intellectually disabled people. Again, I am not suggesting a blanket prohibition on sexual activity but rather a concerned and caring appreciation of the role of their relationship in their respective lives and the need to safeguard and enhance those lives so that their support networks do not have to go into damage-control mode.

I have already noted the vulnerability of the intellectually and physically disabled in virtue of their social and discursive disadvantages. Exploitation trades on the imbalance of power and knowledge between the exploiter and the exploited. It is obvious where caregivers or relatively empowered individuals misuse their positions of trust and their superior knowledge and life skills to gain sexual advantages. We ought to have the strongest safeguards in place to prevent such abuse, and many organizations have rightly adopted a zero-tolerance attitude toward it.

However, there are less-clear situations where a more skilled individual is able to take advantage of a less well-equipped "peer." This can lead to disappointment and abuse even though it is much harder to detect and guard against. Negotiating this delicate area, as I have noted, calls for a sensitive quasi-parental role to be filled. It is also a good reason why peer support and education, from one disabled person to another, ought to be encouraged in sexual matters and life skills generally.

Peers are sensitive to the knowledge and naivete of their fellows in a way that is not easily attained by a person who is differently positioned by the lottery of life. A peer appreciates challenges in everyday life that others may never conceive of, much less have to deal with. This is seen in families, for instance, when siblings share the details of their psychosexual lives (in their context) at a level that they would never share them with their parents. Disability does not exclude such mutuality and may, in fact, mean that there is even more to be gained from encouraging it. For this reason, same-sex buddies or sibling substitutes ought to be encouraged in institutional settings where experiences of sexuality and disability are going to be taken seriously.

The advantage of the same-sex buddy (or "bro") is the relative equality of power and position, despite differences in life skills, between the two people. Such relationships, because of the disabilities of those concerned, may not always function this way, but we ought to be alert to such possibilities and encourage them where feasible. Another positive feature of peer relationships is the development of shared skills rather than control of one party by the other. This approximates normal adolescence in which same-sex friends get together and discuss their emotional and sexual needs, desires, and experiences in ways that can be both empowering and supportive. The sharing of perspectives and information between peers is not happily substituted for by nonpeer (nondisabled) staff workers or counselors, although such players may play useful facilitatory roles in some relationships or groups.

These reflections underscore the need for all of us to have an intersubjective context in which our own vulnerabilities, positionings, needs, hopes, concerns, and so on can be aired and shared. None of us is an island; we all need a place to stand. A place of belonging offers us validation, support, humor, dialogue, and the means to muddle through in authoring or editing the story that emerges from our experiences in life. It is ironic that exactly this kind of context can be left out of the world of those silenced by disability.

Any person uses a range of resources to deal with the challenges of life. They are specially needed when illness intrudes. Some of the resources are discursive and narrative, transforming moments of experience into episodes in a story. In this task the person is constantly gauging what can be said in terms of what is normally said around here and trying to understand what is happening to him or her. Silences impede this task, casting the storyteller adrift in a pathless wasteland. This is particularly true of those whose role as storyteller is constantly being discounted or undermined.

The story of a person's experience with disability or illness is often of this type. Therefore, Hippocratic professionals must share the resources required for encounters to be clothed with meaning and get themselves "storied." We must also give permission for things to be said which otherwise would remain hidden, lost in silence. We can contribute sensitively to stories that can be owned and accepted as authentic by all participants in the partnership of care. Sometimes in such stories we need primarily clinical skill or professionalism, but always what is needed is an admixture of caring. Some times caring will cause pain (but a surgeon is used to that). There are moments in any story (and particularly those of disability) which are intrinsically painful in narrative and emotional terms, but even pain (of whatever kind) and the ways we cause it should be seen with an understanding of its role in the caring process.

My first surgical mentor taught me a profound respect for tissue, for working with the patient's body not against it. That attitude allows one to do surgery in sensitive areas and cause minimal damage. Along with that attitude goes an appreciation that people are wonderfully made—even where we feel and react otherwise. The same attitude should pervade clinical and professional life: respect for the integrity of patients who are doing their best to cope with the challenges of life. When illness occurs, we need a willingness to learn from the patients' expertise: an inside knowledge of that illness so that its true, human dimensions can be appreciated (Balint 1957). This understanding requires a constant to-and-fro between the discourse of medicine and the subjectivity of the patient. As a result the domain of silence shrinks, and, if the job is done with care and attention, the silences left do not hide the keys to the suffering. The nature of the suffering can be spoken or manifest, and we can help the troubled body get about its restorative work. The alternative to listening to the silences is to be confounded by them (as in the case of so many male therapists when they are faced with anorexia). However, some silences can be understood only from certain discursive positions, and some discursive positions are not available to some of us.

Differently abled persons are in just such a position, and our conversations can become so strained and disrupted that the silences are intense. The willingness to see the lived human story behind the misleading mask of apparent less-than-humanity allows the silences to be transcended here as in other areas of clinical life. The doctor-patient hyphen joins and distinguishes the two partners, an important fact when the person it joins one to is a person whom every fiber of one's being strains to remain distinct from.

CHAPTER SIX

Surgeons, Patients, and Unnecessary Holes in the Head

> Where there are procedures which can be right or wrong, a consideration
> of these must constitute a science. I assert that there is no science where
> there is neither a right way nor a wrong way, but science consists in the dis-
> crimination between different procedures.   —SCIENCE

Science, according to the Hippocratics, distinguishes between right and wrong ways of doing things, but this is not always easy, particularly in surgery. Can we ask our patients to undergo procedures that will not do them any good in order to find out what is really effective? Can we ask them to have procedures with unproven efficacy? Can we afford to wait for rigorous evidence when we believe surgery will help a person? These questions clustering around advances in surgery promise insights into important problems in clinical ethics.

Advances in Surgery and the Dogma of the PRDBPCCT

The need for sound evidence about efficacy (implicit in the Hippocratic method) is a major problem for surgery. The metatheory behind orthodox medicine focuses on effective causal interventions and is given "concrete" or "operational" form by clinical epidemiologists as a need for statistically provable efficacy demonstrated in a prospective randomized double-blinded placebo-controlled clinical trial (PRDBPCCT). However, clinical medicine, particularly its surgical arm, is also an *art* involving creativity and imagination. Of course, we need evidence for the efficacy of our procedures, and we need to remove potential biases in gathering that evidence. But surgery, like many human arts, has a history of incremental innovation and refinement of its techniques, much like the crafts practiced by skilled artisans. Two kinds of innovation are found:

1. better ways of doing the job in hand (as, for instance, with modern aneurysm clips or artificial hips compared to their ancestor devices); and

2. interventions based on belief and theory (such as spinal fixation or antibiotic prophylaxis), where the results may be inaccessible to the intuitive judgement of a skilled practitioner.

In between the two, there are changes that should be evaluated a little more thoroughly than by BOGSAT (bunch of guys sitting around a table) methods.

The craft of surgery when faced by the science of medicine calls for a Hippocratic method of evaluating surgical practice. Doing so is difficult because of uncertain baselines against which new techniques are to be assessed and problems in assessing outcomes. We must therefore do what the Hippocratics recommend: document our cases, audit our techniques, and monitor shifts in practice so that, despite historical, nonblinded, non-placebo-controlled methodologies, we do gain cumulative knowledge of our practice. In some areas of surgery, this approach, regardless of its nonconformity to the dogma of the PRDBPCCT, may be the best way to proceed; in other surgical fields the PRDBPCCT is indispensable, and mixed designs are increasingly allowing surgeons to exercise clinical judgment and yet study their techniques for efficacy (Lindley and Warlow, 2000). I argue that there are a number of valid ways of proceeding in this area.

The Art of Surgery

Clinical treatment aims to correct an abnormality producing an illness. Sometimes identifying the abnormality and figuring out how to correct it is easy, as in surgery. Indeed, one could say: *If surgery wasn't simple, surgeons couldn't understand it.*

Where the disorder can be seen and is relatively straightforward, we devise means of correcting it to try to cure the problem. The probabilities of success are sometimes fairly evident (and for that reason easy to explain to a patient). These have, as it were, *an appeal to the educated eye.*

Most interventions of this type are fairly simple-minded: we remove lumps (e.g., removing a tumor from the brain or elsewhere in the body), correct stenoses (or narrowings—such as those in a blocked artery), relieve pressure compromising function or causing pain (such as a disc prolapse in the spinal canal), or drain an abscess (a pool of pus) poisoning the body. In these paradigmatic surgical interventions, anybody can see whether or not we have done what seems to be needed. Even in such cases, though, the long-term efficacy of the procedure requires careful assessment, and some have proved not to be as beneficial as originally thought (e.g., removal of prolactin-secreting adenomas of the pituitary, carotid endarterectomy, removal of the gallbladder, surgical decompression of the spinal cord in cancer, endoscopic removal of bowel polyps, and so on). We could call these widely accepted but unproven interventions.

Some surgical techniques are based on theories that come into question (e.g., gastric ulcer surgery, breast cancer surgery, hysterectomy for CIS [carcinoma in situ] of the cervix, and so on). In such cases, a paradigmatic surgical procedure is actually unproven in its effect on the condition at which it is aimed. Once the question is raised (usually because of evidence apparently conflicting with the theory), clinical trials are needed. Surgeons often participate in such trials only if they still have the option of standard treatment for their patients. A trial using this kind of design is based on what we call the *principle of uncertainty—enter a patient when you are uncertain what to do.*

Quite apart from statistical questions about the efficacy of certain interventions, there are some surgical innovations that are merely technical improvements on accepted methods. In such cases, it is reasonable to consider the impressions of surgeons as to whether the innovation is actually a better way of doing the procedure it supercedes (laying aside questions about the efficacy of surgery as a therapeutic option). However, the impressions of surgeons are not decisive; we ought regularly to audit or review our practice to ensure that modifications or "technical improvements" do not produce unforeseen complications.

So there are a series of question we ought to ask of all surgical innovations.

First, is it a modification (or technical improvement) of an existing technique? For such cases, a technical comparison by the surgeons doing the operation is most appropriate. Provided their judgments are favorable, the technique can be substituted for the existing operation with suitable monitoring of what modifications have been made and any potential problems that might arise.

Second, is it an entirely new approach to a problem? Here, there are two possibilities:

1. the existing surgical treatment is itself well proven to be effective as, say, in removal of a life threatening tumor of the brain; or
2. the existing surgery has never itself been well proven but is a matter of accepted practice.

Given the general principle that any new technique should be compared in some controlled clinical trial against the best available current treatment, in case 2 we need to validate the currently accepted treatment to see whether it is worth doing or merely a sop to clinical activism. If this is not done, then it is unfair to ask those pioneering the new technique to do that more basic investigation because that should be part of a wider study; the most we can ask them is to show statistical equivalence of the new technique to existing methods (unproven as they are).

We can compare the way we look at surgery with the more common clinical trials we find in the various phases of the introduction of drug treatments.

Phase I studies of drugs are comparable to investigations of safety in surgery because we do not do operations on healthy volunteers, and therefore all that can be asked is to show that we are doing no harm. Ancillary investigations for surgical devices—such as mechanical testing or testing in vitro may be required here.

Phase II studies concern efficacy in the clinical situation, and this is where most surgical innovations get stuck. They are often introduced because they appeal to "the educated eye" attuned, as I have noted, to a visible abnormality and its correction. Once it is appealing in those terms surgeons may just get on with it.

The transition from phase II to clinical use often preempts phase III tests in surgery because we do not often take a step back and ask whether correcting the obvious anomaly (in accordance with the educated-eye test) actually helps the patient. (The educated eye has no equivalent in medicine because we cannot survey biochemical and physiological function in an obvious and simple way; therefore, PRDBPCCTs are the only option.) However, some comparable role to a phase III trial might be a surgical audit of large numbers of procedures done in a phase II (safety study) to see what outcomes show up in widespread clinical practice.

Although many surgical techniques often move direct to clinical use on the basis of the educated-eye test, sometimes, as in drug treatment, a trial is undertaken. But even then it is important to "try to pick out serious follow-up work from mere marketing ploys" (Evans and Evans 1996, 27).

In the abstract these issues are simple, but in concrete terms the problems are much more difficult. The first major problem is the very idea of a PRDBPCCT.

Sham Surgery: Unnecessary Holes in the Head

An issue of the *New England Journal of Medicine* canvassed the ethics of placebo-controlled trials of surgery (Freeman 1999; Macklin 1999). The procedure was an operation for the implantation of fetal substantia nigra cells in patients with Parkinson disease. The placebo arm of the study involved fitting a stereotactic frame under general anesthetic, drilling burr holes in the skull (not altogether innocuous), administering cyclosporin for immune suppression, and neurological follow-up assessment. One must ask whether submitting patients to the sham operations (and the cyclosporin) in the placebo arm of such a study can be justified. The first response of every colleague confronted with the issue (myself included) is an emphatic *No!* Even ethicists concur; Macklin claims "it is unethical" to do sham operations that involve cutting into people and sewing them up again (1999, 995). She argues that sham surgery violates the requirement to minimize the risk of harm in research and that informed consent is not an adequate safeguard. Yet is this true?

Macklin suggests "a tension between the highest standard of research design and the highest standard of ethics" (1999, 992). This seems paradoxical. Ethics concerns the making of good decisions in practice and therefore seems to have an inclusive brief, attentive both to scientific merit and to more orthodox ethical concerns, such as *primum non nocere* or the best interests of the individual patient. But we need to think a little more about harms to individuals and to our patients as a target group.

Individual harm arises because any surgical treatment is invasive and, if unproven, may result in no benefit to the patient, but that definition also implies that it is unethical to apply any unproven treatment to any patient. The wound associated with a sham operation is, plausibly, a harm of a different order than that caused by administering an ineffective substance by tablet or injection. However, in clinical life, every harm must be weighed against expected benefits, and this is not easy in the case of a new surgical technique for two reasons.

First, surgery for quality-of-life (QOL) indications is becoming more commonplace. In such surgery, as distinct from rescue or life-saving surgery, we would expect placebo responses to be particularly important. Therefore, controlling for the placebo effect is important in contemporary surgery more than it used to be when surgery was done only in desperate situations. It is far less traumatic—at the beginning of the twenty-first century—to have surgery than it was fifty years ago. Thus, the likely risks or harms from placebo surgery are diminishing. This fact justifies, at least in patients' minds, exploratory surgery where radiological findings are suggestive but inconclusive, for instance, in spinal conditions where it is uncertain whether an operation will significantly improve QOL. The argument that placebo surgery is too risky is therefore weakened. There are, however, more robust arguments against sham surgery.

Vulnerable and Desperate Patients

People with diseases for which there are few effective interventions may be coerced by the hope of treatment, even where that hope is based on speculation or very poor evidence. We see this when cancer patients (and those with AIDS) turn to alternative and unproven treatments, or even bare-faced quackery. However, clinical rigor seems to require that we use sham surgery as a placebo measure in some contexts and therefore that we clarify the ethical constraints on such surgery.

The first requirement is *absolute honesty* about the treatment proposed and the structure of the trial. This is part of the doctor being an expert guide in a health care partnership. In a placebo-controlled study, the patient should understand that the surgery may be "real" or "sham" and the nature of the placebo condition. However, it seems that this is not always well done.

Macklin reports cases in which "researchers performed sham surgery without obtaining informed consent from patients" and that in a trial of coronary artery surgery, "the patients were told only that they were participating in an evaluation of this operation; they were not informed of the double blind nature of the study" (1999, 994). Here it is not the double blinding that is of most concern but the clarity with which they were informed that they might receive placebo rather than active treatment. Macklin notes that "the misconception that research is designed to benefit the patients who are the subjects is difficult to dispel" and concludes that "the protection of human subjects cannot rest solely on the ethical foundation of informed consent" (994, 995).

These concerns do not secure Macklin's conclusion; they merely emphasize the need for a frank conversation rather than a legalistic requirement for a signed consent form. "Studies of informed consent documents show that they sometimes overstate the benefits and understate the risks for research protocols" (1999, 994). Information and consent documents must therefore be read with a critical eye by those of us involved in ethical review. They should allow ordinary people to make reasonable choices on the basis of well-worded information.

In my experience on ethics committees constituted according to New Zealand standards (where half of the members must be lay people), consent forms are often incomprehensible to ordinary people. Therefore, the lay members of the committee play a vital part in ethical review by ensuring that the purposes, the nature of the interventions, and the risks and benefits of participation are all stated clearly and unequivocally in plain language. In some contexts, it is rare to have adequate representation of potential participants on ethics committees but, happily, Australasia is relatively advanced in this area (McNeill 1993).

If the Australasian example is followed, then Macklin's arguments are defused, even though we should note the widespread public perception that if your doctor suggests something it must be good for you. A partnership involving the active participation of doctor and patient in the discussion of any surgical adventure tends to obviate that misconception.

The Reasonableness of Ordinary Folk

Macklin's arguments depend in part on the idea that people should never make other-regarding choices, but this protest is ill thought out. Surgeons often propose surgery that is not backed by rigorous scientific evidence. Most surgical procedures are based on favorable outcomes in historical series and have never been submitted to a PRDBPCCT. Thus, in reality, a number of patients are choosing potentially harmful interventions that have never been proven in terms of their efficacy or benefit. The argument that patients should not be allowed to choose the minimal harm associated with placebo surgery is, in effect, an argument that many patients should undergo possibly ineffective and potentially harmful surgery without there ever being an adequate study of that surgery. This is a weak argument. It is clearly unethical to submit 1,000 people to an unproven and potentially harmful procedure when the merits or otherwise of that procedure might be shown by exposing 100 people (or, more probably, 50) to a much lesser risk. This makes sense not only in terms of the greatest good for the greatest number but also in terms of ethical advice to individuals.

Some thinkers devalue the idea of collective harms and benefits even where they are directly relevant to our ability to benefit identifiable individuals. They protest against utilitarian approaches in an area where the good of the individual is supposed to be our highest motive. Is this good ethics? A narrow focus on the best interests of the individual relies on weighting the relative value of self-interest, autonomy, and paternalism. Yet that balance is internally inconsistent. Take the old chestnut of autonomy, which implies that we ought to respect the reasonable wants and intentions of an individual—those that are rationally endorsable and do not infringe on the rights of others. A more restricted set of altruistic interests value serving others, and they are generally reckoned to be not just endorsable but morally commendable, even where they involve some self-sacrifice for the common good.

On these grounds, participation in a trial of the type being discussed looks reasonable. For any individual with any disorder, a 50 percent chance of a treatment that might help is better than nothing at all. What is more, for most of us, the thought that our present state of ignorance about the efficacy of a potentially helpful treatment would continue to be the case for future sufferers is unreasonable. It is plausible that a statistical opportunity (50%) of possible benefit and also participation in an exercise that will help shape the future treatment of others like me outweighs the 50 percent chance of suffering the relatively insignificant harm of a fairly innocuous surgical intervention. ("Fairly innocuous" should imply no greater statistically validated risks that the normal investigative and preparatory work-up for the condition.)

This consideration also brings us face-to-face with the possibility that altruism is a significant motivation for some people. In the past we have applauded such a motive (particularly when shown by our medical pioneers in experiments on themselves) but we seem to have either forgotten it or become more selfish lately. Denying patients the chance of participating in placebo-controlled surgical research, in effect, says that altruism is no longer endorsable as a rational motive. The narrow self-interest view of human motivation reflected in this ethical stance is lamentable. If a person wants to make a sacrifice and if it is one that a reasonable person might make, then who are the ethics Mafia to deny them that opportunity? Indeed, it seems ironic that ethicists, of all people, should condemn the willingness of some of us to make altruistic choices of the kind that many regard as being a fundamental feature of ethical behavior.

Another problem that arises in PRDBPCCTs is that the clinicians involved may come to believe that one group or the other are doing better or worse. Therefore, they want to break the code and check the results before the agreed end point. The problem is usually managed by having a data monitoring group who can do the necessary analysis without compromising the trial. Code breaking and analysis can then replace the subjective clinical impression that one group or the other are doing better or worse with hard statistical facts about the trial to date and what has happened so that ethical decisions can be made that do not jeopardize a difficult and important exercise.

Safeguards and Provisions for Limitation

Despite the weakness of the arguments against placebo-controlled surgery, there are clearly safeguards that need to be in place. I think that the single most important of these concerns patient information and consent: patients must know that there is a 50 percent chance of undergoing sham surgery, which there is no reason to believe will be of any benefit and which carries certain risks. They should also realize that we do not actually know if the "real surgery" is of any benefit (which is why the study is being done in the first place) and that continuing in ignorance involves everyone in more substantial risks. If, after adequate information, patients decide to participate in the study, then they should be given access to a medical opinion distanced from discussion with the surgical enthusiasts involved. If all these conditions are met, then I see no reason to disallow the altruism of some patients who undergo risks in the hope of advancing the study of their condition and the search for a scientifically proven response to it (given that they also have access to the experimental treatment). Let me flesh out these arguments by considering a real case.

Case Study: A New Treatment for the Cervical Spine

A New Zealand ethics committee was approached by a surgeon (Dr. G) who had developed a device to improve a time-consuming and risky spinal operation. This was a modification of an existing technique, yet it involved the use of a totally new implantable device developed because of worries about the safety of the existing technique (Gillett 1998).

In such a case, should they insist on a randomized controlled trial, ask for an initial demonstration of safety, or ask for a demonstration of equivalence to existing techniques? If the latter is chosen, what safeguards ought to be in place? What should they require in terms of proving efficacy, given that existing techniques are accepted but not proven in any rigorous way?

Dr. G's case ought to remind us that the Hippocratic injunctions about medical knowledge were somewhat less rigid than the current fundamentalism of the PRDBPCCT. We seem to need a refinement of the Hippocratic method of careful investigation whereby "physicians compare the present symptoms with similar cases they have seen in the past, so that they can say how cures were affected then" (HW, 142).

Dr. G's operation was a modification of an existing procedure, incorporating a device designed to have several advantages over other methods: it seemed safer, it did not require a spinal fusion, and it was less painful. These may be relatively unsupported beliefs, but throughout the practice of surgery there is a strong tradition of this kind of innovation by practicing surgeons so that the techniques of surgery develop in a progressive manner (Evans and Evans 1996, 55). Surgical approaches and procedures are refined over time until surgeons can do what is needed safely and well. We are always having to ask whether an innovation requires only the educated-eye test of progressive technical improvement or a more sweeping reevaluation.

It is therefore understandable that Dr. G might do an operation in a way that reflects his attempts to improve on his previous practice, without either rigorous evidence that standard practice is clearly beneficial or that his modification is a genuine improvement. But should a randomized prospective controlled trial be done?

Here Dr. G has a problem in that a PRDBPCCT requires the investigator to be in an equipoised condition. Equipoise exists when the investigator has no valid reason to believe that entering the patient into one or other of two treatments will confer any advantage. Dr. G is not in this position because he (along with many of his fellow specialists) accepts that cervical spinal compression is best treated by surgery rather than conservative means. They might all be wrong, but the question demands a major randomized controlled trial of surgical decompression versus nonsurgical treatment rather than an experiment Dr. G would do on his own limited pool of patients. The problem is that he could not do a PRDBPCCT of his operation versus no treatment because he genuinely believes that surgery is necessary and therefore the only defensible treatment for eligible patients. (He would be guilty of negligence by currently accepted standards if he did not operate.)

Perhaps, however, he should revert to a more conventional type of operation in a control treatment arm and compare his technique to this, or perhaps he should use some more widely used, even if not totally conventional, operation as his control? Again, equipoise fails for reasons already rehearsed—pain, safety as assessed by the educated eye, and intraoperative time (all disturbances of equipoise based on intrinsic features of the surgery rather than on remote clinical outcomes).

So what should Dr. G do about his new technique? To answer this, we need to look at "current best treatment" of cervical spondylosis.

A wide range of results have been reported for the surgical treatment of this problem, but the data are plagued with difficulties. The first is that indications for surgery differ between series and are not always defined in published studies. Second, outcome measures vary from study to study and are often not reported in any detail. Third, the assessment before and after surgery is often carried out by the surgeon doing the procedure or his team, and therefore the results are prone to bias (because the surgeon and his team will look for good results to vindicate their treatment and because patients do not like to disappoint their doctors). Dr. G has his reasons for thinking that his modification is likely to improve the operation by being more efficient and causing less morbidity. This claim should be examined by what is, in effect, an extended safety study involving careful observation of his operative series, specifically looking for evidence of any adverse but unanticipated effects of his technique. For the patients involved, informed consent is extremely important and should cover the points about innovative treatment and surgical research that I have mentioned.

Given the poor evidence about existing treatments, all that we can ask of Dr. G is that he show that his procedure is comparable. If, prima facie, there is no reason to believe otherwise, the patients should be told of their options and of the relation between what is proposed and standard medical treatment for their problem, and be offered a chance to participate. Simple as it seems, many clinicians, and surgeons in particular, are bad at presenting the choices available. They make up their minds about a preferred mode of therapy and do not inform patients about uncertainties or other options. Patients should be empowered to make their own decisions, and they should be told where clinical certainty is not to be had—mastectomy versus lumpectomy in breast cancer, for instance.

If this is done, then patients become participants in the research and design of treatment regimes and learn to monitor their own health outcomes. Such a partnership is very good for medical innovation because the patients feel permitted to contribute their own observations, no matter how odd or unusual these seem to be. This is a rich source of truly Hippocratic data and, as such, is a branch of the tree of knowledge that promises a healthy crop of advances in medicine. However, the possible weakness of this position is the vulnerability of patients and the unequal power relationships in the clinical encounter. Patients can unwittingly be swayed by any bias that colors the advice given them by their surgeon.

Morbidity and mortality are likely to be similar for different ways of doing the same type of operation (all of which pass the educated-eye test), and therefore the reasons why a given surgeon uses one technique rather than another are open to all kinds of influences. A strong financial or research incentive to do things in a certain way, perhaps in a way that brings advantages to himself, can enter this picture, but there are other, less tangible rewards. Therefore, Dr. G's close involvement with this new technique is an important reason to insist on independent monitoring of his results as *the problem of nonblinded assessment of outcomes* is compounded by any bias in favor of the technique. Such an interest is not an absolute reason to refuse Dr. G's request to study the device, but it is a reason to insist on objective and fairly robust standards of impartiality in the gathering and assessment of data.

The Cartwright report in New Zealand, as I have noted, concerned a study in which an in-house university hospital ethics committee performed the ethical review. One of the recommendations to prevent the anomalies arising from such a committee was that review bodies comprise patients and professionals in proportions sufficient to ensure that the lay people were empowered. That was achieved by appointing ethics committees with 50 percent lay and 50 percent professional membership. All research and innovative treatment is reviewed by such committees, and they attempt to strike a balance between the need for innovation and adequate safeguards for patients.

Overall, these groups may be a little conservative in the interest of patient safety, but the lay-professional balance offers an important check on two competing tendencies:

1. a reactionary tendency to revert to received wisdom where innovation may offer new possibilities at the expense of established theory (the case of gastric ulceration and *helicobacter pylori* springs to mind); or
2. a rather bullish enthusiasm for new technology that may be costly and relatively untried.

Ethics committees must be aware of these two sources of bias but also should find out whether the new technique has been presented at professional meetings and has been reviewed by colleagues of the surgeon concerned. The downside is that some major medical advances might never have been made (as would surely have been the case with early kidney transplants and open-heart surgery [Jennett 1986, 244]) because of dangers they posed to patients before they were perfected.

Ethics committees should also be equipped to check regularly the studies they have approved. At the very least, they should get self-reports by the investigators, but ideally they will also do spot checks of adherence to the protocol (much more costly and time-consuming to implement) and have access to external data review by an independent data-monitoring group.

I can now return to the question "Should Dr. G do a PRDBCCT?"

1. Dr. G is not in an equipoise condition because he has a reason to believe that the new technique causes lower morbidity, gives shorter operating time, and is a technically superior way of achieving the desired result.

2. The practice of "blinding" of participants is not appropriate because patients should know what surgery they have had and the surgeon necessarily knows what he has done even though "blinded" assessment of clinical outcomes may be achievable.

3. Some patients may have particular problems that make Dr. G. think them especially suitable for the new procedure rather than the old ones, and, in all conscience, he may find it hard to advise them that he believes the two ways of doing things to be equivalent.

Some of these problems are ameliorated by careful attention to case mix in reported clinical series, standardized questionnaires and instruments for measuring indications and outcomes, and careful assessment of diagnostic and other parameters used. They are also mitigated by the uncertainty principle (Lindley and Warlow 2000). This principle, as I have noted, provides for the doctor to be genuinely reflective about the standard of evidence he has for his beliefs and, where he is uncertain or the evidence is inconclusive about the best treatment for his patient, to take part in a well-designed trial to address that uncertainty. The resulting approach holds great promise in many areas of surgical research.

A Wrinkle: New Indications

The case of Dr. G has a twist because of a Hippocratic development. Some of Dr. G's patients showed entirely unconventional indications for such major surgery, and the Hippocratic practice of careful observation leading to empirically grounded conclusions produced a problem. Many of the patients had a pleasing and somewhat surprising result in terms of relief from their headaches and neck stiffness from cervical spondylotic stenosis. Dr. G, who operated for standard reasons but gave patients the chance to talk about their disease and their operations, was surprised to hear this repeated story. He noted that the resolution of tension-type headaches was, for some patients, the most significant single change after surgery. He began to regard headache as worth considering among the complex of indications for surgery. Eventually the resolution of headache after surgery became so commonplace that he was prepared to operate for patients who wanted the procedure mainly in the hope of getting rid of their headaches (with due warnings about the uncertainties and their entitlement to an alternative opinion quite possibly differing from his own). Increasingly, patients were referred as "domino" cases: they or their doctor had heard of somebody with a similar syndrome who had been dramatically relieved. Of course, there is no reason to believe that Dr. G's device differed from any other decompressive technique in this effect, but the word got around that he had a "magic cure" for this troublesome problem.

What should he do at this point? A number of people seem to have had a significant change in morbidity and quality of life by opting for a relatively novel operation for controversial indications. He cannot therefore, in service of his Hippocratic duty to benefit his patients, just ignore that fact. It seems, at the very least, that he should monitor the cumulative results from his invasive and (transiently) painful surgery to check for safety and efficacy so that he takes reasonable steps to make sure that he does no harm. It also seems that the hypothesis that symptom relief is truly related to surgery ought to be submitted to rigorous statistical testing.

What Should a Patient/Participant Be Told?

If we take seriously the model of consent and medical advice in which patients are empowered to make intelligent choices about their own care, it follows that Dr. G must outline the options available. In doing so, he should portray as accurately as he can the relative merits of different options and the morbidity to be expected with each. He should also mention the uncertainties surrounding his innovation and offer patients an alternative, independent, and perhaps more conventional opinion from another specialist.

When all is said and done, Dr. G has a prima facie duty to do an operation that he believes to be the most cost-effective and the least likely to cause complications. If he uses his new technique, he is bound to audit his results carefully and attempt some kind of valid clinical comparison that will yield good evidence as to the relative merits of his and other techniques.

That he does not have a satisfying theoretical basis for his observations about cervical spondylotic headache should not stop him from doing the procedure on empirical grounds because theory often lags behind data (indeed, scientific or Hippocratic thinking would have it no other way). However, because the results of his surgery are partly assessed on the basis of quality-of-life criteria and for that reason are susceptible to the biases that a PRDBPCCT is designed to eliminate, he must do something like a PRDBPCCT. Yet in the area where Dr. G is working, we should note that, as in many areas of surgery, there is a need for a comprehensive clinical trial of surgery versus no surgery, perhaps based on something like the uncertainty principle.

The Creeping Inflation of Best Practice

I ought finally to turn to a worrying fact of clinical life in the context of Western medicine. New advances in surgery are more expensive than those they replace, and they are often not validated as being superior to more established (and cheaper) techniques in rigorous clinical trials. Thus, to take but one example, we are tending to apply more and more complex instrumentation and implants in spinal surgery. These are justified on the basis that they provide more rigid fixation of the spine and thereby (allegedly) are more robust in terms of spinal function and stability. However, it has never been proven that they are advantageous, even though that is claimed on the basis of anecdotal reports and small retrospective series. The problem is exacerbated when the uncritical use of new technology (which has a rationale justifying it but no evidence that it is better) sets new standards for adequate or best practice so that those using older techniques are made to look as if they are not providing the best treatment. Given that operations and the associated technology can become definitive of best practice by this evidentially flawed route, there is inevitably an upward spiral of medical costs driven by the technological takeover that leaves clinicians frightened of being left behind or considered out of date.

In such an environment, it is important to pay attention to evidence-based medicine (EBM), which gives little weight to the unsupported opinions of doctors about interventions and advances. EBM provides a way to resist the trend in public debate and courtroom practice. In both settings, Cochrane (the founder of EBM) notices the following trends: "the upgrading of 'opinion' in comparison with other types of evidence and the downgrading of the word 'experiment' . . . The general scientific problem with which we are primarily concerned is that of testing a hypothesis that a certain treatment alters the natural history of a disease for the better" (1989, 20).

The "brief, dramatic, black and white" and poorly supported opinions he objects to are not in accordance with the Hippocratic tradition where reason and observation work together and clinical practice is based on sound empirical evidence as to the efficacy of interventions. I will later develop the reservations expressed in chapter 3 about the general applicability of positivistic science thinking about complex and holistically balanced systems. For now, Cochrane is worth heeding because surgical techniques are central to that type of inquiry. A bunch of guys sitting around a table, often at a very expensive conference (BOGSAT evidence where the gender *is* important), can be young technophiles or old Luddites, but in either case we need careful Hippocratic appraisal of what is best to do, and that appraisal needs to take account of well-compiled evidence in cases similar to the one under consideration. Particularly, where a clinician's practice is subject to appraisal by an expert witness, that expert witness ought to be expected to base his or her opinions on such evidence.

We need innovation in surgery to make techniques safer. Therefore, we need good research to check on what we are doing and to refine our indications for surgery. Surgeons and the patients consulting them need to go into their respective roles in these developments with an open mind and a careful attention to the need for good observations in a primarily healing art. Therefore, we need a spirit of open and informed partnership addressing the imbalances that exist in the clinical setting so that the patient is a partner and co-investigator. When significant innovation is in the offing, an independent ethical review ought to oversee the trials required to develop and test that innovation.

Despite all this, there are reasons why we ought not delay or unnecessarily obstruct surgical innovation by insisting on orthodox and rigid adherence to the tenets of the PRDBPCCT, especially when the educated eye might inform us that a procedural variation is better than the existing method of doing the required surgery. There may be some cases where a placebo operation not only has a place in surgical trials but also is mandatory, but there are far more where a mixed methodology is the appropriate way to assess our techniques and innovations. In this open-minded spirit, I can now look at areas where evidence-based medicine may have things to learn from other orientations.

CHAPTER SEVEN

When Good Doctors Do Bad Things

> Although the art of healing is the most noble of all the arts, yet, because of the ignorance both of its professors and of their rash critics, it has at this time fallen into the least repute of them all. The chief cause of this seems to me to be that it is the only science for which states have laid down no penalties for malpractice. Ill repute is the only punishment and this does little to harm the quacks who are compounded of nothing else. Such men resemble dumb characters on the stage who, bearing the dress and appearance of actors yet are not so. It is the same with the physicians; there are many in name, few in fact. —THE CANON

These Hippocratic words have a contemporary ring to those accustomed to reading the popular press and the complaints of patient's groups. Those create an unbalanced impression because, along with all the weeping and wailing and gnashing of teeth, patients commonly say, "Of course, you can't trust doctors, but mine is OK." Although most doctors are virtuous and dedicated professionals, things go wrong in clinical life and for a number of reasons. We have always dealt with these as failings of the individual professional and focused on liability for damage to a patient. The presumption is that patients suffer harm in clinical settings as a result of negligence or incompetence and that these problems are attributable to the professional concerned. In fact, every doctor I know lives in constant apprehension that he or she will fail in some way and fall foul of this punitive system. Yet we are increasingly realizing that many of the things that go wrong are not a result of individual failing but of systems faults or even just statistical outliers. As a result, this aspect of our lives as professionals is now increasingly being addressed at the level at which it should be (Leape and Berwick 2000; Malcolm 2000).

The Hippocratic attitude (with a New Zealand twist) involves treating our colleagues as whanau, or "kith and kin." Part of this approach is to honestly confront the causes of those clinical events that harm patients, some of which do arise from our failures. A healthy start to that task is to acknowledge the reasons why a doctor can fail to do what he or she knows perfectly well how to do. Once we have dealt with the causes within each of us, as it were, we can turn our gaze on the context within which we work.

The Problems that Occur

Patients worldwide suffer harms in medical settings. They affect up to 5 percent of cases in reputable hospitals (Brennan et al. 1991; Davis 2001; Vincent, Neale, and Woloshynowych 2001), and they include drug complications, wound infections, technical complications of procedures, diagnostic mishaps, and so on. About one-quarter are due to clinical negligence and another quarter to errors of other kinds (Leape et al. 1991). Sometimes these harms are associated with or even exacerbated by the ill-advised use of complex medical technology, but always they represent a compound of individual failing and other factors.

The class of events where clinical care harms a patient is called *medical misadventure*. It is made up of events of two different types; call them *medical mishaps* and *medical errors* (a terminology used in New Zealand which captures one important distinction). A *mishap* is an event in which every health care professional acts as we would expect of a professional of his or her type in a situation where the adverse event happened. An *error* means that a health care professional has not performed adequately and has caused harm. Events of both types may be avoidable according to the Swedish system of dealing with iatrogenic harm, but only the latter type is compensable under tort law as it exists in the United States (Fitzjohn and Studdert 2001). Health care professionals constantly deal with risky interventions in the lives of others, thereby putting themselves in the way of causing such harm because the word *risky* implies that a possibility of harm is built into the intervention. Thus, there is a statistical rate of adverse outcomes to be expected even where the intervention is carried out by a person who is a competent, perhaps even excellent, exponent of the techniques involved and who is conscientious in performing the particular intervention that goes wrong. A physician dealing with life-and-death surgery (such as neurosurgery) lives with this reality all the time. It is a basic principle of natural justice that one should not be held accountable for any event in which one's action (or negligent inaction) was not causally related to the harm. Thus, in reviewing what has happened, one must assess the likelihood of what did happen against the base expectation of that event happening and the occurrence or otherwise of an error. Traditionally, we do this badly and tend to think "I screwed up" or "I could have done better." In fact, given that doctors are committed to trying to make a difference to the well-being of their patients, this pattern of thought comes with the territory, however well- or ill-grounded it may be on a given occasion. Moreover, what one traditionally thinks in one's own case is transmuted in interesting ways into a judgment on the actions of a colleague.

When faced by a calamity in the practice of another or a colleague, one thinks either "I would have done it better" or "There but for the grace of God go I." The former tends to be the reaction of a young doctor. As time goes by and experience makes its mark, the reaction increasingly takes the latter form.

The surgeon breezed into the operating room, psyched up for the scheduled operation, knowing that it was one of the most demanding he had performed for some time. The patient was a relatively well young man with a huge tumor, probably benign, sitting underneath the brain and stretching the major cerebral arteries over its surface. The patient and his wife, an operating theater nurse, had traveled some distance to come to this surgeon for this operation. The likelihood of failure was quite high, and if something went wrong in the operation, the patient could well be left with disfiguring and disabling neurological deficits. On entering the theater, the surgeon noted that the patient had been positioned ready for him to operate and that the patient's head had been shaved in preparation for the incision. Determined to impose the optimal working conditions on the OR, the surgeon exchanged pleasantries with the staff, started a Mozart recording, and went to the scrub bay. He started the procedure, and all went well. The incision was well planned and its position ideal for the removal of the tumor. He opened the coverings of the brain, half expecting to see the tumor peering out at him. It was not evident. He gently retracted the brain. It was still not visible. At that moment a sinking, sickening feeling swept over him, and he turned to the X-ray screen, confirming that he had opened the skull on the wrong side. As he assessed the situation and prepared to close his incision and reposition the patient to operate on the correct side (actually the left), it flashed through his mind how, recently, in thinking about a colleague who had done the same thing, he had thought, "How could he have been so dumb?"

I could dissect this case at length in terms of the personal pressures on the surgeon, the procedures in place for ensuring that something as basic as opening the head on the correct side would be checked, the extent to which basic checks are part of the duty of every surgeon, and so on, but I would still be left wondering about what had happened. In any event, the operation went well, and the patient and his wife, much relieved that he had survived intact, were completely supportive and understanding when the surgeon shamefacedly confessed the mistake. However, that does not answer the difficult audit and quality question as to how this event, which was clearly a result of error, should be responded to.

Assessing the performance of any doctor calls for sophisticated judgments about whether he or she is practicing well and whether a misadventure can justly be attributed to features that are characteristic of the doctor's clinical practice as a whole or are isolated events arising from an unfortunate combination of circumstances. Even though the difference between mishap and error seems pellucidly clear, it is not so in practice. We need to look at case mix, track record, and peer review.

Case mix: Any doctor who routinely deals with cases that colleagues regard as complex, difficult, or dangerous would be expected to have more adverse outcomes than somebody with a much less demanding scope of practice. Thus, we should assess, in looking at adverse outcomes, a statistical rate of expected bad outcome relativized to the type of patient being treated. This makes the audit or track record of doctors extremely important.

Track record/audit: Doctors are increasingly required to keep an audit of their practice and the morbidity and mortality of their case management. This audit allows a particular question or complaint to be assessed against a more adequate framework rather than being subject to a one-time, ad hoc judgement based on sometimes conflicting opinions about what happened and what should have happened. (I have already noted this in discussing informed consent.)

Peer review: This process supplements clinical audit with ongoing reflection and conversation designed to help clinicians reflect on their practice. It is light years away from expert opinions in an adversarial setting. The latter can often be akin to the work of credible "hired guns" whose contract is to support one side or the other of a case in which there has got to be a winner and a loser. Peer review is supportive, critical, and aimed at quality improvement.

I argue that even when litigation is resorted to, we must get away from the expert witness as currently conceived and move toward assessments by panels of respected experts. Such a panel provides the considered opinion that one cannot hope to get from "the expert witness" acting within the "hired-gun" model. I also urge that a systematic audit, perhaps enhanced by critical incident reports and conducted in association with peer review, is vital in coming to a balanced assessment of any clinician's practice and assisting his or her own reflection on that practice. I finally suggest that an atmosphere of safety, care for one another as professionals and colleagues, and humility—rather than power, competition, and abuse—is essential in delivering good clinical care to patients and communities.

Personal Failings

When a person who can act well does not, it is a personal failing. This phenomenon has attracted philosophical attention for more than 2,000 years. As traditionally discussed by philosophers, it is normally taken to mean weakness of the will (or *akrasia*). Both Plato and Aristotle puzzled over it in its pure form when an agent acted in a way that he knew he should not (all things considered), but I will include all types of failures of action and belief.

I have, in outlining the Hippocratic tradition, related it to the work of Aristotle, an astute commentator on the human condition. His discussion of akrasia is classic (*Nicomachean Ethics,* Book 7.2). He discusses the man who cannot benefit by reason because even though he knows all the reasons to act well, he still does what, all things considered, he knows he should not. Aristotle says that he lacks phronesis, or practical wisdom, the ability to act according to one's best reasons. Practical wisdom arises from training in which one is taught how to respond to a variety of actual situations. In some situations one has the opportunity to observe the conduct of a wise teacher and in others one benefits from that teacher's correction of one's own responses. Such supervision and shaping results in phronesis. There is, however, a kind of trainee who knows how to talk about excellence but does not exhibit it. Reasoning with or instructing such a person is of no avail because, as Aristotle so nicely puts it, "If water makes a man choke, what can you give him to wash it down?" (ibid.). It is not words (in the form of injunctions, instruction, or regulation) that such people need because their defect is in the translation of reason into action.

This kind of failure is evident in certain typical surgical situations. The first that always springs to mind in relation to the abandonment of reason involves a flood of passion—the heat of the moment. The second is when I find myself saying, "Why am I doing this operation?" and the third when I think to myself "Why did I do that?" during an operation.

The *overwhelming of reason by passion* can and does happen in clinical life. It most often happens to surgeons who lose their tempers (other fleshly failings are more common in other specialties). When one considers the tension that is sometimes found in an operating room, it is not surprising that emotions can boil over and conflicts that have simmered below the surface, either between different people or within the surgeon himself, can precipitate a ridiculous incident. I have seen a surgeon throw instruments on the floor like a child in a tantrum, shout at a scrub nurse until she was so upset she had to leave the operating theater, and even humiliate a resident in front of staff in such a way that the resident could neither answer nor remain in the situation and, again, had to leave the room. There is no credible defense for such behavior, and most of us, once the moment has gone, do apologize for acting in such immature ways. This first form of action failure, occurring in the heat of the moment, should give the reflective surgeon cause to undertake a process of self-understanding and training in virtue that will make such events less likely. Yet temperament and heated moments are not the whole problem.

I sometimes find myself doing an operation knowing that I am far more likely to regret it than to be glad afterward. On such occasions, I can usually identify the weakness in myself that has made me more ready to operate (with a small chance of improving things, a lot of expense, and an increase of the patient's dependence on the medical system) than to bite the bullet and confront the patient with the fact that surgery cannot help him or her. I am not alone in this. Many patients have had multiple laparotomies for abdominal pain, or back fusions for long-standing back pain ("perhaps due to mechanical instability"). During the operation, the decision reveals itself to have been ill advised, and you find yourself just wanting to be somewhere else, or you realize that you will find it hard to justify the operation in your audit or review meeting with your colleagues. What is even worse, as you turn your mind back on the operation and its sequelae, you yourself would justifiably pour scorn on it if it had been done by somebody else. However, there are patterns to be found here.

Some patients manage to isolate you from your colleagues, perhaps by singling you out as the only doctor who has really understood them, by playing on a sense of rivalry with some other doctor who has attended them, or by just mentioning to you some reason why you are uniquely whom they want to treat them. These are all danger signs—you should ask "What am I being set up for, and why?" Often when you do something you wish you had not done, there is some other factor that has made you vulnerable at the time; you are tired or feeling other pressures in your life, you are going through a period of doubt about your own abilities, your bank account is a bit thin that month, and so it goes on. None of these should have any bearing on how the patient is treated, but they do, and you find yourself doing that which you have no good reason to do.

Some things just happen. Recreating the events surrounding them often allows you to understand why; perhaps a fleeting thought or impulsive movement precipitated the ill-advised action. Sometimes your instinct tells you that something is not a good thing to do, but reason says otherwise. Some factor may have come to dominate your thinking—the image of the miraculous surgical result that has obliterated the real difficulties you are likely to face doing the operation, or the thought of solving the problem with a single stroke. A cool calculation about real probabilities and the likelihood of success is hard to translate into actual images of what one is likely to strike during the operation. An older and wiser surgeon than myself, my mentor at the time, once said to me "Surgery is not about what you can get away with, it is about what you can do safely every time." The ability to distil and act on reflective lessons learned from experience is part of what Aristotle calls *phronesis,* and it tells you when to act on your intuitions and when to be suspicious of them. Sometimes, though, you ought to heed intuitive thoughts—a topic to which I shall return.

Surgeons deceive themselves despite that in their more reflective and melancholy moments, perhaps when some operation or intervention has gone badly, they may vividly recall the occasions on which they have done so and the results to which that led. We are all susceptible to "the recency effect," where we gauge the likelihood of success or otherwise of what we are about to do by thinking back to *our last case.* Surgery is also a sanguine discipline in which many of us are convinced that we can boldly go where no surgeon has been before and escape, with ourselves and the patient unscathed. When we are wrong, neither we nor our patients escape unscathed. The tragedy or disappointment can provoke denial or sober reflection. In the one case the surgeon becomes a more damaged person and less of a reflective practitioner, and in the other he or she learns something ultimately of benefit to both surgeon and patients but at a significant cost. It does require a certain optimism and courage to persist in taking up cold steel against the ravages of time and disease, and therefore the sanguine temperament, perhaps tempered by a realistic sense of what one can achieve based on a growing experience of having achieved it, is an indispensable part of clinical surgery.

We do neither ourselves nor our patients any good at all when we act with good intentions but poor judgment because then the collected folly of wishful thinking, self-deception, impulsive action, and idiosyncrasy or narcissism combine to lead us into bad actions. We need to be optimistic, we need to give hope to those who desperately need it, and we need to avoid the kind of fatalism or inertia that condemns our patients to outdated and inferior treatment. Nevertheless, we also need to have a canny eye for what is genuinely worthwhile rather than be credulous or deceived about our capabilities. As surgeons, indeed as healers of any kind, we need the humility to work with the body, contributing what we can to its attempts to cope with dysfunction. The right balance between activism and quietism is hard to define but can be sensed by those attentive enough to themselves and their patients to appreciate and master the art that is clinical medicine.

The art of surgery requires the capacity for judicious action and the ability to reflect on what one has done. Young surgeons are exposed to a rich variety of clinical experiences, but sometimes the attitudes that our trainees encounter are not at all enriching. They encounter arrogance, bigotry, immaturity, and insensitivity, and therefore many of the lessons that experience would otherwise teach are eclipsed. Well-honed clinical skills are the right breeding ground for good attitudes, but they need to be allied with good mentoring. When one denies one's own deficiencies because of misbegotten attitudes about one's own superiority and worth, the result is defensiveness and insecurity. Both are antithetical to the open-mindedness required for learning and the grounded self-confidence that leads to good interpersonal relations. What is more, the person who is constantly trying to prove him or herself is *driven* in a way that is ultimately destructive to the clinical partnership. Our stories are messed up by people like that, and when they wield the powerful tools of medicine, we can emerge severely wounded from encounters with them. Ideally, a mentor should train one not only in surgical technique but also in the techniques of the self and the development of phronesis.

In trying to address the sometimes dysfunctional culture of clinical medicine, one needs to develop a nose for the attitudes that perpetuate dysfunction and a heart for genuine and caring (if mildly subversive) reform. Balloons, in the form of overinflated egos, need pricking, and some statuesque figures need to have their attention drawn to their own feet of clay. A spirit of debate and irreverence (which can distinguish genuinely hallowed ground from that which should be demythologized) is indispensable for the well-balanced clinician. We should, among other things, learn to laugh at ourselves and expose our illusions. Medical jokes are a vital part of training, particularly in the fraught and dramatic world of surgeons who may actually regard all the world as a stage on which they should be lead actors. The best source of surgeon jokes is anesthetists, and they make for interesting reflection. For instance, an anesthetist adjusting the light during an operation conveyed the reason why the wound was not well illuminated by saying: "The most opaque substance known to man is the head of a surgeon."

A related story has a jumbo-jet flight attendant come breathlessly down the aisle asking, "Is there an anesthetist on board?" Puzzled, a woman anesthetist responds and is taken forward to first class. There she finds a distinguished-looking man reading a book who turns to her and says, "Oh, hello, I am a surgeon. Could you adjust the light for me?" There is also the story about two surgeons' wives, the younger of whom complains that her husband is overly amorous and she does not know what to do about his unwanted advances. The older one says, "I solved that one years ago, dear. Forget headaches and tiredness. When he is getting overheated, you say, 'Cut it out,' and then a different light comes into his eyes, his nostrils flare, and he looks around saying, 'Where, where?'" Perhaps both the need for ego deflation and its basis are illustrated in this joke about ward rounds. The team is gathered around the bed, and the discussion turns to what is wrong with the patient. Learned opinions are offered and rejected until the frustrated junior resident asks, "So what the hell is wrong with the patient?" The senior resident mutters, quite audibly because of a momentary hush, "God only knows." The chief resident, not missing a beat, turns to the professor and remarks, "And you're not telling, are you, sir?"

Impaired Doctors

Apart from the personal failings that we all show from time to time, there are doctors who slide into dangerous professional territory and show disturbing trends in their practice. In the past we may have tended to overlook these trends and to close ranks, with the result that the public often believes that doctors are as thick as thieves, more ready to stand by their colleagues than to see patients protected or justice done. Indeed, the Hippocratic oath is blamed for this ethos.

"I will pay the same respect to my master in the Science as to my parents and share my life with him and pay all my debts to him. I will regard his sons as my brothers and teach them the Science, if they desire to learn it, without fee or contract. I will hand on precepts, lectures and all other learning to my sons, to those of my master and to those pupils duly apprenticed and sworn, and to none other" (The Oath, 67).

It is not clear that this passage, in the context of the other writings, supports any form of professional protectionism. The Hippocratics conceived of the profession as an extended family with its own traditions and sense of honor. In contemporary New Zealand terms this means that we should treat our colleagues as whanau, an attitude with important implications for our conduct toward those who are impaired or fall short of the standards of the profession, and for clinical institutions.

Your whanau is many things. It is the ground on which you are nurtured, it is the source of your name and identity, it is the fabric of traditions that give you roots for your own being and for your destiny, it is the context in which you have honor and a place to stand in the presence of others, and it is a hallowed organic being to which your own deeds will bring either honor or shame. Within it, you can hold your head high and learn how to conduct yourself. Within it, you are emotionally rooted and can find counsel and support when you need them. This concept offers important guidance with respect to both the impaired doctor and the work of professional disciplinary mechanisms.

Treating colleagues as whanau therefore means that we should have an attitude of care rather than judgment. We care for members of our families, and we have an eye to their best interests, but our attitude is not uncritical. We care for their well being in moral and spiritual as well as material terms. Impaired colleagues run the risk of moral harm, the harm that arises for a person from having harmed somebody else, and we have a duty, as family, to keep them safe in their practice. We cannot stand aside and indulge a colleague in such a way as to allow more serious harm to occur than the damage that has already been done. Impairment is bad enough, but it is even worse when our complicity or indulgence leads to errors that any person would find difficult to live with. For that reason alone, we must be vigilant in the caring way that family are vigilant about the lives of each other.

Aside from this watchfulness, there is the tradition of honor and standing in the community associated with any whanau. The medical profession is well aware of its public face; it commands a certain respect because of its long tradition that implies a distinct standing and role in relation to the health of the community. This status is eroded by those who practice when impaired or who do dishonorable and disgraceful things. Their actions affect the whole family, and the family must call them to account and exercise its powers to bring them back on track. Therefore, our conception that we are bound together by family-like ties has significant implications for the ways in which we regard professionals who are impaired. A mixture of indulgence and refusal to face the issue, followed by abandonment when things get so bad that somebody has to be called to account, is not a proper part of the attitude to our colleagues as whanau.

Doctors can be impaired for personal, social, financial, alcohol- and drug-related, marital, sexual, or illness-related reasons. Impairment refers to anything that makes the doctor unable to exercise reasonable care, skill, and judgment in treating a patient. The problem is usually recognized when things start going wrong and are noticed by a colleague or another health care professional such as a local pharmacist, a nurse, or social worker. Some of the problems that lead to impairment are inherently liable to occur in the medical lifestyle, and they all have a direct impact on competence.

Important problems arise when young people are taken from high-pressure schooling to a high-pressure university course without being given the breathing space to develop as persons who can cope with the emotional and other traumas of everyday life. Within a few short years, these fresh-faced adolescents are plunged into fraught and demanding life-and-death situations where they must work alongside other colleagues of many different ages, each with their own balanced or unbalanced approach to life, death, career, and relationships. Some of these colleagues are idealistic, some perfectionistic, some cynical, and there are complex technical and intellectual challenges, emotional demands, exhaustion, narcissism, and nepotism, all served up with generous helpings of black and sometimes vicious humor.

These pressures on young doctors are accentuated in countries where qualifying as a doctor involves incurring a large debt that must be repaid when you start working. The financial insecurity of a large educational debt, when added to the many other sources of stress and tension on a young medic make it nothing short of amazing that any physician emerges with their idealism and humanity intact. This particular problem is worsened by the socialization of a doctor to expect a certain standard of living and develop a set of social aspirations that create their own financial demands.

Marital and sexual problems tend to abound because doctors are often busy and career oriented. At home, they can be quite demanding and needy because of the emotional drain of their professional lives, and they may find it difficult to set aside quality time for relationships. They are also constantly in contact with a variety of people toward whom they are sympathetic, with whom they have close daily personal contact, and who share some deeply emotional highs and lows. On top of all that, they meet patients by whom they are seen as helpful, caring, sometimes heroic, and who often idolize them. The resulting pressures on close personal relationships, an emotionally charged working environment, and a ready set of contacts available to start new relationships is dynamite, not only for the young but also for the restless—those facing the difficult years of middle-aged doubt, disillusionment, adventure seeking, and prosperity.

The need for escape and the combination of factors already identified can be important in disrupting relationships as well in drug- and alcohol-related problems (which are exacerbated by failing relationships). Both areas require special vigilance within the profession for a number of reasons. For instance, a number of interested parties (social and commercial) will woo doctors by using alcohol-related events, and a ready source of various drugs with potential for abuse goes with the territory.

As if all that were not enough, there is the old and wise saying, "The man who treats himself has a fool for a doctor." Doctors are often very poor at diagnosing illness in themselves, and often, particularly with illnesses that affect judgment and performance of a skilled professional task, they are the last to realize what is happening to them. Busy doctors are bad at self-care. They procrastinate and put their own health low on their list of priorities, often driving themselves mercilessly in service of their career or their perceived duties to others—patients, colleagues, trainees, students, professional organizations, institutions, and so on.

Unfortunately, overwork can also make its own contribution to incompetence as doctors cut corners to get everything done and, despite their considerable skill and intelligence, fail in basic aspects of their clinical practice. All these factors compound and interact with each other and can go undetected because of the background noise created by genuinely hard problems and the constant risk that a given case will have a bad outcome, all worsened when our clinical skills and judgment are stretched. Of course, the hard cases arise far more often for those who are incompetent for any reason. The Hippocratic writings identify "sorry doctors who . . . cure men but slightly ill . . . [and] their errors are unperceived . . . but when they have to treat a serious and dangerous case, a mistake or lack of skill is obvious to all" (Tradition, 75).

When things go wrong, we do make excuses for ourselves, and considerable reflective skills on the part of doctors are needed to realize the extent to which they are deceiving themselves. Every patient is a one-time problem in some respect or other, and so many of the contributing factors to bad outcomes are difficult to identify. The surgeon who is perfectly good at what he does but who is "unlucky" is well known. We always used to say during our surgical training that the most important thing if you were admitted to hospital was to get a lucky surgeon. One is reminded of the golfer who said, "I'll tell you one thing I've noticed: the more I practice, the luckier I get." The Hippocratics figured out this tendency years ago: "Even I do not exclude the operations of fortune, but I think that those who have received bad attention usually have bad luck, and those who have good attention good luck" (Science, 140).

In reality, there is too much in the way of confounding detail and complex multiple causation for any of us to be completely accurate in reflecting on our own competence. Therefore, it is important to have close and open working relationships with other colleagues who can, in a nonconfrontational way, help us deal with our own shortcomings (which we all have). This occurs when we do foster the idea of colleagues as whanau, diligent about the honor of the family but also supportive of one another in adversity.

Moral harm matters in families because it is hard to live with and cannot be readily healed. It affects the honor of the family because an outsider has also been harmed in ways that a compassionate person cannot easily put behind them and an honorable person cannot overlook. Sometimes, though, the harm has occurred because a combination of circumstances conspires to make doctors do things they would not do if they were situated differently or not themselves impaired in some way. We therefore have a further reason, for the sake of doctors themselves, to put in place the supports that minimize the likelihood of them suffering the sometimes catastrophic effects of impairment in their and their patients' lives.

Quite apart from all this is the genuinely bad doctor who abuses his power to exploit patients or conceal his own inadequacies. It is in the interest of all professions to deal harshly with this kind of person, and most of us feel no moral qualms about doing so. We have no inclination to close ranks with predatory creatures such as those who abuse the trust of their patients, just as such abuse is not tolerated in good and well-functioning families.

What We Have Now:
Three Ways of Dealing with Bad Things

Given that bad events are going to occur even in the best of circles, there are three ways of dealing with the problem:

1. litigation;
2. discipline;
3. clinical governance and safety.

I can take these in turn, evaluating their relative merits in terms of how they deal with the needs of patients, their effect on the quality of medical practice, and their efficacy in detecting and correcting the failings of clinicians who make errors.

The Role of Litigation

There are a number of justifications for civil litigation as the means of responding to medical negligence. They can be summarized as follows:

a. it directly penalizes those who have been negligent;
b. it imposes liability on the more knowledgeable and powerful party;
c. it is less restrictive than government regulation;
d. it deals with minor as well as major negligence where that leads to harm. (Whelan 1988)

These justifications seem sound. Many of the harms befalling patients are definitely caused by medical error (as defined above; see Leape et al. 1991), and it is reasonable to penalize doctors who cause harm. Thus, the patient should be able to sue the doctor rather than the fault going unpunished and the remedy or compensation coming from somebody else entirely—a third party insurance provider or the community acting through some other agency. Moreover, doctors are the ones who ought to be responsible for stopping these things happening because they have the power in the clinical relationship. Putting the responsibility on doctors to avoid litigation also means that the cumbersome and expensive process of government regulation and compliance is kept out of clinical practice, which, even without it, can often become overly bureaucratic and paper bound. And it is true that mistakes not serious enough to call for the heavy hand of regulation are still subject to complaint and remedy through litigation so that there are incentives to eliminate them. Unfortunately these justifications, though plausible, do not stand up to scrutiny.

First, the penalty does not fall on the doctor causing the harm for two independent but important reasons: (1) *court settlements do not track errors* but tend to be driven by the extent of patient harm, and (2) *the doctor is insured for malpractice liability.*

The first of these problems is revealed by empirical evidence about misadventure and the results of litigation. "In a multivariate analysis, disability (permanent vs. temporary or none) was the only significant predictor of payment . . . There was no association between the occurrence of an adverse event due to negligence . . . and payment" (Brennan et al. 1996). In fact, not only is there little connection between genuine malpractice and settlements, but also there is no consistent connection between negligence or incompetence and claims against doctors (Studdert et al. 2000). "Medical malpractice litigation infrequently compensates patients injured by medical negligence and rarely identifies, and holds providers accountable for, substandard care" (Localio et al. 1991).

The second problem is obvious after a moment's reflection on the first. Doctors are insured against the damages awarded in malpractice suits so that settlement for those damages is made by a third party—the company indemnifying the doctor. Such companies recognize perfectly well that bad things can happen which are subject to awards of damages but which are not straightforwardly attributable to negligence or incompetence, and therefore they attract clients by risk sharing rather than punitive premium adjustments after law suits. Thus, the effect of a settlement is to cause the insurance premiums paid by all doctors to increase. Such premiums are legitimate overheads of clinical practice, and therefore, inevitably, they have a domino effect of increasing doctors' fees.

The net result is that bad doctors are not necessarily punished, and all patients end up paying more so that settlements for the "lucky" patients who get compensated can be paid out. This outcome is captured by the phrase "the multimillion dollar medical malpractice lottery"—a gruesome sweepstake that offers some patients the chance of becoming fabulously wealthy at the cost of their health and well being and on the basis of increased medical costs to everybody else.

There are a number of positive reasons for not buying into the malpractice/ litigation myth.

It is *unfair* to those patients who suffer serious harms but cannot prove fault.

Their needs may be as great as those who do "prove fault" (according to the suspect standards that prevail in such actions), but those needs unjustly go unmet.

It wrongly *isolates the doctor* as the causative agent when, for the reasons I
have discussed, mistakes can have complex causes so that good doctors, acting
well within the standards of professional care that we want to enforce, can be
caught up in a chain of events with a bad or even disastrous outcome.

It encourages *defensive medicine* and *adversarial attitudes* in what I have argued
should be a partnership with the patient. Defensive medicine means that the
costs of medical care and the standard of best practice are continually being
redefined according to what could possibly have been done that was not done
rather than what, in the light of good evidence, is likely to secure a good outcome for the patient. There are always more tests and more checks that can be
built into the management of any case; many of these add small but discernible
risks to the clinical course, and all of them add costs. Adversarial attitudes are,
however, more damaging to the conduct of medicine as a whole. Clinical medicine ought to be a mutual problem-solving exercise in which an informed
patient works with a clinician to try to produce an outcome or solution to the
clinical problem that is the best that can be achieved and that both can live with.
Unfortunately, these problems are not really solved by the other traditional
response to malpractice—medical discipline—although it is better than the
multimillion dollar medical malpractice lottery.

Medical Discipline for Malpractice

A doctor who falls short of professional standards is dealt with by the disciplinary mechanism established by his community. This mechanism generally
takes the form of a set of provisions that control who gets a license to practice
medicine, and a complaints procedure whereby doctors who have caused harm
or been guilty of substandard practice can be assessed according to professional
standards and a suitable disciplinary action can be taken. The disciplinary mechanism generally upholds the same sort of guidelines as medical litigation.

According to these guidelines, a doctor has a duty of care based on certain
requirements: "(1) he must possess the degree of professional learning, skill, and
ability that others similarly situated possess; (2) he must exercise reasonable care
and diligence in the application of his knowledge and skill to the patient's case;
and (3) he must use his best judgment in the treatment and care of his patient"
(Warren 1980, 125). Traditionally, care alleged to be negligent is brought to the

attention of the licensing or disciplinary body by a patient, but in some places (in fact, in New Zealand and Sweden) there is mandatory reporting of medical misadventure and other routes through which defective treatment is referred to the regulatory authorities.

In general, the disciplinary process works as follows.

1. A complaint is received by the disciplinary body of the profession.
2. The complaint will usually be reported to the doctor concerned.
3. The complaint is considered by the medical disciplinary process, and some attempt is made to mediate between the doctor and the complainant.
4. The case goes to a quasi-judicial hearing, where the existence or otherwise of malpractice is determined according to widely accepted professional standards.

This process can happen to any doctor at any time, and in many settings it is supplemented by an impaired doctor scheme of the type discussed above, which, ideally, prevents too much (actual and moral) harm being done. The ultimate outcome of a disciplinary process may be that the doctor is struck off the list of qualified medical practitioners and has to give up practice, but lesser penalties/remedies such as supervised practice can be imposed. In fact, most countries have bodies (with either state or national jurisdiction) able to use a range of remedies similar to the U.S. state medical examining boards. These can "issue reprimands, limit a physician's license to practice, or place a physician on probation . . . require a physician to receive additional medical education or to submit to a professional competency exam before a suspension or probation will be terminated . . . or suspend or revoke a license" (Warren 1980, 155–56).

Critics of the system have various gripes with it. It can seem to fail the test of "Who watches the watch?" (Juvenal: *Sed quis custodiet ipsos custodes?*) For some members of the public, the whole problem is that doctors close ranks and protect their colleagues when something goes wrong, an approach that will not wash with a public that is increasingly knowledgeable about the profession and its conduct (Coates 2000). Conversely, we say, "Set a thief to catch a thief," which certainly seems apt when one testifies before and serves on disciplinary bodies, in that doctors are the best placed and best informed monitors to catch out other doctors who are pulling tricks on the credulous. On reflection, it seems that regulatory bodies ought to have professional and lay representation so as to be both well informed and open to the voice of those outside the medical ethos. If they are constituted to be that way, such bodies are seen to be open to scrutiny from outside the profession and not to be in-house arrangements.

Three further problems are not addressed by disciplinary mechanisms per se, although many communities have provisions in place to address them.

1. Disciplinary and complaints mechanisms do not alert us to problems until somebody is so seriously harmed that a complaint occurs.
2. Quasi-judicial frameworks support a "blame-and-shame" culture for medical misadventure.
3. Such an ethos does not carry within itself a presupposition of safety and support for the practitioner who has erred or been caught up in unfortunate events.

We therefore need to create a better context for good professional practice than either litigation or a diligent and significantly punitive disciplinary framework can provide.

Clinical Governance: Where Can We Go from Here?

The third response to medical misadventure is to promote a climate where patients are safer because errors are prevented. The Harvard study reckoned that 58 percent of adverse events were due to faulty management and therefore preventable (Leape et al. 1991). A New Zealand study indicated that nearly 40 percent of adverse events were "highly preventable" (Davis et al. 2000, 205). It is easy to see why throughout the world there is current or pending legislation and health policy initiatives aimed at a more intellectually sustainable framework for regulation of the profession as well as at safeguarding and providing for the maintenance of competence (Malcolm 2000). Delivered into the hands of bureaucrats, this kind of policy can have the feel of what Charlotte Paul termed *External Morality* (with a big *E* and a big *M*) even though it should facilitate the traditional relationship between the health professions and the society in which they work by establishing procedures in relation to adequate clinical practice within government or other health care institutions.

In general, clinical governance focuses on methods of audit and collaborative consultation whereby the standards of every practitioner are improved through involvement in a structured process. Wherever it is practiced, this initiative involves clinical staff in management decisions so that clinicians and administrators learn to appreciate the strengths that each bring to clinical care and service delivery (Heyssel et al. 1984). This approach has tremendous promise in terms of ensuring that we develop workable professional standards relating clinical practice to medical research (Scally and Donaldson 1998). The development of clinical practice contexts in which all health care professionals can have an active and engaged part in the design of their working environment is a huge step toward implementing quality measures and practices that tend to avoid misadventure.

One of the most important single changes in such projects is the creation of an atmosphere in which any members of staff can speak out on any issue that worries them.

> The surgeon was just about to close the wound, having decompressed the levels at which the patient appeared to have a significant cervical spinal stenosis. He was a little puzzled, as his original operative intention was to do a wider decompression from that which the scans had indicated was necessary. A nurse, who was looking at the scans and just getting the clinical notes ready for sending back to the ward with the patient after the operation, suddenly remarked, "That's funny; the name on these scans is not the same as the name of the patient." It was rapidly ascertained that the films of another patient with a very similar cervical spinal condition had found their way into the packet of the patient being operated on, the only difference being that the other patient had less extensive disease. Needless to say, the operation was then extended and completed as required.

Now, this could not have happened unless a relatively junior member of the operating team had felt empowered to speak up and voice a concern. This incident then initiated a wider discussion so that some minor changes were made to prevent such an error in future.

Outcomes and outcome statistics are easily accessible for the purposes of audit in some areas of medicine but are not universally so. The areas where review is more difficult are those in which scientifically measurable outcomes and easily documented endpoints are not to be found (as is the case in alternative and complementary medicine but also in many areas of primary care or community medicine and nursing).

Nonetheless, the process of clinical review and the empowerment of clinicians to take part in decisions affecting their working environments so that they can suggest initiatives, institute practices that are conducive to safe patient care, and provide a supportive working environment for staff are possible in these less cut-and-dried areas of practice. What is more, the interdisciplinary exchange facilitated within such a shared framework is likely to benefit all the Hippocratic professions. As one who has experienced the process firsthand, I can testify to the improvements that result. But whatever one thinks of clinical governance, some professionally based and workable quality and surveillance mechanism must be put in place in contemporary clinical medicine.

In health care generally, the caveat emptor rule is either irrelevant or inadequate as a means of quality control. Patients (or clients) are highly dependent on health care professionals for their regimes of management, and, as the Hippocratic writings note, actual clinical outcomes (even in well-managed cases) vary a great deal from case to case despite superficial resemblances. The professional must therefore be trustworthy in making an initial diagnosis, interpreting any investigations, embarking on appropriate management, and being honest about prognoses. The complexity of human disease and recovery, and the variability of natural history in almost every condition that we treat, combine to confound any but the most sophisticated analyses of outcome so that patients are in no position to monitor the quality of the treatment they receive. Two things then become extremely important: the first is the partnership model of clinical care that I have discussed, and the second is the integrity of the profession. Therefore, we must revisit the issue of an External Morality for clinical practice as it occurs in relation to nonvocational institutions and mechanisms of control.

External Morality relies on control and surveillance as opposed to the personal vocation and dedication to self-improvement that are inherent in an internal morality. I have noted, however, that the Hippocratic professional takes on not only a set of duties but also, in fact, a way of being. The features of this way of being involve striving for excellence, an astute eye toward the realities of complex health care situations and what can be achieved, and a commitment to life-long learning. One enters this practice in partnership with others and with one's patients, but it is not something that anybody in their right mind would ever *contract* into. Unfortunately, we are increasingly being taught to see our standards as professionals in the light of generic contractual obligations rather than such vocational desiderata.

Seen as aspects of a contractual obligation, what we are asked to do is daunting and potentially unlimited. Therefore, it is likely to foster an adversarial climate, and it is also going to cost a great deal. The imposition of external standards therefore goes along with the provision of external rewards—rewards other than the personal satisfaction of having fulfilled one's vocation in a way conducive to a sense of well-being or eudaemonia. For a doctor, eudaemonia arises, in part, from having lived well in one's calling and having done well as a person with that calling. In a climate of external morality and adversarial attitudes toward one's failings, these satisfactions are blunted and often obscured by other considerations—such as the thought that one is under surveillance and constantly trying to meet somebody else's standards. We must be alert to anything that tends to accentuate those alienating aspects of the clinical environment.

One must therefore beware of systems that tend toward mandatory reporting of medically adverse events and the suspected incompetence of one's colleagues because the good effects of such a provision can be easily outweighed by its undesirable consequences. How the mandatory reporting requirement is seen depends on what we put in place around it. In the "support and safety" environment that is fostered by clinical governance measures, it provides protection for professionals as well as the public. If one is prevented from practicing badly and can, after a period of remedy and correction, be rehabilitated back into useful clinical or vocational work, then that is one thing. But if this effort is allied to a consumerist, adversarial, and litigious orientation in which grievances rule and those baying for blood are the major voices, then things are going to go from bad to worse. We could end up in the ridiculous situation that prevails where any settlement for misadventure is forestalled by evasion and noncooperation with the pursuit of clinical improvement through audit and corrective planning, due to fear of litigation. To some extent avoiding the harmful effects of misadventure depends not on legislation but on education, public attitudes, and the sociopolitical climate that is generated around health care. In fact, this climate has a profound effect at many levels.

The Hippocratic Duties and Liabilities of Nonphysicians

For clinicians, the ethical framework of their work is clear: they have a duty to provide effective health care at an appropriate standard within the resources available. That care should be scientifically informed and benefit from the competent exercise of clinical judgment focused on the individual patient's condition. However, there are other players in the delivery of health care, and they affect clinicians' ability to carry out that duty. All health care professionals work within constraints imposed by resources and the management of health care services, but the ethical duties of the relevant funders and managers are much less well defined than those of clinicians. Perhaps it is time for policy makers to generate duties and codes of practice that reflect the role that such people play.

Health care managers have a duty to provide the conditions in which clinical activity can flourish and provide the most benefit to the maximum number of consumers within certain fiscal constraints. Their duties should be entirely supportive to the highly qualified professionals their organization employs, and they must always bear in mind that their salaries are drawn from the revenue generated by those people. Yet often the whole deal seems to get reversed, and clinicians find that they end up spending a greater and greater proportion of their time fulfilling bureaucratic requirements. When this happens, I sympathize with the comment made by one frustrated clinician: "To err is human, but to create an absolutely impenetrable, mind-numbing, hog-snarling, paperbound, foul-up requires a bureaucrat who has at least a passing acquaintance with health care management."

Health care enterprises use money taken from a community or from patients within that community for the purpose of providing good health care. Thus, they have a duty in terms of the informed administration of the moneys that sustain their activity. Competition and secrecy is unhelpful in that we need sustainable standards striking an acceptable balance between service provision and safety, and all providers should be held accountable to those standards. The sharing of methods, practice guidelines, audit procedures and protocols, and the free flow of information should therefore be as much the norm in health provision as it is in the science of medicine in general. In such a context, corporate values are likely to be counterproductive and to produce distortions in health care provision which have, in some well-documented cases, demonstrably led to a loss of focus on the patient's good and a decline in service delivery relationships between management and clinicians (Stent 1998).

Such a dysfunctional context of health care provision is impossible for the clinician in that he or she has a duty to patients and the community over and above any loyalty to an employer. The Hippocratic ethos implies that clinicians must exercise responsibility first and foremost to those who need their care rather than to any corporate entity. In this uneasy position, the imposition of corporate mentality and misguided notions of corporate loyalty can only be destructive to the responsible practice of medicine. But our response to this danger should not be legalistic. Only if the profession and the management of health care institutions work together can serious problems be addressed in a way that avoids unfairly apportioning blame to any party and that protects patients from harm. This patently did not happen in the case of a British O & G (ob/gyn) consultant who continued to practice long after it should have come to light that he was not only harming but also abusing his patients (Roach 2000). Such cases show how much work, both by clinicians and managers, needs to be done.

Loose Ends and Loose Cannons

I hope to have made the case that clinical governance, audit, ethics education (involving training in virtue), and mentoring are the way to make health care safer and better. Nevertheless, whatever we do, clinicians will sometimes act badly and people will be harmed. Therefore, some form of remedy or redress will always be required, and the foregoing arguments suggest it should be based on a robust reporting system and a means of making distinctions between malpractice (error and negligence) and misadventure as a supplement to a system of clinical governance. This system is not well served by suing doctors and is much more defensible when it involves expert panels and audit considerations. Such a system should be allied to a compensation scheme for patients which does not require the patient to prove fault and which limits settlements. If a set of provisions of this kind is in place, then the community can justifiably feel that it is served by a profession governed and held accountable in the way most likely to protect patients from harm and to remedy the causes of bad clinical management.

In the present crisis in medical insurance, caused by an out-of-control malpractice industry and somewhat haphazard professional regulation, it is imperative that we take the practical and legislative steps required to regain what we have lost—a vocation with an internal morality that is conducive to safety in practice, effective self-regulation in partnership with our patients, and realistic support for one another as professionals. Only within such a climate of practice and the collegial relationships that sustain it can the moral tools of the profession hope to be adequate to the task for which they have been crafted. When we contemplate some of the dire medical challenges of the twenty-first century, we find that those tools are needed as never before.

CHAPTER EIGHT

Is AIDS the Postmodern Illness?

> Whoever would study medicine aright must learn of the following subjects
> . . . the seasons of the year, . . . the warm and cold winds, . . . the effect of
> water on the health, the effect of any town on the health of its population,
> . . . the life of the inhabitants themselves.   —AIRS, WATERS, PLACES

These Hippocratic remarks urge a broad perspective and diverse knowledge in understanding health, illness, and disease. Postmodern thought makes a similar demand, urging us to be aware that all illness is "situated at the crossroads of biology and culture" (Morris 1998, 71). That message implies that HIV/AIDS is a strong candidate for the title "the postmodern illness," in that it ended the life of Michel Foucault, the leading poststructuralist, and also mirrors the essential features of postmodern thought.

- It is fraught with uncertainties and contradictions.
- It provokes a reevaluation of values and epistemic paradigms.
- It confronts technology with its own limitations and the reality of suffering.
- It foregrounds the complex relations between sex, death, and culture.
- It locates people in discursive networks holistically related to the states of their bodies.

Uncertainty

HIV/AIDS abounds with uncertainties and contradictions. In an age celebrating life, diversity, and liberation from constricting mores, it confronts us with death and our mortal limitations, provoking widespread reactions recalling our responses to the plagues of history (Pinching 1996). "But there have been epidemics, even pandemics, before. Why should AIDS be seen as such a special case? . . . The first ground of its uniqueness is that it combines two features not previously found together in quite such stark and absolute terms . . . it is most prominently a sexually transmitted complaint and . . . it is a deadly disease lacking at present any medical means of prevention or cure" (Almond 1996, 3).

Postmodernity was born in a climate that questioned whether Western society constrained and repressed many aspects of individuality in lifestyle choices. What was considered "natural" or "normal" by our forbears was problematized and deconstructed, and many conventional truths, such as the naturalness of monogamous heterosexual relationships, were seen to incorporate tendentious social constructions and political agendas. Getting over these constraints was required so that we could recreate human life and society in ways that reconceptualized our sexuality, the idea of illness, and so on. But HIV/AIDS confronts us with grim facts that induce a kind of humility before the power of nature that is out of kilter with postmodern, post-Nietzschean thinking.

Nietzsche, the iconoclast, inspires the deconstructive project culminating in postmodernism, arguing that "natural" things and universal truths are open to the kind of critique that exposes their roots in the exercise of power by some human beings over the subjective bodies of other human beings. In this vein, he railed against the settled morality of the herd: "The strange narrowness of human evolution, its hesitations, its delays, its frequent retrogressions and rotations, are due to the fact that the herd instinct of obedience has been inherited best and at the expense of the art of commanding" ([1886] 1975, 102). The herd endorses decency, order, patience, tolerance, and platitudes about the good life constructed from ideas about human nature, civilization, and our superiority over the beasts. Yet the good life so described seems unutterably boring, even if each of us has an "authentic" version to live out that seems to give adequate expression to one's individual character.

The malleability and habitability of the Western world conduce to a kind of easygoing, do-your-own-thing, popular "philosophy," which, along with polite eclecticism and liberalism (like Jane Austen without the edge), welcomes the freedom offered by existentialist questioning of the moral order. By the late 1970s, gay sexuality was becoming destigmatized, and those pillars of society formed by stable dyadic relationships (around which primary social groupings of whatever form could cluster) were under threat. HIV/AIDS gave a new health-based impetus to the moral stance of the "gay bashers" and those wanting a return to what was "natural" (for reasonable, middle-class, urban people) because it was seen, quintessentially, as a disease confined to gays and drug abusers. It is no longer so confined, and the horrific worldwide carnage is predominately among the underprivileged and oppressed—women and children in Third World countries. This new wave of death and disease prompts a search into what used to be dismissed as a marginal problem, or a disease confined to those who lived unnatural lives and therefore (apart from sympathetic and sincere feelings for those who suffered) a disease irrelevant to the vast majority of humankind. "AIDS is in many ways a mirror of postmodern uncertainties. There is, most important, no cure. The human immunodeficiency virus (HIV) that causes AIDS has a long latency period, symptoms vary, function is unpredictable, and experimental therapies abound. Its once irreversible power to kill (now slowed by drugs) and its association with changing sexual behaviour and gender roles give it a prime claim to be the master illness of our time" (Morris 1998, 59).

Morris summarizes the ways in which uncertainty is a hallmark of HIV/AIDS. Sexual contact is dangerous but not invariably so. The easy sexuality of that late twentieth century has had to negotiate a new set of hurdles—protection from infection, concerns about the sexual history of one's partner (and how should these be acted on), and a good reason why sexual choices can no longer be regarded as private and casual in that there is always the potential (even if remote and unlikely to eventuate) of a lethal outcome. Furthermore, what does HIV mean? If one finds out that one is HIV positive, it transforms one's life—affecting all intimate relationships, giving a meaning to apparently minor health problems that may be ultimate, indicating a shadow that cannot be banished by any known intervention. Life with HIV is lived in the presence of mortality and finitude—it is postexistentialist life, and in that life, health and disease are deeply relevant.

In the normal world, only some people are preoccupied with health and disease, and many of us, even health professionals, turn to art, literature, educated company, and life as it should be lived, rather than allowing "shop" to intrude any more than it has to. (It is worth preserving the boundary even though the Hippocratic self is always co-present with one's alter egos.) Once you learn that you are HIV positive, however, there is no longer a choice; the mind is sensitized to and colonized by an area of medical knowledge. One's fate is decided in this arena quite apart from one's own life story, which, until the diagnosis, may have remained independent of the health care juggernaut.

What is more, the knowledge that comes to dominate one's life (biomedical knowledge) is itself incomplete and elusive. There are promises and the expected faith in the methods and truths of biomedical orthodoxy, but the message, despite all the "razzamatazz" it occasionally drums up, is sobering. There are many dissenting voices that may trade in the uncertainties surrounding this devastating disease or may contain genuine insights about the delicate balance between disease and the subjective body. Of course, for orthodoxy these voices do trade in uncertainty, but the open-minded also welcome attempts to understand more fully—perhaps through unorthodox, subversive, and resistant discourses—more things in human life and well-being than are dreamt of in a biomedical philosophy (to borrow from Shakespeare's *Hamlet*).

Therefore, uncertainty and vulnerability abound for the HIV/AIDS patient and undermine the cut-and-dried requirements of contemporary evidence-based biomedicine, so we do have to consider broad social trends and educated extrapolations from what we know. The case of HIV/AIDS shows that "illness is no longer a purely biological state—no longer a brute fact of nature—but rather something in part created or interpenetrated by culture" (Morris 1998, 71). This idea holds even though death from AIDS is a hard bottom line on which conceptualization and intervention converge. Death, one might say, is the one certainty of life, even postmodern life.

Yet even the end points are chimeras because biomedical knowledge can deflect our attention from a significant feature of the postmodern conception of medicine. "Illness in the postmodern age is understood as fragmentation, and what we seek from the process of healing is to be made whole" (Morris 1998, 67). This wholeness that AIDS asks the Hippocratic professions to concern themselves with, like so many other topics that I have addressed, is a function of life stories and the ways in which they are constructed, lived, told, and brought to a close.

Values, Consent, and Empowerment

The uncertainties surrounding the clinical profile and natural history of AIDS infect the knowledge that should accompany a positive test result, so testing for HIV does need to be linked to a means of access to counseling. "Through individual counselling, people can be helped to relate the generalities about HIV infection to their own personal situation and can be empowered, through support and the acquisition of life skills, to reduce risk of transmission to or from others in the future" (Pinching 1994, 907).

Psychological responses to HIV/AIDS "profoundly affect people and their relationships and lives, and their consequences are as appalling in the social and economic spheres as they are in the medical (Coxon 1996, 137). Gay communities increasingly provide the support and the scripts for a number of alternative lived realities for people who are HIV positive. "An emerging solidarity, reinforced by the cumulative personal losses, soon led to action to protect each other through prevention programmes, based on peer-based education and influence" (Pinching, Higgs, and Boyd 2000, 5). Here again the medical facts about HIV/AIDS are problematized—affected communities, their structures and stories, and the discourse of the subjugated all bear on the lived reality of a phenomenon that is often regarded as falling squarely within the domain of biomedical knowledge and power.

In HIV/AIDS the hegemony of medical power/knowledge is seriously challenged by a group of patients and potential patients who are used to fighting the establishment on behalf of their lifestyle. The members of this group are, by and large, well educated and pay little regard to conventional hierarchies. They understand that HIV/AIDS is quintessentially a problem in which culture and biology have intersected to define the epidemiological and personal parameters of the disease and its effects. The denizens of Clinicum, when they came into close contact with AIDS and begin to explore the reality that is the lives of sufferers and those at risk, discover that working with individuals within the at-risk subculture is the only way to make progress in understanding and controlling the disease. A genuine partnership between doctors and their patients in which the patients play a full and intelligent part, is a sine qua non of good practice. "AIDS and HIV have caused a major acceleration in the previously gradual shift from an outmoded medical paternalism to a more contemporary model in which patients are empowered to take a central role in determining their own treatment" (Pinching 1994, 911).

Because a positive HIV test has a significant impact on an individual's life, even "tame" medical ethics recognizes that the test itself requires explicit consent. This has led, however, to problems for epidemiologists and the practice of screening at-risk individuals in order to obtain an objective profile of the biomedical parameters of disease. The need for consent implies that the management of those who may be HIV positive demands that medical caregivers show mutuality, information sharing, empowerment, and partnership. These demands have been seriously problematic for some doctors.

For those convinced that we cannot discriminate against HIV/AIDS patients, there began a long conversation, with many twists and turns, as doctors faced the new reality. Even the surgical fraternity eventually recognized that this disorder presented a challenge that could be met only by getting engaged with patients' stories, values, lifestyle choices, and need for participation in their treatment. This realization has made HIV/AIDS a flagship area for responsible twenty-first-century medicine.

Technology in the Context of Sex, Death, and Culture

In many of the countries where HIV/AIDS is most prevalent, there are problems that preclude narrowly biomedical constructions of what is going on in terms of infective agents and allopathic remedies designed to combat the infecting organisms. In the Third World countries where HIV is rampant, the social inequity between men and women and between different sectors of society put effective and proven drugs out of the reach of most affected people (Cochrane 2000). Julie Hamblin, a lawyer writing on this topic, remarks, "For me it was not possible to comprehend the true enormity of the HIV epidemic in the developing world until I visited East Africa. In countries such as Kenya and Uganda, it has pervaded every level of society . . . and it is literally true to say that no family remains untouched" (1994, 35).

The aggravating factors in the Third World are predictable against the background of an informed understanding of the real gains that have been made in the West where affected groups have become educated and empowered in relation to the disease. In sub-Saharan Africa, though, the systematic repression of women and their exclusion from any kind of power over their own life choices has made them helpless victims of what should not be a plague but has reached those proportions. "There is nothing more poignant than talking to an African woman who knows all about HIV . . . but who says: I know my husband has other women but what can I do? If I suggest that he use a condom, he will assume that I must have had other lovers and tell me to leave. There is nowhere else for my children and me to go" (Hamblin 1994, 37–38).

Here stories seen through postmodern, discursively informed eyes hold the key to a clinical phenomenon. But to change these life stories, we need to think carefully about the issues raised at the beginning of this book: when and how do we decide that a society is in need of moral reform? Stemming the tide of HIV/AIDS in the Third World means that certain traditional mores must come under pressure, but how else do we respect Hippocratic values? In this work, biomedicine does not guide us to the required interventions, and it distorts the real issues by recasting them in its own terms. Perhaps in the foreseeable future, we will have drugs to treat AIDS or mitigate its onset, but the patient group concerned does not play the game by the rules of Clinicum and its orthodoxy: evidence-based medicine. AZT, or other drugs like it, need to be tested. Yet here, once again, human stories undermine research protocols.

> Jon has recently learned that his partner Dwayne has been infected with HIV. Dwayne is in a clinical trial of a new drug, XCT, which is supposed to slow the progress of HIV from time of infection to the first clinical manifestations of AIDS and also to attenuate the course of clinical AIDS. The word is going around in the gay community that XCT has a dramatic effect on the disease and that you know if you are on the real thing because XCT produces a strange rancid odor in the urine. Although many of the trialist know this fact, they have not told the doctors. Therefore they can tell who is in the experimental group and, small groups of trialists who are known to each other are even sharing the active drug.

Now, in one sense these individuals are acting irrationally because we need sound clinical trials of new and untried therapies (as outlined in relation to surgery). However, there are ties that bind us together when we face a common threat, and this drug might make the difference between life and death in HIV/AIDS. Unless the representatives of Clinicum understand the human reality out there, then the clinical trial as it actually happens (not as it is planned and statistically structured) will not work. If XCT saves lives, then the affected community may realize that its availability, after trial, is going to be limited by expense and opportunity, which are governed by the same biotech industry that resides over differential insurance cover and other injustices. They are not likely to cooperate with this faction despite its usefulness to them. The proof that everybody should have been treated with XCT is poor consolation for survivors whose lost lovers and friends complied with the biomedical authorities and did not seize the opportunities to share the drug.

What about the doctors? The challenge to the health care professions is manifold but, in part, concerns the myths that define HIV/AIDS. To dispel these myths, we have to work with those who have little in common with us to change society and its stereotypes. AIDS victims have been fired from their jobs, abandoned by health care professionals, and rejected by frightened family and lovers. The near hysteria found in some circles can be offset only by inclusion, the sharing of stories and problems, and a harmony between the people at risk and the clinicians urging education and reform of public, professional, and legal attitudes. Only so can we hope to find research solutions, adequate responses to stigmatization, and a true partnership in addressing this multifaceted problem.

The worldwide problem of AIDS has now (geographically speaking) come back to its beginnings in the Third World, so the debate has shifted yet again. Three major issues have been raised about AIDS in Third World countries. The first is the evident link between legislative and societal discrimination and AIDS. "The three parameters that ethical and compassionate consideration jointly suggest for any proposed AIDS legislation are: (1) it should guarantee strong action against discrimination where this is appropriate, (2) it should promote essential measures to protect public health, and (3) it should free from legislative control aspects of life that it has seemed immoral for society to recognize, in order to bring them within the orbit of health promotion measures" (Almond 1988, 152).

If we want to address the issue of AIDS in Africa, we need to acknowledge that a large subset of African men expect to achieve sexual gratification whether or not the woman concerned is willing or prepared to have intercourse. That women are disempowered and politically repressed, uneducated about the risks of AIDS, and unable to take control over their own sexual activity for societal and micropolitical reasons is directly correlated with the spread of disease. Attending to these problems is to some extent legislative, even though the sex lives of women in that part of the world evince problems that are not amenable to legislation. Almond's "essential measures to protect public health" are inseparable from these stories and remain largely untouched by the tools of biomedicine and the techniques of the clinic.

A narrative orientation can also help us sort out the ethical tangles in drug-related research and the availability of expensive HIV/AIDS drugs in the Third World. Jon and Dwayne vividly illustrate the problem of placebo-controlled trials of anti-AIDS drugs in many Western countries (Mirkin 1995). Third World countries have two advantages (in terms of such research): they have large numbers of patients, and the access to the drugs concerned is often limited to the context of a funded research. Yet should we do this research, given that the trial demands that a number of people will be denied access to potentially effective medication and that the population as a whole may not have access to the drugs even if they prove beneficial? Paternalistic debates by Western ethicists have raged to and fro on the issue (Angell 1997; Lurie and Wolfe 1997; Resnick 1998). Here a realistic story can help us greatly.

> Then Nkami Mbutu spoke: "We must think on this quite carefully. Of course, Caltizech want to do this trial here for their own benefit, and when I talked to Father O'Hara he said they cannot make sure that only some people get the drugs in America where they have their factory. The trial means that only half of our people with bad blood will get the drug, and half will not. So, if this is a good drug, some of us will die and not be given it. But I know that many of our local people already die from this disease. And many die badly because they do not have other things— good water, good food, health checks, and nurses. But I visited my relatives near Dakar, and they have a drug trial happening there. In their town they have a clinic paid for by the drug company. They all use that clinic whether or not they are in the trial—the local elders insisted on that. There, even if people do have the disease and they do not get better, they are more healthy, and they do not die so quickly. But also not so many people are getting sick because they talk to the clinic doctors, and the doctors tell them things about the disease and what causes it. My relatives say that before they had no hope, they would all die from this, mothers and babies most of all, but now they have hope. Think carefully, but, for me, I would have the clinic.

Nkami is absolutely right: people are dying in large numbers in sub-Saharan Africa, and their deaths are made worse because of associated untreated STDs, poor health care when they are sick, fear of infection, lack of knowledge about prevention, and the list goes on. Most of these things are changed merely by being included in a trial whether or not you get the "active treatment." Only the blinders of biomedical science prevent ethicists from seeing this fact, so they focus on the all-or-nothing stand of possibly beneficial full treatment for all or complete neglect quite apart from the general health care measures that are part of the package that comes with the trial.

Even a 50 percent chance of effective medication, when combined with 100 percent access to better health care services, may be manna from heaven for communities where HIV-related diseases are rife and there is no treatment at all for the co-morbid conditions that make it such a potent killer of the underprivileged. By contrast with the ethical arguments emerging from the hegemony of medical science, narratively informed ethical arguments grapple with the reality of the lived human suffering and forget the moral high ground of principles like beneficence and justice. The ethics are found best in the business of trying to understand the predicament of those affected by the disease.

What about the fact that the treatment, once trialed, will not then be available to those whose bodies have demonstrated its effectiveness? Can this be ethical? We can, of course, lament the glaring evidence of double standards in health care throughout the world, but this dichotomy exists in our own communities in the name of abstract principles like liberty and freedom of choice. We should also note that, whereas we feel we ought to protect the "poor natives" who may not have access to high-tech health care, we would balk at placing serious restrictions on those who sell arms to those same countries so that petty wars and political differences cause the death (through war or resulting malnutrition) of thousands. Just where do ethical stances begin and end in this mess? There is global injustice, and it allows differences in health status to be perpetuated by corrupt governments, Western greed, and multinational profiteering and, of course, that ought to be addressed. It is one thing to sound the ethical trumpets from the comfort of an assured health care system where most things can be treated in a well-appointed clinic and quite another to allow the same clarion calls to deprive a tribe or community of a venereal health clinic. Whether or not that Third World setting can afford the drugs that are developed from work in that clinic is, to some extent, irrelevant in view of their clear and present danger. Nevertheless, one might insist that the provision of that clinic, for the purposes of the drug company, also resulted in a lasting gain in expertise and services for a local setting, but that would be a matter for negotiation after one has secured the unqualified good that is being offered to some very needy people.

HIV/AIDS and the Networks of Life

Information, empowerment of the patient, a partnership in health care, all these imply that what is somewhat inadequately called informed consent is important when we are doing HIV tests on individual patients and that we cannot force any person to have an HIV test. However, that partnership, like all such arrangements, is subject to significant strains in certain situations.

One concern is the procedure to be adopted if a health professional suffers a penetrating injury while looking after a person at risk. Many have debated the issues surrounding routine or mandatory testing of surgical patients so that surgeons can be protected from infection (Zuger and Miles 1987; O'Connor 1991), but that policy is unnecessary and ineffective. First, the likelihood of transmission of HIV is slight even when the patient is HIV positive; second, the status of the patient at the time of the injury is not an infallible guide to the risk to the health care worker; third, there are no recorded cases of patients refusing consent to HIV testing under those circumstances; and, finally, it is unwise to base general policies on difficult cases.

The risk to a health care worker from exposure to body fluids from a patient with HIV infection is about 0.4 percent (O'Connor 1991). Thus, most of the time, even if the patient is HIV positive, and there has been a penetrating injury with blood or body fluids, the health care worker has nothing to fear. What is more, there is a window period before antibodies to the disease can be detected (Pinching 1996). Therefore, decisions ought not to be based on the result of an antibody test but on some better indicator of risk of infectivity. Given that the at-risk community is relatively knowledgeable and that patients, by and large, appreciate the attention they get and the concerns of health professionals, the rules about informed consent should hold even in the area of risk exposure in health care settings. Patients who refuse testing are giving a much clearer indication that they are at risk than a test (taken without consent) could ever do. Thus, the importance of an intelligent partnership and an informed and sensitive appreciation of the whole picture comes to the fore yet again.

Doctors and other health care workers who encounter new cases of AIDS need (and generally do develop) an understanding of the patient's journey that earns trust from the individuals and groups concerned. People at risk of AIDS are, potentially, allies in the fight against the disease, but they may feel insecure because of mixed feelings about their sexuality, their lifestyle, and about the reactions of those they love and among whom they need to feel they belong. Thus, patients may well be alienated, so the doctor and other health care professionals have to try to make the problems of HIV/AIDS intelligible and negotiable. The physician's most important assistants in this task are members of the community that HIV/AIDS sufferers will enter if they are diagnosed, and it is within this community's interpersonal bonds that choices about the disease need to be made.

Finding out that one is HIV positive always occurs within a narrative context, and the doctor must try and discover what that is. That story will include important personal relationships in which HIV positivity is relevant in some way or another. The most common problem that arises is whether to tell one's partner, and here the last fifteen years have seen an increasingly clear consensus emerge. "It appears that American homosexuals have recently been striving for more intimate and permanent relationships, or for the establishment of small groups of friends and acquaintances who have sex only with others in the group, so that they can be knowledgeable about the health of their partners" (Deuchar 1984, 614).

At the time when this was fiercely debated, the standard arguments about disclosure concerned the duty of confidentiality to the patient and the consequences of a policy of informing established sexual partners (Gillett 1987). These arguments were inconclusive. To me it seemed clear that the arguments could not be separated from the increasing need for the at-risk community to encourage and foster the development of forms of relationship that would be more caring, fulfilling, and committed. The relevant communities in many countries converged on the same realization and began widely to accept the following approach.

If the patient is in an active sexual relationship with a regular partner, there is an identifiable risk to the partner. To ignore this risk is to deny the presumption that, where they can, doctors will keep other people from harm, whether or not those people are their own patients. But patients are caring participants in dealing with HIV/AIDS, and they have a need for and commitment to their partners' trust and reciprocal commitment. It is inimical to this kind of relationship to deceive or deny partners knowledge directly relevant to their own well-being.

It follows that the doctor who has an HIV-positive patient ought first to counsel the patient about the meaning of that result and discuss its implications for his or her sexual partner. The doctor should then help the patient see that the partner needs to be told.

It is clear that the risk of an uninfected person developing AIDS is not something to which any person would willingly expose any other person for whom they care. To do so would be to act in bad faith—to rely on a certain moral or ethical stance while cynically acting in a way that pays no regard to it. The most important resource that anyone has in dealing with HIV/AIDS is a caring network of relationships or whanau (in the broadest sense of that word). Bad faith of the type shown by patients who try to hold doctors to a duty of confidentiality when their partners are at risk is unsustainable. The deceit involved and the complacency about the fate of someone for whom one is supposed to care destroy the trust and mutual concern on which control of HIV/AIDS and the change in risk behavior has been built. We have therefore converged on a practice of counsel, support, and openness in dealing with HIV infection within settled sexual relationships.

It is worth noting that the honesty that results from taking this stance is likely to produce a more constructive, cooperative, and caring approach on behalf of the doctor, the patient, and those vital others who must share the burden should the patient develop the full manifestations of AIDS. We could say that the patient's story, within the context of a policy of caring and supported disclosure of HIV status, is likely to be very different from that told in an alternative context.

AIDS has taught us, in a way that nothing else could have, that medicine within the limits of biomedicine alone is insufficient to meet the challenge of postmodern disease. It has also taught us that if ethics defers to the hegemony of biomedicine, it is also inadequate for the challenges we face. These are important lessons and reinforce that ethics should be subversive and yet supportive to the world of the clinic. The only way to fill both of those prima facie incompatible roles is to remain in close critical dialogue with medicine but never subordinate to it. This is an important realization in the face of alternative medicine.

CHAPTER NINE

Healthy Bodies, the Medical Panopticon, and Alternative Medicine

> The various forces in the body become milder and more health-giving when they are adjusted to one another. A man is healthiest when these factors are co-ordinated and no particular force dominates. —TRADITION

The unique challenges presented by HIV/AIDS and the empowerment of patients as individuals and a group has forced the profession to broaden its gaze to take in the interface between biology and culture. This is a hard ask because it undermines the dominant discourse of biomedicine and makes the issues of health and illness more complex. Yet at least the move can be accommodated by the establishment in terms of the general relevance of contextual and other factors in management of disease. As regards what is going on in the patient, viewed as a biological organism, medicine can still maintain that it holds the epistemological keys that are required to unlock that puzzle. However, holistic therapists object, arguing that the medical gaze is like a basilisk; it transforms the objects it targets so that they lose their own internal life or spirit and conform to the terms in which medicine constructs them. Holistic medicine argues for the law of the life of the whole organism so that a more subtle appreciation of its delicate inner balance can take precedence over the reduction of that thing to a mechanism, the parts of which function according to the determinations of biomedical science. The former approach aims to work within that inner balance, but the latter aims to override any abnormalities by introducing counter-agents that have their own effects on biological functions (*contraria contrariis curantor*). For a holistic therapist using such agents to cure disease is akin to adding one insult to another.

Orthodoxy and Heresy in Medicine

We can see this conflict writ large in the way the profession has dealt with the surge in public demand for alternative approaches to health and healing. "Physicians have struggled to defeat alternative medicine and to obtain monopoly over the health care of their patients since physicians began systematically organizing in the United States" (Boozang 1998, 185).

Almost as soon as the topic of alternative approaches to health and disease is mooted, the cry from the profession focuses on evidence, conveniently forgetting how much of what passes as good medicine does not itself shape up in those terms. "There cannot be two kinds of medicine—conventional and alternative. There is only medicine that has been adequately tested and medicine that has not, medicine that works and medicine that may or may not work . . . Alternative treatments should be subjected to scientific testing no less rigorous than that required for conventional treatments" (Angell and Kassirer 1998).

I have given numerous examples where the idea that every human illness event can be transparently illuminated by scientific medicine is obviously inadequate to deal with what is happening. Yet this falls far short of opening the door to alternative medicine methods by those who are dissatisfied with medical orthodoxy.

> All therapeutic avenues meet at life's innate healing or destructive processes. So direct study of human healing might serve as a unifying focus, bridging disparate worlds of care—a truly integrated medicine. In recent decades orthodox medicine's successful focus on specific disease interventions has meant relative neglect of self-healing and holism, and from this shadow complementary medicine has emerged with its counterpointing biases. The gap between them is however, narrowing with the emerging view, backed by the study of placebo and psychoneuroimmunology, that to ignore whole person factors is unscientific and less successful. (Reilly 2001)

This tolerant and inclusive attitude, hinted at when I discussed the dissenting voices to the dominant evidence-based model, asks more subtle questions of the healing professions than can be framed by orthodox allopathic medicine. It asks, for instance, whether those many conditions that do not kill nor produce any objectively identifiable disease process but do make for illness and unhappiness are best regarded according to the traditional positivistic model or best regarded as some kind of imbalance of the human organism as a whole in which adjustments toward health are more likely to be required than a heavy-handed attack with a chemical agent that is supposed to counter the ill effects of the disease process (if only they could be biochemically defined).

Orthodox Medicine as a Discursive Regime

To understand why such an open position is hard to get to from here, we need to look a little closer at the culture of subjugation that is biomedicine and the episteme that serves it. We can begin by examining the way that Foucault explored the general relationships between social, political, and economic power and Truth or Knowledge (the capitalization is important).

> In societies like ours, the "political economy" of truth is characterized by five important traits. "Truth" is centered on the form of scientific discourse and the institutions which produce it; it is subject to constant economic and political incitement (the demand for truth, as much for economic production as for political power): it is the object, under diverse forms, of immense diffusion and consumption (circulating through apparatuses of education and information whose extent is relatively broad in the social body, notwithstanding certain strict limitations); it is produced and transmitted under the control, dominant if not exclusive, of a few great political and economic apparatuses (university, army, writing, media); last, it is the issue of a whole political debate and social confrontation ("ideological" struggles). (Foucault 1984, 73)

His thoughts about truth and power can be applied directly to modern medicine, its institutions, its knowledge, and its many alliances.

Medicine clearly locates its truth within scientific discourse.

The entire move toward evidence-based medicine (EBM), laudable as it is, has forced us to recast medical knowledge such that experimental studies designed to isolate single effective interventions (perhaps acting in combination) take on the highest level of credibility and lock in place the allopathic model.

It is incited to further efforts to expand and use that truth from within and without.

The focus on this kind of evidence means that all real knowledge of health and disease becomes constructed in terms of what can be used to devise effective causal interventions that reliably affect the human body in certain ways (regardless of what else is going on). This then becomes the norm for clinical explanation and the end toward which diagnosis is oriented.

It is diffused and consumed in a huge number of different ways.

Medical thinking (and low-level medically influenced advice and "wisdom") can be found everywhere in contemporary Western society—magazines, television, films, and advertising. All these sources are poorly placed to undertake deconstruction or critique—they evince the sound-bite mentality eminently suited to the propagation of the "X is the problem and Y is the answer" approach to health and disease. "Give me the bug and we'll give you the drug" is the style of orthodoxy and the reason why any map of the health care terrain is "dumbed down" into similar terms for the purposes of dissemination.

The knowledge of medicine and its practice is dominated by methodologies that are likely to make money for the big players.

The alliance between major medical and pharmaceutical concerns, the institutions performing medical research, government regulatory bodies setting standards for health care, and the organized profession surely conforms to what Foucault calls a political and economic apparatus, and it reinforces the reductive or positivistic view of health and disease. There is, of course, a good reason for favoring this view: it has led to most major advances in health care that we have seen, particularly in the twentieth century. The other result of these alliances has been the identification of good quality care with the use of the latest and most expensive medical technology and the undermining of clinical acumen in favor of objective indicators necessarily based on the general features of the case rather than a particular clinical synthesis by an experienced physician. This upping of the ante in what counts as good clinical practice drags physicians willy-nilly into the use of the latest technology because reliance on their own, perhaps very experienced, judgment could leave them exposed to medicolegal risk on those occasions when, as is bound to happen at least sometimes, things do not turn out well.

It is a major focus of political and social debate.

Modern medicine is thus part of a discursive regime in which those who live within it and all the multiplicities of their lives are measured and mapped in relation to Clinicum's validated methodologies. Validation is dispensed according to the reductive, mechanistic model of the body as a complex machine rather than the less well-marked and scientifically self-righteous lines followed by holistic practitioners. The voice of medicine, arm in arm with the voice of science and the political weight of the profession, dominates the political and social debate about how much and what type of health care should be provided by any society for its members. This is hotly debated because the quality or otherwise of the health care provided within it has symbolic significance for any caring society, political relevance to the controllers of that society, and a huge economic impact on the resources it controls.

Orthodox Medical Science and Its Frayed Edges

Orthodox medicine, as I have outlined, has tried to follow the Hippocratic model of science and gain its knowledge from a careful and cumulative experience of the phenomena that make up the domain of clinical practice. However, given the intrinsic power that has become attached to academic and institutional medicine, it has become theory bound and paradigm dominated in a highly positivistic mode of scientific practice. The knowledge that is gained as a result of these trends has a tendency to occupy the epistemic high ground and back its assumption of power by appeals to its demonstrated efficacy within the context of the healing ethos (as is evident in an editorial by Angell and Kassirer from the *New England Journal of Medicine*).

In innumerable areas, medicine has succeeded by imposing the rigid and positivist model on those ideas that it accepts as true. Yet it has also ruled deviant ideas that have later proved to be important in understanding a given problem. I have already noted the shift in thinking about cancer toward what looks like a position congenial to limited holism. In the past, if one had classified cancer among the immunological disorders, this would have been clearly wrong, but now that possibility is at the heart of a huge number of research programs investigating cancer etiology. A further example is the theory of gastric ulcer formation. When I graduated from medical school, a multiple choice answer that offered the view that gastric ulceration was a disease involving bacterial infection would be marked *false* with all the assurance of a positivist representation of reality. Now, however, an answer of that type would be marked *true* because we have discovered that an infective process is critical in the development of gastric ulceration. However, one can reply that these changes in perspective have taken place within orthodoxy and therefore, to some extent at least, have vindicated its claim to be a critical and evolving system that relies on scientific understanding and not ideology or power.

Given the value of standards for effective practice, it sometimes seems that the holistic condemnation of reductive medical science opens the city gates to all the "wild things" that howl out in the badlands at the edge of Clinicum, making promises that are unproven and often costly. To those of a reflective bent these facts seem to point not to an "après moi, le deluge" mentality but to the need for renewed Hippocratic and critical openness to clinical experience on both sides of the orthodox-holistic debate. "A more moderate holist view might not suggest the need to eliminate mechanistic analysis, but that organized wholes occur at various levels, so mechanistic explanations must be given at that level. This demonstrates that mechanism and reductionism are different concepts, although almost always confused in holistic medicine" (Saunders 1996, 117).

Saunders later remarks that "biological systems have no vital force or principle but do have properties not predicted or predictable from chemical laws or theory (117). This statement seems profound until one realizes that a higher level mode of functioning engendered by the system as a whole might be just what is meant by "vital force or principle" in holistic writing (unless that writing is explicitly linked to a mystical theory that cannot be given a naturalistic reading). I would extend this type of thinking beyond the accumulation of the type of data traditionally legitimated by the natural sciences such as physiology and pathology to the clinical situation in all its aspects.

Spinal Epidural Empyemas

Over the last year we have managed in our service a number of cases of spinal epidural empyema. In each case, we have done the right and rational thing by extracting infected tissue (or "laudable pus"), culturing it, and devising a drug regime according to the sensitivities and resistances of the cultured organisms. In a significant number of those cases, the patient has not gotten better until we have resorted to old-fashioned antibiotics in old-fashioned doses (despite the laboratory findings). Now, this method is contrary to those in the best practice guidelines, but it works. Until recently, I regarded this result as a curious but inexplicable fact that, as a crusty old clinician, I found strangely satisfying. I have now been informed by one of my research students that microorganisms form "films" in natural situations with emergent properties that do not show up in the reductive context of laboratory cultures and therefore have a profile of responsiveness to antibacterial agents in the clinical situation that may not be reflected by what we learn from the objective and validated methods of biomedical laboratory science.

The Powerful Placebo

I was recently consulted about a patient who had a long-standing and refractory clinical depression. She had tried most of the available antidepressants but had not really had any good relief from her depression until she had been enrolled in a trial of a new drug. Her improvement since starting the new treatment had been dramatic and sustained, much to the relief of her clinical caregivers. She had, however, been in the placebo group in this trial. I was asked what her treating clinicians should tell her.

The Postponed Craniotomy

I was in the operating theater on a Sunday afternoon, about to do a craniotomy for a cerebral aneurysm that had caused a subarachnoid hemorrhage. As I was about to scrub up and start the operation, the anesthetist mentioned that the patient had been responding strangely during anesthetic induction (in fact, this had been true of him throughout the forty-eight hours since his hemorrhage). As the images of my discussions with him and his facial expressions and responses passed before my mind, I became convinced that he would suffer severe cerebral vasospasm and a stroke if I proceeded with the operation and that I should delay it. I said to the OR team that I did not feel right about doing the operation despite all the preparations that had been made. The senior operating theater nurse who was to scrub for the operation said to me, "If you don't feel right about it, you should not go ahead." I pulled myself up with the admonition that I was a good evidence-based practitioner and that this kind of thing was not part of rational clinical conduct, but I eventually bowed to my misgivings and cancelled the operation. Twenty-four hours later, having woken from his anesthetic, he was a different man and went ahead to have his surgery with no complications (which, as far as I know, might have happened anyway).

In each of these cases, we are not merely broadening our medical understanding to include the human element involved in the understanding of suffering. In fact, we enter a domain in which complex, intuitive pattern recognition is able, perhaps, to alert us to an underlying reality about the patient as a subjective body that reductive biomedicine could easily overlook. This means, as the case of the eighty-three-year-old lady who has said good-bye to her loved ones and the case of HIV in the developing world have tended to show, that we need to include varieties of knowledge that are quite conscious of their historical situation and that count as a virtue the detailed and unrepeatable observation of particular episodes. The rigor attached to this kind of knowledge cannot possibly be a result of double-blind controlled trials because its aim is to grasp the wholeness of a specific and perhaps unique problem.

This elusive knowledge arises at the microlevel between individual patient and care team, and at the macrolevel between communities and researchers trying to understand patterns of disease and illness. Experiments cannot be done which cover the whole gamut of factors important in health and disease, although the results of certain experiments may be useful in analyzing these patterns (as the Hippocratics realized). Reflection on the particular case (be it a community or an individual patient case) is indispensable and needs to be informed by critical thinking about biology, pathology, culture, value, and social structure. This kind of inclusive knowledge cannot arise if we insist that all new ideas and their method of investigation must be procedurally sound according to a narrow positivist interpretation of the Hippocratic method. We cannot, however, just throw up our hands and allow anything at all to count as a valid perspective on the problem. The tests we should apply are intrinsic to the values inherent in the health care enterprise. We need researchers to be self-critical, sensitive, caring, systematic, and open to the multiple subjective realities that constitute the situation. To encompass this diverse set of virtues we might need to enlarge our research teams in ways suggested by HIV/AIDS so as to include members conversant with the discourses informing the participants and not just the highly abstract discourse of contemporary medical orthodoxy.

My next task is to explore the ways in which the medical gaze, as restricted by conventional medical science according to the biomedical and statistical model, may prevent us from seeing important features that become evident only to a richer, more tolerant, or more radical epistemology of health and disease.

The Medical Panopticon and Its Unbounded World of Inmates

In a series of works dealing with prisons, madhouses, the clinic, and the intrusion of government into the life and health of citizens, Foucault developed a set of ideas that examine the predicament of the individual in the context of a discursive regime that determines the Truths affecting our lives and well-being. We can draw many of these observations and insights together by discussing "the medical panopticon."

The mechanism of power according to which society controls its members in significant areas of life is rendered visible by an analogy with Bentham's panopticon—a radical form of imprisonment. The panopticon is basically a tower with the function to "reduce in the inmate a state of conscious and permanent visibility that assures the automatic functioning of power" (Foucault 1977, 201). It is constructed as follows:

> at the periphery, an annular building; at the centre, a tower; this tower is pierced with wide windows which open onto the inner side of the ring; the peripheric building is divided into cells, each of which extends the whole width of the building; they have two windows, one on the inside, corresponding to the windows of the tower; the other, on the outside, allows the light to cross the cell from one end to the other. All that is needed, then, is to place a supervisor in a central tower and to shut up in each cell a madman, a patient, a condemned man, a worker or a schoolboy. By the effect of the backlighting, one can observe from the tower, standing out precisely against the light, the small captive shadows in the cells of the periphery. (201)

Unlike the effect of confinement in a dungeon—an exclusion from visibility—in the panopticon every movement is observed. "Visibility is a trap . . . He is seen, but he does not see. He is the object of information, but never the subject of communication" (201). The arrangement of the divisions between the cells separates one inmate from the other and creates isolation, but the inmate is, subjectively at least, always visible to surveillance from the tower.

Similarly, a patient with hypertension has a silent disease until it manifests itself through cardiac failure, bleeding in the urine, a stroke, headaches, or some other indicator. Then, from the moment the diagnosis has been made, the patient is in no doubt that he or she ought to be under medical surveillance because of its "prophylactic power" (Jay 1986, 192). To the extent that one has brought into the myth/reality of the protective power of the medical gaze, the panopticon is therefore immensely reassuring. Its real power, though, is the induction of the supervisory function in the inmate himself. The inmate (or subject of the medical gaze) makes himself into a self-monitoring medical object whose dimensions are measured according to medical classifications and judgments. The result of the medical panopticon is the discipline of bodies so that they reproduce in themselves the normative judgments of clinical biopower at the microlevel. (*Biopower* is the general term used to denote the control of governments over the biological functions of the populace.) The activities of bodies that violate the norms set by clinical discourse are a legitimate focus of concern for the scientific discourse of contemporary medical surveillance. The aim of the unbounded medical panopticon is to get the inmates—patients at large—to impose on the body the disciplines that orthodox medicine demands of them. But how is this done?

Foucault identifies certain modes of productive power which take our disorganized or free-ranging bodies and turn them into docile bodies "that may be subjected, used, transformed, and improved: hierarchical observation; normalizing judgment; and the examination (1984, 180).

Hierarchical observation coerces by means of observation; the gaze that falls on one defines in its own terms certain values and an order to which things ought to conform. One becomes subjectively constrained by that gaze to think of oneself in certain ways and act accordingly (1984, 189). Thus, I ought to observe my blood pressure (or have it observed), and there it sits, waiting to be taken at any moment. In fact, if I do not know what it is, I am already lacking some property that I ought to have. I am complete only when I know my blood pressure, it is normal, and the figures can be made available to those who have power over it (so they can validate the observation and its significance).

Normalizing judgment implicitly imposes a rebuke or penalty for falling short of what one feels to be an adequate standard, and therefore it implicitly teaches me to refer myself to a certain standard, to differentiate my own position vis-à-vis that standard, to measure it, to aspire to conformity, and to avoid straying beyond the frontier of acceptability (1984, 195). Thus, my blood pressure becomes an indicator of the state of my being in relation to something central and significant in my life, and I ought to want to remain within the boundaries set for it and not be excluded from the benefits that are promised by docile behavior.

The examination makes me into "a case . . . the individual as he may be described, judged, measured, compared with others, . . . corrected, classified, normalized" (1984, 203). The case record summarizes me and tells the story of my illness in terms of an alienated gaze whose terms now define my moral status. The morality is that of Clinicum—compliance and responsiveness to the interventions of the physicians. How is my heart? What does my echocardiogram show, my ECG, my blood pressure? How is my diet, my alcohol intake, my lifestyle? I am now a medicalized soul configured by the disciplines of the medical machinery and its corpus of knowledge (177).

These modes of discourse shape subjectivities according to relations of power and create historically situated knowledges about health, disease, and the story of a relation between the person and the medical system. The knowledge is generated by the system, and through correction and discipline I become a docile body understanding myself in the light of the medical gaze. A prominent feature of the genealogy of myself as a docile (medicalized) soul is fear. Fear locks me into the medical discourse as much as the invisible, intangible operation of the power of the medical panopticon, even though it is required only when my guilt leads me to stray near the uncontrolled and frightening borders of the state of being that the laws of Clinicum have ordained for me.

Organized, politicized, legitimated medicine tends to discount other knowledge, including intimate knowledge of one's own body. That knowledge is not of the right quality and therefore distracts one from the truth of one's medical being. This condemnation is felt acutely by midwives and their clients, for instance, but there are other knowledges out there. They interact with Clinicum but necessarily must draw on the resistance of the subjugated to the dominant epistemic mores of medicine. In this mode, they appeal to "local memories," such as abnormal stories of healing and struggles against institutions, that have broken through a seemingly impassable barrier to health. From the hierarchy of Clinicum, though, such knowledge (as all subjugated knowledge) is seen as naive, "located low down in the hierarchy, beneath the required level of cognition or scientificity" (Kelly 1994, 21). This knowledge is not allowed to affect the structure and regime of truth in Clinicum because it has opposed the modes of exclusion, confinement, control, discipline, punishment, docility, and surveillance which operate there.

The outer darkness, where mythical and mystical beasts lurk to prey on unwary patients who have lost their way, is a scary place. The certainties of the panopticon and the protection of its surveillance is on the near side of the boundary, and they discourage adventurous digression from the disciplines one has been taught. If one transgresses, then exclusion, subjectively felt within one's soul, has made one, metaphorically, a leper (Foucault 1967, 7). "Sacred distances" kept the lepers housed on the peripheries of society, their salvation attained by accepting the responsibility for their own exclusion. Their contribution to the "unity" of society was to take individual responsibility for maintaining their abandonment and its legitimacy. This exclusion was not perceived as a method of suppression but as segregation, an action participated in by those who were segregated and those who demanded it of them. Yet one "crosses the boundary" when, as a patient or doctor, one participates in the discourse of unorthodox or heretical medicine.

The images and values attached to lepers validated the discourse of the normal world by making vivid the outer boundary that ensured that the normal could think of themselves as well within the domain of order and reason. The medical world defines that boundary in terms of tradition, effective intervention, and science, all cast in terms that exclude the "follies" and "great unreason" of folk, traditional, and nonbiomedically validated approaches to healing. To say that there is truth beyond the borders which ought to affect what we do within the borders is heresy. A practitioner, an official of Clinicum, who hints that "the leper colony" may offer things of value to those who never need to go there can provoke a very threatening conversation. The discourse of Clinicum portrays itself (to itself and others) as a complete globally sufficient discourse about health and disease. Foucault describes at length how the discursive regime bolsters itself so that the local discourses of the excluded would not challenge the "globalizing discourses with their hierarchy and all their privileges" (1994, 22). Most of these involve power that is productive in that it operates on the subjectivity of those within the ambit of the regime.

The interest of my three stories (Spinal Epidural Empyemas, The Powerful Placebo, and The Postponed Craniotomy) is that in each case the kind of thinking that goes on outside the boundaries of scientific reason needs to be taken seriously and be investigated. These kinds of responses to clinical reality, in which the subjectivities of individuals encourage a microdiscourse and minor knowledge, collectively subvert the dominant discourse. "In the end we are judged, condemned, classified, determined in our undertakings, destined to a certain mode of living or dying, as a function of the true discourses which are the bearers of specific effects of power" (Foucault 1994, 32).

Foucault here draws our attention to the subjective determinations that govern our positioning within or without the realm of the normal as defined by the dominant discourse. These determine our modes of practice and, if one is a patient, one's mode of living and dying. How do they do this? How can people, through their thoughts, determine the modes of living and dying of themselves and others. The unbounded panopticon and its mechanisms of power hold the key.

In the domain of Clinicum we are increasingly under surveillance, and biopower enforces documentation to articulate the incidents of our lives as part of a compendious casebook constructed according to certain norms. (I have discussed some of the beneficial effects of this under the title of clinical governance.) The invisible "gaze" of surveillance through the compilation and collation of information, and subsequent (often computerized) assessments and recordings, are as effective in the monitoring and control of physicians and patients as was the combination of transillumination and the supervisor in the panopticon.

Yet the real trick of the panopticon, as Foucault observed, was the production of truly pervasive surveillance by the self-directed transformed gaze that is the subjectivity of the inmate. The "unbounded panopticon" and the subjectivity it exploits ensures its function as a mechanism of control because, as in the transformation of the asylum from a place of cells and chains to a place of discipline, it takes away the possibility of focusing any articulate resistance. I turn a medicalized gaze on myself as a physician and myself as a patient, and the very possibility of resistance becomes alien or unthinkable.

The medical gaze (conformed so as to meet certain standards) and the case information recorded by it define the case. The discursive functions served by the mechanism of surveillance, judgment, and discipline may not be visible to the person, who is both object and subject in the "unbounded panoptican" because it is so vast in its complexity. The subjective correlate is likely to be that everybody knows they ought to "improve" themselves by taking steps to look after their health, it is just that the dimensions of improvement are dimensions of docility.

Once one has entered Clinicum, the healthy body is already compromised because it is no longer defining and pursuing its own proper function but has become a machine whose function is measured by alien standards. According to these alien standards, the ills that flesh is heir to are not ills that flesh can address or hope to understand because flesh (and its self-knowledge) is now subjugated to the discursive regime of medicine. To espouse another discourse is to rebel, to align oneself with the "lepers" those excluded from rational healthy society. What is more, it is well known that the problems of health in the realm of the excluded are not like those on the right side of the boundary that demarcates the outer darkness. Out there are degenerate minds and bodies that have escaped the order of Clinicum and are dissolute both epistemically and morally. Such bodies pursue their own courses, which deviate from our norms of reason and fall in the way of diverse sources of dysfunction because they have strayed off the path of goodness and right-thinking. That, at least, is the position of the orthodox, but it does not satisfy subversives and skeptics such as myself.

Outside the Walls: Other Systems of Healing

In North America and Europe, large numbers of people are turning to alternative, complementary, and holistic healing systems to find what they cannot find in orthodox medicine (Smith 1983; Pietroni 1992; Monaco and Green 1993). The traditional and alternative healing systems (as I have noted) tend to share that aspect of the Hippocratic belief which holds that health is a harmony in the holistic function of the organism and that disorders arise when this integration and balance is upset. Thus, they see the ailing organism as a system that is failing to deal with a challenge to its proper function. Foucault contrasts the two conceptions as follows.

(a) "illness is . . . a specific entity that can be mapped by the symptoms that manifest it, but that is anterior to them, and to a certain extent independent of them" (Foucault [1954] 1987, 6);

(b) "the illness concerns the overall situation of the individual in the world; instead of being a physiological or psychological essence, the illness is a general reaction of the individual taken in his psychological and physiological totality." ([1954] 1987, 9).

The latter view points toward the postmodern conception of healing as restoring a totality that has been fragmented and tends away from the view that illness is a specific entity that can be attacked by an agent acting within the body but somewhat independently of bodily forces. We can illustrate the contrast in these two general views by comparing orthodox (allopathic) medicine to home-opathy. The biomedical community requires that conventional allopathic med-icines have both demonstrated empirical effectiveness and "theoretical support by deduction from accepted scientific laws" (Saunders 1996, 113). In this way, they become rigorously proved (Ellis et al. 1995). I have already noted that the type of evidence and proof implicitly validated here suits an intervention that has a relatively uniform and measurable causal effect in whatever patient it is applied to, no matter what unique configuration of "internal forces" comprises that patient's inner disharmony. It is clear that any minor adjustments of such disharmony which may not have uniform effects across all individuals with sim-ilar symptoms or manifestations of disease are not going to show up well in such testing.

Hahnemann, the founder of homeopathy, believed that, "no external mal-ady . . . can arise, persist, or even grow worse without some internal cause, with-out the cooperation of the whole organism, which must consequently be in a diseased state" ([1833] 1993, 234). Hahnemann urged physicians to work with "the vital force," which, if prompted to mount the right response, will then "effect complete recovery" of the affected individual (153). Homeopathy is not alone, as is evident from the Hippocratic writings, in seeing the cause of illness as a disturbance of that (inner harmony or ordering principle of life) which pro-duces health. However, this kind of view has corollaries that are problematic for reductive biomedical science and its approved methods.

1. A sensitive characterization of the individual derangement of health must be made.
2. An individual remedy must be devised.
3. The healing systems of the person must be assisted to restore the per-son to health.
4. A successful remedy might illuminate the internal state of the person concerned.
5. A successful treatment course may be the first step on a path of restora-tion to true health.

Taken together, these points are crucial in trying to understand holistic healing systems.

Alternative healing systems do not aim at the disease considered as a classi-fiable entity apart from the unique system of the individual patient who is in a dysfunctional state. This means that the response an alternative healer makes to a presenting complaint is to look at the person who has fallen ill and ask "What is it about you that has led to this imbalance in your vital forces?" This question may suggest a variety of different answers to what looks like the same question. For instance, say that the question concerns migraine headaches. The alternative healer will question the patient (seen as an integrated and situated organism that is producing a certain distressing phenomenon) and ask what combination of forces allows this phenomenon to arise in this person? A conventional physician will ask, "At which point in the characteristic and perfectly general biological process that is a migraine can I intervene to stop the events pursuing their usual course?" The one response is individual and contextual within the function of the whole organism; the other is reductive and looks for a general remedy that does not take account of individual differences (except as they fall under broad types). In that sense, they are "cross-grained": the former—holistic—response is not amenable to the kind of testing that investigates the dimensions of inherently general biological phenomena that are measured in a way designed to "smooth out" or "see through" the individual variations (which are conceptualized as producing statistical "noise").

This problem is completely overlooked by most critics but evident to anyone after considering the philosophy of science as it applies to medicine (see chapter 3). I have already considered some of the points made by Saunders, Boozang, and Angell (who do exactly this), but the arguments can usefully be revisited at this point.

Alternative medicine has often arisen in the semimythical thinking of *outmoded systems of scientific thought* (like vitalism, mesmerism, animism, and botanicals). Saunders and Boozang argue that many of these systems are implausible because they appeal to the type of events and processes that have no established place in contemporary scientific theory (204). But this argument depends on the ideology that our science, as far as it currently goes, is complete enough to allow us to make principled decisions about all clinical phenomena. Discursive regimes do produce this kind of sanguine claim, but in medicine it looks to be very shaky in the face of the many events that have proven it wrong in the past.

There is *no evidence* that most alternative medicine works according to "adequately controlled outcome research" (Boozang 1998, 204). I have noted that holistic approaches to health and disease may be "cross-grained" with respect to orthodox medicine and that therefore they may be bound to fail the kind of evidence-based tests we impose using orthodox medical categories. The migraine problem demonstrates very well how typical clinical interventional trials looking for general effects regard individual variations as statistical noise, whereas case studies in which individual responses and their variations are of profound interest are unlikely to come up with general conclusions apart from a much deeper and more comprehensive understanding of the system as a whole. This point is sometimes expressed by remarking that there are *no widely acknowledged tests* by which alternative medicine can be assessed (Saunders 1996, 112). Here the effects of the discursive regime are striking in that acknowledgment is of a piece with validation, or what Foucault calls the set of rules by which statements are judged and allowed to govern what counts as truth (1984, 54). The regime of science has conditioned us to believe that only biomedical statements have a proper place in our system of thought and that any system of thought that does not structure itself in the same kind of way is to be discarded or relegated to the outer darkness of unreason. Similar arguments are pertinent to the metatheoretical objection to holistic medicine.

There is *no scientific theory* (or rationale, according to Boozang) to support the practices concerned. This metatheoretical complaint undermines the aspirations of most alternative or holistic systems to any scientific status by pointing out that they have no theoretical coherence with the rest of our thinking about the natural order. Yet I have already indicated a number of clinical facts that suggest that our thinking about the world of illness and disease, as sophisticated as it is, is still very "gappy," in that there are holes where the observed findings do not fit neatly into current theory. Kuhn, Feyerabend, and Foucault, among others that I have already discussed, alerted us to the ways in which paradigms normalize thought and dictate what will count as a respectable way of asking questions, doing experiments, and so on. Holistic medicine has a number of techniques and orientations that eschew generalizing in favor of trying to discover the singularity of the suffering human being and thereby including in the understanding of illness the person's context of life and unique responses to the challenges he or she encounters, some of which conceptually escape reductive accounts and simple powerful remedies. It is not to be expected that the patterns and relationships that are posited in such systems would be transparent or even accessible to the biomedical model.

We need, as in the Hippocratic writings, to retain a critical stance toward the explanations we are offered and to use our reason to weigh competing accounts of disease and healing, but we should be aware of the extent to which that stance is affected by biomedical training and what it considers scientific (although in some types of holistic medicine the ideas appealed to sound like complete nonsense). Within each tradition the evidence of systematicity and reflective practice may or may not be found. Where it is found, we need to take note of what is turned up, and where it is not, we ought to insist that something beyond anecdotal impression is essential to any healing system that strives for credibility.

There is a view in alternative systems that *individuals are responsible* for their own health (Saunders 1996, 113). I have already observed that this belief is also part of the medical panopticon and therefore not unique to the dark side. In holistic medicine the emphasis is on treating the person as a whole subjective body internally responsive as a psychosomatic unity to what is done to it. Given this attitude, one might not want to alienate a person from the workings of his or her own body by conceptually rendering aspects of its function out of the reach of that individual. The medical gaze objectifies and alienates the individual so that the key forces operating on the body can be measured and manipulated by experts working according to general specifications, but that is no longer as acceptable as it was in a more paternalistic era. Holistic systems of healing tend to return the knowledge and understanding of the case, as far as it goes, to the person who is the body and has lived through it since birth. The dominant regime regards bodily changes as being outside the possibility of any kind of internal or organic control or influence by the individual. Therefore, the influence of the patient as an integrated being is, perhaps, being constantly underplayed and undermined by the agents of Clinicum who thereby lose a potent source of co-therapeutic endeavor. Of course, this does not mean that the occurrence of disease can be tied to a moral or spiritual failing in the patient or that the patient can serve as a ready sop for absorbing any blame for failure of therapy.

There is *no reason to despair* of reductive medical science: It may find answers for problems in the complex integrated human system without resorting to holism. This is possible, but I have given a number of reasons for believing that it is likely to be severely limited by its own discursive apparatus for measuring and delineating the nature of the case. Therefore, we can say that there is *a reason to think that reductive medical science will not find all the answers* for malfunctions in the complex integrated human system because it is possible that a delicate and holistic balance of competing and complementary factors in the individual may be vitally important in some illnesses. These by their very nature may not be able to be affected by externally imposed remedies but may rather require a responsive working with the patient as a whole being. If anything like this is true, as it might be, it is also true that we understand very little about it and that only a diligent application of the Hippocratic method and the doctrine of harmony will teach us more.

People can be put off effective therapy for their ills. It is sadly true that therapists and patients adopt and persist with inappropriate treatment in the belief that it will work. This, however, is a failure engendered by a poor diagnostician and an opinionated rather than reflective practitioner, and it is aggravated in an oppositional climate of health care in which the exercise of power is pervasive. Thus, the phenomenon, when it occurs, is not a good reason to reject an otherwise plausible method or a whole school of thought to which a practitioner might happen to belong.

The defenders of orthodoxy are quick to mention that bogus remedies, fakery, and charlatanism abound in the areas broadly considered under alternative, holistic, and complementary medicine. But orthodox practitioners have a role in this confused situation in that many of them do treat knowledge about the patient's ills as privileged knowledge that properly belongs to and should be controlled by doctors and the medical system. That is not in the spirit of this book.

When patients are alienated from their own bodies by the discursive regime of medicine and made to think that their own local, intuitive, minor knowledge about their condition is irrelevant, they are not well equipped to sort through the various promises of cure and relief that they are offered (Boozang 1998, 199). However, alongside the rogues, there do seem to be holistic methods and practitioners that are dedicated to ideals that place them well within the Hippocratic tradition. Indeed, the corollaries of the holistic view (diagnosis of the deeper derangement, a remedy directed to the deeper problem, working with the healing systems of the ill person, altering the capacity of the person to deal with illness, and suspicion about superficial remedies) are independently admirable and continuous with some of the best attitudes of that tradition.

We can also concur with a general suspicion of those who hide behind mysticism to defuse any systematic investigation of their claims. Here the clinical stories I have mentioned are highly relevant. The problem of the spinal epidural empyema treatment that confounded our laboratory methods is susceptible to further investigation by biomedicine. There is a perfectly understandable reason why the unique interaction between mixed infections of bacteria and particular patients cannot be dealt with according to tests done on the bacteria that will grow for us outside the body of the patient and in a laboratory. I once published a paper on pyogenic brain abscesses in which the harder we looked, the more contributors to the abscess we found. Thus, the "give me the bug, I'll give you the drug" approach might be a little cocky in the face of clinical reality. It is likely that years of learning to deal with such things without the sophisticated and reductive techniques of the modern microbiological lab have allowed the recognition of patterns based on clinical presentation and anatomical location that correlate directly with the kind of remedy that works (for reasons we do not fully understand). We may find out more about this, although the complex interaction between infecting organisms and the techniques we use to sample, isolate, identify, and test them may keep that knowledge from us.

The puzzle of the powerful placebo was created by the idea that every effective treatment must be a bioactive substance introduced into the patient's body. We now have good reason to believe that this kind of thinking is deeply misleading in medicine in general and does not have the kind of scientific support that it is supposed to have (Kienle and Kiene 1997). The placebo is defined by contrast with the intervention that is theoretically supposed to do all the work in the clinical situation, but, given that we do not always understand the complex situation in which we are intervening, it is evident that we do not always understand what will alter it. Only when we allow the allopathic insistence that all the effective treatments fall within the category of externally identifiable chemical agents are we misled into thinking that the placebo myth is as true as we take it to be. The depressed patient who found relief in the placebo arm of an antidepressant trial is a vivid demonstration of the complexity of treating any psychiatric disorder and the superficiality involved in biologizing such things.

The intuitive cancelling of the aneurysm surgery further supports the suggestion that there may be complex patterns that experienced clinicians notice and respond to but that they cannot name in statements that conform to the norms of medical discourse. It may be that the patient who is prone to cerebral vasospasm exhibits a "look" or "habitus" and that the neurosurgeon picks this up. The dominant discourse of EBM can conceptualize this phenomenon only as an unscientific clinical intuition. Yet my unease about proceeding and my vivid set of images (or premonitions) about what would happen if I did may have reflected exactly the associations that a pattern recognition mode of cognition caused in my brain and therefore may represent a sophisticated distillate of scattered clinical observations. These things are worth noting if only to realize that the discursive regime of biomedicine, with its normalized classifications and recognized phenomena, is not the sole source of truth about health and illness.

I began trying to understand the challenge of holistic, alternative, or complementary medicine and have been led deeper into thinking about medical orthodoxy and its epistemic basis. That inquiry has taken us into strange Foucauldian and postmodern territory. It has emerged that postmodernism and the questioning of the regime of truth that is biomedicine is an iconoclastic and deeply unsettling exercise. However, we are not bereft of guidance in this situation because we have at hand the sound advice Hippocrates gave to his students. The way forward would seem to lie in a careful documentation of cases and outcomes. This practice may become part of the regime of truth that governs medical statements in our society just as biomedicine has. We may end up with audits of clinical management patterns and an independent licensing body, much as we seem to be moving toward. Rather than being captured by the medical panopticon and its regime of truth, it is to be hoped that any such mechanism will examine what is going on to see whether it is being conducted systematically and with due attention to reflective and critical scrutiny within the understanding fundamental to the healing system itself. If they function in the right spirit, such bodies will be attentive to stories of the kind I have mentioned and to the wider orientation toward health and illness that was spurred by HIV/AIDS and sharpened by our need to deal evenhandedly with complementary medicine.

Part III / The Endings of Life

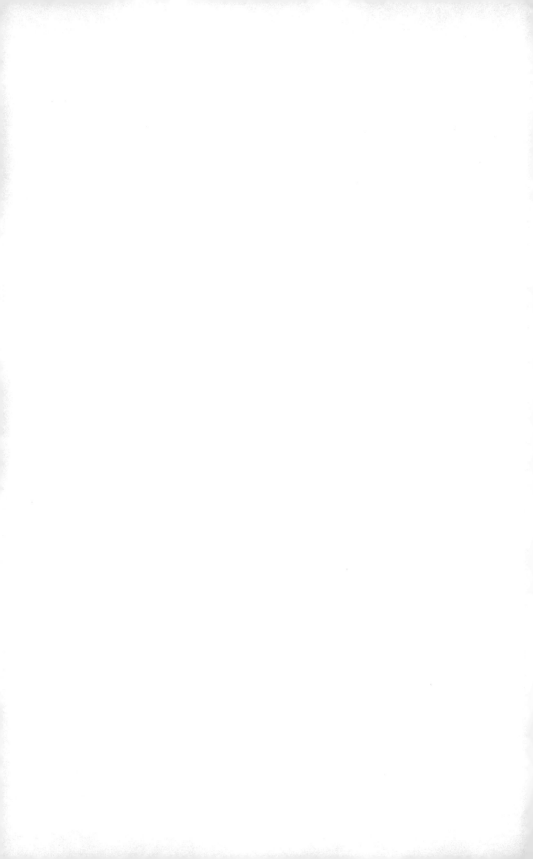

CHAPTER TEN

The Endings of Life

It ought to be generally known that the source of our pleasure, merriment, laughter and amusement, as of our grief, pain, anxiety, and tears, is none other than the brain. It is specially the organ which enables us to think, see and hear, and to distinguish the ugly and the beautiful, the bad and the good, pleasant and unpleasant. —THE SACRED DISEASE, 248

When does a human life end? The answer seems obvious, and most people would say it is when the heart stops beating. But that answer must be wrong. Every day in hospitals throughout the world, patients' hearts stop beating without their dying because cardiac resuscitation means that the person goes on living. Indeed, if the decision to initiate resuscitation were wisely made, that would be the norm, but often it is not. Nevertheless, it is clear that the stopping of the heart is not death, and some other condition—irreversibility or some such—must be added so that we encounter the troublesome questions about cardiorespiratory death and brain death (Youngner, Arnold, and Schapiro 1999).

Two Kinds of Death?

The issue is made vivid by "the Pittsburgh paradox" (arising from the Pittsburgh protocol). "In this protocol, patients are taken to an operating room, where the ventilator is removed and, after a few minutes of asystole . . . the patient is declared dead and the organs are removed" (Youngner, Arnold, and Schapiro 1999, xvi).

Now, as a means of effective donor heart retrieval, this protocol looks suboptimal, but as a means of giving death a robust and intuitive validity, it looks hopeless. Imagine the following conversation.

The mother of a youth shot through the head is informed about her son's eligibility to be an organ donor and asked to agree, given that he, like many students at his college has indicated in writing that this was their wish. The following conversation ensues.

> Mother: Yes, doctor, I think that was what he would want. He was always a generous boy.
>
> Doctor: Well, it's good to be able to honor his wishes in this way.
>
> Mother: But tell me, doc, how are you going to decide he is dead when all those machines are keeping his breathing going and his blood going round and all?
>
> Doctor: Well, ma'am, we will take him to a special OR and take away the artificial supports. His heart will stop, and then we will know he is dead.
>
> Mother: Oh! So you are not going to use his heart for a transplant, then? Funny, he always said he wondered what it would be like to have his heart beating in somebody else; he saw that in the movies, you see.
>
> Doctor: Yes, ma'am, we are going to use his heart.
>
> Mother: How are you going to do that when it is stopped?
>
> Doctor: Well, we can start it up again.
>
> Mother: Now hold on. Run this by me again. You say he's dead because his heart has stopped?
>
> Doctor: Yes.
>
> Mother: And you say you are going to give it to someone else and then start it up again?
>
> Doctor: That's right.
>
> Mother: Well, why don't you start it up in him?

She has a point (so much for the untutored lay public). To answer her, the doctor has to come clean about the real reason why we say that her son is dead— it clearly has nothing to do with the heart or its future function. Just such reflection, throughout the world, favors a brain-death criterion of death as the only philosophically, ethically, and clinically sustainable criterion. But why should we regard irreversible cessation of integrated brain functioning as a suitable criterion for death (rather than, for instance, irreversible cessation of kidney or any other vital function)? What is the link that seems intuitively obvious to us between brain death and the death of a person?

The answer involves intuitions about well-being and personal identity, both of which are grounded in the moral foundations sketched at the outset of this book.

Well-being (Aristotle's eudaemonia) is excellence of human function. Many of us live quite satisfactorily at a somewhat lower level, but nevertheless an adequate level of functioning requires a reasonable standard of health and physical comfort, a mental life that one finds meaningful in some significant way, and a sense of who one is that is commensurate with personal dignity or worth. I have argued that such a life is grounded in a place to stand (captured in the Maori term, *turangawaewae*) and having an individual story to live (closely related to *tino rangatiratanga*). In many countries we recognize that a patient who is of sound mind has the right to refuse any treatment whatsoever according to the values evident in this personal narrative. Thus, if a person finds that ongoing medically maintained life is more of a burden than a blessing, he or she does not have to undergo any treatment to prolong that life just because their doctor so orders. This principle has been implicitly endorsed in the cases of at least two patients with high spinal injuries who have requested that their ventilators be withdrawn, and it relies on the idea (deeply rooted in our philosophical understanding of persons, human lives, and personal identity) that any treatment applied to any person must be commensurate with that person's values and life story. This principle—that any treatment administered should be treatment to which that person would consent if, per impossibile, he or she could—is difficult when the patient is in an irreversible coma of a more or less profound type.

Persons, Identities, Narratives

I have argued that an individual's narrative and life project determine what counts as doing the right thing for that person in a way commensurate with the continuing identity of a person as an individual with a unique and longitudinally integrated mind-life. Locke states the case as follows: "For it being the same consciousness that makes a Man be himself to himself, personal Identity depends on that only . . . For it is by the consciousness it has of its present Thoughts and Actions that it is self to itself now" ([1689] 1975, 336).

For Locke, the mind and its conscious life—or lived narrative—is what makes a person's life the same life at different points in time. We can, in fact, make this vivid with the aid of a well-developed imagination. Imagine that it becomes possible to ensure yourself against a catastrophic brain injury by having a regular total brain information download (TOBID) (like saving up-to-date files on your computer). The relevant medical insurance packages ensure that if you do have such an injury then you lose only the chunk of your life between the download and the accident.

> Two individuals, Jose and Mario, are in an accident. Both have had TOBIDs done before this happened, so although both their brains are hopelessly scrambled, the read-out could be read back in to restore their normal mental functions after the injury. The problem is that the brain care institution doing the read-in is staffed by a worker who has problems with foreign names and therefore reads Mario's mind into Jose's brain and vice versa. Now, who wakes up when Mario's body stirs into consciousness? Whatever we think here, we must note that we are going to encounter a person who has Jose's memory, attitudes, subjective relationships, moral commitments, desires, idiosyncrasies of character, tastes in music, and so on, even though it is Mario's body. Most of us are inclined at this point to waver in our thinking but come down on the side of a body switching having occurred and Mario's body now being inhabited, for all intents and purposes, by Jose and vice versa. If it makes it easier, you could think of them as being identical twins, in which case people certainly would treat Jose as Mario and vice versa.

If we would come to this conclusion about Jose and Mario, then Locke has discerned the intuitions of normal folk. That conclusion is even more compelling in a further thought experiment.

> A young man, Nigel, is admitted to hospital to investigate headaches and epilepsy. He has a CT scan and an MRI scan and is told he has a malignant brain tumor. He is told that with that diagnosis he has a life expectancy of a few months. He is naturally shattered by the news, and the neurosurgeon suggests that he talk to a nurse or the chaplain.
>
> Two days later the neurosurgeon comes back, saying he has very good news. He tells Nigel that they have been working on brain transplants for some years and that he has just learnt about another young man whose motorbike has been mangled under a train. They have managed to keep his brain alive, but the rest of his body is damaged beyond hope. Nigel is told that he can have a brain transplant and will not need to die from his malignant brain tumor after all. Nigel is momentarily overjoyed. However, as the neurosurgeon goes to leave, Nigel suddenly says, "Hold it, who is going to wake up from this operation?

Now you and I know that, on reflection, we do not believe it will be Nigel who wakes up, and, if that is so, Locke receives further support. It seems that most of us do believe that the brain is the seat of the life of the person as a person rather than any other part of the living human body.

It is quite uncontentious that an adequate level of brain function is required both to support conscious life and to keep a cumulative record of any individual's life experiences so that a lived narrative can be inscribed in that person in some relatively durable form. As long as this lived experience can be activated, there seems to be a continuation of the life of the person as a person rather than merely as what Helmut Thielicke calls "the biological remnant of a person" (1970).

When we reflect on this, some prominent themes emerge which I have discussed elsewhere (Gillett 1992, 1999a). They include *personal identity* or a story that is one's own, *conscious awareness* of the world around one, and *intentional action* and interaction with others.

Personal identity is, I have argued, an autobiographical feature whereby an individual constructs a life story for him or herself. This story may not be a particularly original or deliberate affair but has a narrative structure and weaves a life together as an integrated whole. As the individual living *this* life story among *these* people, I am who I am. In our realistic moments we may recognize that the narrative is more often edited than authored. Nevertheless, it remains the sometimes haphazard creation and property of the person whose name it bears. It is open-ended and continually being updated in the light of everything that is happening to one. Therefore (as Aristotle, Kierkegaard, and Jean Paul Sartre, among others, remarked), one's lived autobiography is not finished until one is dead because everything that happens up to that point will ultimately be part of the remembered (perhaps by self and definitely by others) story of the lived life.

Second, *conscious awareness or lived experience* is the person's response to the world and others. Here films such as *My Left Foot* warn us against a certain cognitive (or able-bodied) elitism by reminding us that defects in communication do not, particularly in the context of neurological damage, always indicate a lack of (or deficiency in) conscious awareness. The possibility of a person being a passive observer among other people entails that the position of a moral patient who is reliant on others for the quality of their experiences must be considered when we debate the ethics of end-of-life decisions. We have now got the technology available to detect whether patients are in the awake but incommunicative state that is envisaged here. (The locked-in syndrome is such a state.) Yet I have argued elsewhere that there are philosophical reasons to doubt the Cartesian idea that passive self-contained inner awareness is possible (except where there is a specific interruption of the normal pathways connecting awareness to responsiveness). Human consciousness is an active, interactive, and exploratory function of the whole organism (Gillett 2001).

This brings us to *intentional action and interaction,* by which a person expresses him or herself in relation to others. Intentional action implies conscious purpose because the simple or stimulus-driven responses of lower animals cannot be said to have the same content as superficially similar human acts (Gillett 1999b). An intentional action, as Sartre famously noted (1958, 433), is based on a human perception of how a given situation could be changed in line with the conceptions and interests of the individual concerned. We normally regard a person's life as, in a sense, constituted by the actions they perform along with the attitudes and dispositions those actions reveal. Even where the individual concerned is severely disabled, there can be a quality of interaction that those who know the person can discern and respond to in a complex and nuanced way. Once the possibility of any such action or interaction is irrevocably lost because of severe and widespread brain damage, there is no person as an engaged participant in human discourse. Therefore, except in those cases where some critical injury has interrupted the normal channels of intrapersonal and interpersonal communication (as in locked-in syndrome), the person's life as a person has ended.

I can usefully at this point revisit Aristotle and Locke. Aristotle noted that the human soul is best thought of as a holistic set of functions and capacities realized in the human body through its interaction in rational and social/political (discursive) life. Locke concurs from a post-Cartesian stance in which the mind is seen as something distinct from the body. Dualism aside, we can affirm the close link between brain function and one's integrity as a unique psychological being. The continuity and ongoing activity of the mind (by which the human body is integrated in its function and the person enjoys an ongoing narrative identity, consciousness of his or her surroundings, and the ability to respond to things that happen) seem to underpin the special value of a human life. We could recall Aristotle's *psyche* and refer to these functions as jointly comprising the soul of the person concerned. It would follow that once the functions crucially supporting the soul are destroyed, then the life of the person *as a person* has also been destroyed. If bodily life as a biological remnant of a fully human life is then continued, it does not have the same significance as the life of a person. This philosophical conclusion has profound practical implications.

The RUB: The Worst Possible End to the Story

Difficult ethical issues arise when a human life is under mortal threat. How should we decide about withholding or withdrawing lifesaving treatment from a patient when a human life is at stake. The patient has usually been admitted relatively acutely, having suffered a medical catastrophe so that rescue treatment or a decision about cardiopulmonary resuscitation (CPR) is required. At this point we often think of only the simple alternatives—life and death—but there is another significant category: survival in an unacceptably bad state for the patient concerned. There is, in a word, the RUB (an acronym for the risk of unacceptable badness). The RUB is drawn from a soliloquy during which Shakespeare's Hamlet muses, "To sleep, perchance to dream, Aye, there's the rub."

He is contemplating suicide, having been told by a ghost (purporting to be the ghost of his father, the recently deceased king of Denmark) that his uncle (who has since married his mother) murdered his father. Should he take revenge on the basis of this possibly suspect information or just exit? If he acts on demonic information and commits a mortal sin, he will be damned, but if he fails to avenge his father, he cannot live with himself. In this quandary (contributed to, according to some commentators, by a Freudian Oedipal conflict) he thinks about suicide and the release of eternal sleep. But he is arrested by the possibility that in death, as in sleep, one dreams. The prospect of spending eternity dead and, therefore, impotent but wracked with the moral torments that have provoked his suicidal thoughts is, to him, an unacceptably bad prospect. He recognizes that his desperate situation has posed a risk of his falling into this unacceptably bad state at his own hands. "Aye, there's the RUB."

Shakespeare's Hamlet faces the RUB at a morally challenging point in his life story, and doctors face the problem time and again if they work in rescue medicine. Patients and relatives often have to weigh a probabilistic chance of surviving a serious catastrophe if rescue treatment is begun. We speak of a small chance of life on the one hand and a black hole—death—on the other, and, faced with this stark choice, we often hear "Well, Doc, go for it. After all, any chance is better than none." But is that so? The person, if saved, may be left in an unacceptably bad state. The RUB expresses the probability of survival in such an unacceptable state of "living."

For instance, a patient with a severe brain injury may have a 5 percent chance of survival but, given brain scans and other evidence, only a 10 percent chance of an acceptable life and a 90 percent chance of an unacceptably bad survival. The RUB acknowledges the small chance of survival but then says, "The reality is, that if he does survive, there is a nine to one chance that he will not thank us for having saved his life." In these terms, the wager is sobering. It is hard to imagine a telling analogy, but let me try.

You are standing in front of a pair of doors. You are told that if you choose the left door, you will die. If you choose the right door, you will immediately be tipped into one of ten chutes. Nine of these will leave you demented, bedridden, with tubes in your nose and veins and bladder, and unable to do anything for yourself, and you could remain this way indefinitely. One chute will allow you to recover to something like your normal self. Which door do you choose: right or left?

This is a stark and taxing choice, and it is very hard to make, but one hopes that the person making it on one's behalf has a clear idea of what one would feel about it. In fact, the proper role of relatives or other surrogate decision makers is not widely appreciated among doctors. In most jurisdictions, the relatives have some say, whether binding or not, about the treatment given to an incompetent patient suffering a medical catastrophe. Yet those making the decision ought to try and do what the person at risk would have wanted to happen to him or her and not what the relatives or anybody else think should happen. This applies as much to medical staff (and the whole clinical team) as to relatives. The role of anybody making such a decision is to try and do what would be of substantial benefit to the person concerned where that is best defined as an outcome that now or in the future the patient would consider worthwhile.

The role of the relatives, in ethical terms, is therefore solely to inform the decision makers of what the person is like and what they think he or she would have wanted. This information allows the caregiving team to form their own opinion of what is best to do, considering the clinical realities and their own experience. That approach avoids potential conflicts of interest (perhaps over property or perhaps for some other reason) and emotional factors that may confound the decision. The ethical responsibility of the health care team is to make the best decision in light of what the patient would have wanted, acknowledging that there is uncertainty both about the clinical course and what the patient would actually want if, per impossibile, he or she could be consulted. The medical uncertainty about the unfolding clinical reality in an acute care situation is an important part of these scenarios.

As a profession, we are bad at admitting uncertainty, fearing that patients will lose confidence in us if we do so. There is, however, little cause for that worry and much anecdotal evidence to support the opposite view. If one is uncertain, one should say so, because that initial openness is important in acute care as well as emergency or rescue medicine where a period of intervention may be required to gather the information required for a firm prognosis. Expressing that uncertainty explains why one might not want to rush into a binding decision about future therapy, and it also sets up the expectation that the relatives will be involved in ongoing discussion at critical points in the clinical course.

The worry about patient confidence relates to the further widespread and rationally unsustainable belief among doctors that beginning treatment and then stopping it is worse than not beginning it at all. A moment of reflection clarifies the issue: the need for the best information—for instance, about the severity of the initial insult and about its response to treatment—implies that a trial of treatment rather than absolute withholding is the correct way to go. It is important that clear signals are given that treatment is being trialed and that the patient's response is an important indicator of how long the treatment should continue. If the uncertainties of acute care are acknowledged, and the idea of a trial of treatment is communicated, then withdrawing treatment that has been intense and vigorous is not seen as a "bolt from the blue" (signaling to the uninformed an inexplicable change in clinical management). People are generally good at coping with this kind of thing if they know what is going on. Relatives who understand the rationale for a trial of treatment are aware that the withdrawal of that possibly lifesaving treatment is an issue to be revisited once its likely effect has been gauged and that it is not part of a clandestine medical process from which they are excluded. In this context, the RUB can be realistically considered by all parties.

The RUB cuts out the simplistic "two options" approach to life-and-death situations and lets everybody see that the chance of survival might be bought only at the cost of a very high risk of an unacceptably bad outcome. Anybody with the best interests of the patient at heart then takes stock and faces their responsibility to do what the patient would want if he or she were able to choose. By questioning relatives and friends facing this uncertainty, the team can try to discover the values and interests that the patient had before the catastrophe that put his or her life in danger and show their respect for the more or less integrated story that is their patient's life. Taking this approach into a rescue situation obviates many problems in clinical and emergency care. Even if there is not an explicit advanced directive, there is usually enough evidence to form some judgment about the fittingness of certain possible endings to that story. In an entirely analogous way we can, in a discussion of CPR with the patient him or herself, convey the reality captured by the RUB, and when we do that, the "any chance is better than none" line becomes much less attractive than it seems at first blush. Paying attention to the RUB entails that life-and-death decisions in critical and other situations are seen for what they truly are in that the two alternatives, life (to be valued positively) and death (to be valued negatively) are joined by the third alternative: *life to be valued negatively.* Putting the third alternative into the moral balance along with the other two radically changes that balance.

The RUB may not be explicitly used with patients and relatives, but it should inform the ethical advice given by clinicians (and, where appropriate, clinical ethicists) dealing with the life-and-death decisions that are all too common in clinical practice. It does not make such decision making easier and may even make it harder, but it does make it more responsive to the hopes and fears of any person faced with the mortal perils that wait behind a hospital door. As a result, it becomes more likely that what we decide on that person's behalf at the threshold of life is in keeping with what that person would have written into the story.

Story's End and Its Look-alikes: PVS and Locked-in Syndrome

At this point it is useful to notice the convergence between the view that I have suggested and Wittgenstein's thoughts about mind and consciousness. Wittgenstein constantly debunks the idea that consciousness and thought are anything less than active, responsive, and engaged modes of interaction with the environment around us. In this respect, his views are entirely convergent with the phenomenological tradition according to which consciousness is essentially intentional or world involving (Gillett and McMillan 2001). The implication is that the holistic and many-faceted reactions and responses that go to make up my many experiences of being *conscious of* a given thing or person are exactly the kinds of thing that constitute and are not just evidence for consciousness per se (or my consciousness as a person). In other words, the relevant patterns of behavior and reactivity that we are used to recognizing in others (but may be bad at describing in any convincing way) jointly comprise what we call consciousness. They normally strike us as a whole or we intuitively get the picture rather than having to infer consciousness from a list of features that we can individually check off. (Though a checklist—such as the Glasgow Coma Scale—may be an invaluable clinical tool in measuring levels of consciousness.)

This holistic sense of the consciousness or presence of another person with whom we are in contact shows itself in many ways. For instance, I might say, "He strikes me as being shy" or "It seems that he has a romantic interest in her." If I were a woman and were asked to justify my statement, I would say, "woman's intuition," but as a man I am forced to say something like "multiple subliminal cues" or, if less articulate, I might say, "I bet I'm right." In this type of case, we pick up on features of our environment that we have been learning to "read" since we were a few hours old. It is therefore not surprising that they are as little susceptible to justification or supportive descriptive evidence as statements like "That is red" or "I smell milk"; these things we know but not by a process of inference and reason. The ability to detect such things is, in one sense, inscribed in us by experience and not usually learned by conscious effort. They ground what I have called "Wittgenstein's startling claim"—"consciousness is as clear in his face and behaviour as it is in my own case" (1967, 221). As we think about this and how good we are at picking up myriad things that we just recognize as we get older and more savvy, this claim looks more and more plausible—consciousness may be the kind of thing we can *just see*.

The implications for the patient in a persistent vegetative state (PVS) are clear but, I think, can do with some articulation in the context of the present discussion. In PVS the higher levels of the brain have been devastated, usually by a combination of shearing stress injury to neurons and global cerebral anoxia. Both of these selectively damage the higher brain—the cortical system and its ramified connectedness within itself and to lower brain centers and pathways. The result is that there are no longer enough informational "megabytes" to do the work required for conscious experience. If consciousness genuinely involves a ramified set of cognitive operations on data gathered from the environment and if these make use of the extensive processing capacity that the human brain affords, then consciousness does not reside in a single locus of activation in the brain but in the holistic functioning of widespread and articulated loci of information processing. This includes selective attention and directedness toward the objects, conceptualized experiences, and feelings that make up my conscious mental life. The richness of that activity entails that processing carried out in relatively primitive centers such as the brainstem or isolated subcortical areas does not even get close to conscious activity in the subject concerned. We can therefore say that a patient in PVS no longer has a conscious mind of the type essential to the human psyche; there is insufficient and insufficiently integrated activity in the brain to support those functions we call "mental" or "conscious" in the being concerned. The person is not *conscious* because he or she is not in that complex state that comprises the many acts of being *conscious of* the things that go on around him or her.

We can contrast this with the locked-in syndrome, a problem case for clinicians and, as it turns out, for our normal epistemic practices in relation to the mind (or the human *psyche*). In locked-in syndrome, patients are conscious but cannot signal it by any responses or activity because not only have they lost the ability to voluntarily direct any of their bodily activities (except, in most cases, the ability to move the eyes up and down) but also the cortical areas of the brain are disconnected from their normal bodily manifestations. Patients may also have lost some of the sensory inputs to their brains. This state therefore removes all the normal bodily cues that go with widespread higher brain activity and makes the person inaccessible to others unless those others realize the predicament and use some ingenious system (such as yes-no eye movements) to open up lines of communication. If communication is established, then others can discern that the patient is conscious of what is going on. This is exactly as a Wittgensteinian account says it should be. To clarify the point, we can ask: If consciousness is essentially a matter of responsiveness, how can there be consciousness in *coma vigilante* or locked-in syndrome?

This paradox is resolved when we notice that Wittgenstein establishes the meaning of a term through its use in a sufficient range of typical or paradigmatic cases. Where the normal conditions underlying that practice do not hold, our normal criteria may not work. Thus, if I normally judge that something is a cat (and therefore an animal) on the basis of its being a warm, furry, purry creature that looks like a cat, then I will make mistakes in a world where robocats (who are also warm, furry, and purry) abound. In the same way, if consciousness is typically recognized on the basis of an intact CNS, then certain kinds of damage to the CNS will preclude our normal practice. This does not undermine the claim that a state of responsiveness and so on is actually what we are talking about when we talk about consciousness, it just implies that there are clinical conditions in which that state is unrecognizable to everybody but the subject concerned. In the locked-in case, the cognitive capacities of the individual are fully developed, but the connection between those capacities and the integrated functioning of the body is disturbed: connecting lines are cut even though the internal hard drive is more or less intact. Therefore, as in other cases such as profound cerebral palsy, the cognitive capacity of the person may be completely misjudged because it is not manifest to us.

When we understand the problem, we can see exactly how it comes about that the experience of consciousness is, in some sense, still present whereas the manifestations are grossly altered. The person is still interacting with the world but it is all one way and therefore he or she cannot show it. Our ability to recognize consciousness and the "presence" to us of other people depends on their being manifest to us, and therefore we make a mistake. On the basis of natural history (a knowledge of the importance of the brain and the integrity of the nervous system for conscious life to be present and noticed), we would conclude that the physiological situation in locked-in syndrome is the kind of state that would defeat our epistemic capacities even though they are normally quite sufficient to detect the presence of consciousness.

Notice that the same strategy defeats any attempt to argue for an abiding worry that often affects the care of PVS patients. *The abiding worry* is that there is enduring consciousness in PVS patients but that it is not communicated to "us outside." Here, however, the biology leads us to the opposite conclusion to that which is forced on us in locked-in syndrome. In patients with PVS, the *capacity to be conscious* has been destroyed. In that sense, the PVS case is the exact reverse of locked-in syndrome: the cognitive or experiential core of consciousness is gone in PVS even though some fragmentary vestiges of what would ordinarily be manifestations of consciousness remain as an expression of activity in other parts of the brain.

In summary, we can conclude that the kind of information-processing activity needed for consciousness requires a high order of interconnectedness and complexity in the nervous system. Where the system has been seriously damaged and is unlikely to be able to sustain integrated conceptual activity then, on any broadly Aristotelian account, we can be reassured that the psyche (or soul) of the person has been destroyed. Thus, it seems that we can, by careful argumentation, establish the factual basis on which our ethical thinking about PVS and other brain-injured states can be firmly grounded.

1. Consciousness (simpliciter) is a complex of cognitive abilities that are severally captured in ascriptions of the form "A is conscious of X."
2. In the normal case these abilities are manifest.
3. Therefore, generally we can tell that someone is conscious.
4. In odd cases, such as locked-in syndrome, we cannot tell because of the abnormality involved in the case.
5. PVS is not such a case; here the equipment needed for consciousness has been destroyed.
6. The abiding worry that a PVS patient may be conscious "in there" is based on a mistake.

Ending the Narrative in a Fitting Way

The person in PVS has stopped telling the story of his or her life or even experiencing it as a lived life. It therefore remains for those of us who know and love that person to try to ensure that the life story is ended in a way that is fitting, but medical ethics and medical law have to combine forces to make that possible.

The ethical issues surrounding PVS came to the fore in the case of Tony Bland, the young man injured in the Hillsborough stadium disaster. His plight was considered in *Airedale NHS Trust v. Bland,* and the judges concerned felt that the issue should be resolved by respecting the hypothetical wishes of Tony Bland himself, thus implicitly endorsing the view that his death ought to fit the whole context of his life. They debated the removal of the gastric feeding tube keeping him alive, and their opinion on the subject echoes similar reasoning as was expressed in the United States cases of Brophy and Quinlan (Schrode 1995). The judges remarked that

> if Anthony Bland were to be momentarily restored to consciousness with full knowledge that he would shortly revert to his PVS, and if he were to instruct those caring for him that he no longer wanted artificially to be kept alive, the doctors and nurses would be obliged to respect his wishes . . . The horror of his situation is such that few would not think it perfectly reasonable for him to decide that, as he has already lost all sense and consciousness, he would prefer to die . . . Anthony Bland is an individual human being and the principle of self-determination says he should be allowed to choose for himself and that, if he is unable to express his choice, we should try our honest best to do what we think he would have chosen. (Hoffman L.J. [Airedale NHS Trust v. Bland (1993)])

In such cases, some choice must be made whether to continue treatment or discontinue it, and we should ask, "Why would a PVS patient choose a lifetime of unconsciousness and futile medical treatment?" If, in asking this question, we attend to the patient's life and attitudes, then we can do our best to make the decision that the patient would have made had that been possible. In fact, I would go further and argue that, because it is a basic feature of the life of any person that he or she should live and experience his or her own life story, it is not just futile to keep an irreversibly comatose body alive in PVS but it does that person a certain kind of violence.

A similar line of reasoning led a New Zealand court to decide that the termination of an Auckland patient's life would not be unlawful (Auckland Area Health Board v. Attorney General [1993]). Mr. L, a man of fifty-nine years, had been totally paralyzed by Guillain-Barré syndrome (which strips away the coverings of the nerves), so he was in the locked-in syndrome. The unanimous opinion of all the specialists who saw him was that there was no hope of him recovering. He had expressed informally that he did not ever want to be left in such a state, and his wife supported the medical team in their request to terminate his ventilator treatment. The court ruled that it would not be unlawful for the medical team in charge of Mr. L to terminate his life support, and, that having been done, he died within thirty minutes (Gillett, Goddard, and Webb 1995). Here again the decision was made in accordance with the principle that his wishes would prevail because the court determined that Mr. L would not want his life to be indefinitely sustained in the ventilator dependent, locked-in state that had befallen him.

Two recent cases, one from Ireland and one from New Zealand, have confirmed the applicability in law of these general ethical considerations in end-of-life decisions.

The Irish case concerned a woman aged forty-three who had been severely brain injured at the age of twenty-two during a gynecological operation. She was, at the time of the judgment,

> spastic, her jaws were clenched, she could not swallow, she was incontinent and bedridden . . . For 20 years she received nutrition and hydration through a naso-gastric tube. This caused her some distress and she pulled it out on many occasions . . . [She] was unable to speak and attempts by a speech therapist to establish some form of communication proved unsuccessful. [She] appeared . . . able to recognise members of her nursing staff, and reacted to strangers by showing distress. She

could follow people with her eyes and reacted to noise, although this appeared to be mostly by way of reflex action. (Re a Ward of Court [1995], 401–2)

The high court, per Lynch J, consented to the withdrawal of artificial nutrition and hydration and this decision was upheld by the Irish Supreme Court. The main points of the judgment were:

1. the ward's best interests should prevail over other considerations,
2. the court exercised a parens patriae jurisdiction to ensure that those interests were protected,
3. the right to life includes a right to a dignified death,
4. the provision of nourishment through a gastric tube was intrusive,
5. the right to self-determination means that a competent adult has the right to refuse any medical treatment whatsoever,
6. this right should not be denied a person who does not have the mental capacity to exercise it, and
7. in this case, the ward should be allowed to die a natural death.

The reasoning of the judgment is made clear by these seven points, and the obvious links to the Bland case are noted in the text of the judgment. It is striking that the right to life is, in this case, linked to the right to a dignified death in keeping with that life. Absent this connection, we run the risk of employing life-prolonging treatments without any ethical or juridical constraint on their proper use. Here that is done by invoking a "right to a dignified death," but it can also be done by invoking the idea of substantial benefit (as I have defined it) or a sense of what is fitting in the whole context of the person's life story.

The New Zealand case, concerning sixty-nine-year-old Mr. G, was heard in the high court in Dunedin on 6 December 1996 (Re G [1996]). Mr. G had suffered severe brain injury in a road accident some sixteen months previously and was in an almost identical condition to the Irish ward of court. "He is totally immobile, is unable to talk or otherwise communicate in any meaningful way and is incontinent of urine and faeces. His CT scans and EEG show severe brain damage. Every effort has been made to rehabilitate him but to no avail. He has remained in the same state and there is no prospect of recovery. He is kept alive by food and fluids through a gastrostomy tube and is provided with all necessary and appropriate medical and nursing care" (Judgment of Fraser J [Re G (1996)], p. 2).

In this case, the judge also consented to the removal of gastric food and fluid and in coming to that judgment took note of the Mr. L case, the Bland case, and the Irish case already described. He identified the following important considerations with respect to Mr. G:

1. Mr. G's injuries and his present condition,
2. specialist opinions that artificial feeding and fluid be withdrawn,
3. the fact that the prospect of meaningful recovery was "virtually nil,"
4. the ethics committee's unanimous decision that they had no objection to withdrawal of treatment,
5. the application for withdrawal by Mr. G's family,
6. the evidence that Mr. G's wishes if they could be ascertained would be to have treatment withdrawn,
7. the fact that withdrawal of treatment would not cause pain and suffering.

On each of these points the judge took detailed expert evidence before he ruled that consent should be given for treatment to be withdrawn and measures should be used which would allow Mr. G "to end his life and die peacefully with the greatest dignity and the least distress" (17).

Once we accept that life need not be preserved at all costs or, in other words, that there is a link between the right to life and the right to a dignified death, we can acknowledge that there are conditions in which continued life is an intolerable burden. It then becomes possible to decide on somebody's behalf that that person would regard his or her present existence in that way. The concept of the RUB (the risk of unacceptable badness) suggests that a person facing this risk ought to be reassured that if a state he or she would regard as unacceptably bad eventuated, then health care professionals would not keep him or her alive by intrusive medical means. This I believe to have been the situation in the case of Mr. L. He had indicated that a state such as the one into which he was tragically plunged was unacceptably bad in his eyes. If that is true, then we can no longer presume that we have consent to treat and must withdraw life-prolonging treatment if we wish to respect the dignity and integrity of the patient.

I can now move on to the even more tricky problems that arise when patients are in limbo—they are at the end of their lives hovering at the borderline between life and death.

CHAPTER ELEVEN

Ethics in Limbo

> When a man is attacked by a disease more powerful than the instruments of
> medicine, it must not be expected that medicine should prove victorious.
>
> —SCIENCE OF MEDICINE

The Hippocratics clearly recognized their limitations but also their need to learn
as much as they could, even where a disease was too powerful for them to defeat.
I have used the Hippocratic approach (interpreted in the light of virtue ethics
and a sense of the patient's narrative) to explore decisions at the end of a person's life, but other distinct issues arise in the "limbo zone" of an intensive care
unit (ICU) where patients are struggling with diseases that threaten to over-
whelm them. Such a person cannot take an empowered part in clinical decision
making, but, as I have argued in the case of PVS, considerations of narrative and
the patient's values require us to do some hard thinking.

What we should do in ICU situations about research, transplant decisions,
and treatment alternatives can be deduced from a few simple premises.

1. Each person ought to be treated in a way commensurate with his or her
    own life story and its values.
2. Medicine can do only those things that have a realistic chance of bring-
    ing about a substantial benefit to patients.
3. The clinical team has the most complete information about prognosis,
    modes of treatment, and the current clinical needs of the patient.

4. There is always uncertainty.
5. In a case of uncertainty, a person should be treated in a way most likely to conform to his or her wishes.
6. Where nothing is known about the patient's wishes, a person ought to be treated in ways that correspond to the wishes of a reasonable person.

If we are armed with these premises, issues in the limbo zone become quite tractable.

ICU Research Ethics

In intensive care, there are standard practices that, as is the case throughout medicine, outstrip the best evidence for their efficacy in the conditions they are used for (Moore et al., in press). ICU specialists are activists (and therefore, in one important respect, like surgeons). ICU requires rapid definitive intervention, often under extreme time pressure and despite considerable uncertainties about the clinical situation. Therefore, it is not surprising that many of our treatments, as in surgery, are based on current theories about the human body and its workings. In ICU we have near-total control over what goes on in the body, we have drugs to manipulate bodily physiology, we regulate breathing patterns, and so on. We are not working by guesswork any more than in any other complex area of science, but the complexities of holistic human function can sometimes confound the "knowledge" that our theories endorse (as I have argued in the case of alternative healing methods).

Two examples help to make the point.

It is reasonable to believe that because blood carries oxygen and nutrients around the body and nature has designed the human blood system to work with a certain hemoglobin (Hb) level then maintaining a level close to that would provide optimal conditions for healing and recovery from major trauma or illness. Not so. An important recent study found that patients maintained at a hemoglobin level of 10–12 g/l (close to the normal values of 12–18 g/l) did worse than those who were transfused only when they dropped below 7g/l (Hebert et al. 1999).

It is plausible that patients who have cardiac arrhythmias after heart attacks are at greater risk of death than others and therefore that antiarrythmic drugs would mitigate this risk. Indeed, it seems almost unethical not to give such drugs to patients after heart attacks. However, a PRCCT (prospective randomized controlled clinical trial) of antiarrythmics against placebos showed an increased death rate in the actively treated group. (Ruskin 1989)

In each of these cases, we see that plausible theories about the human body and how it works can mislead us about whether this or that intervention is beneficial. Thus, there is a real need in ICU care (as there is in surgery) to do the trials that will show us what should be done in a given clinical situation.

Yet this immediately provokes a set of questions about the need for informed consent to medical research. I discuss this in the light of the premises above, which ground a number of substantial conclusions about research on those who cannot give consent. In fact, those conclusions are predictable from the discussion of advances in surgery, the need for PRDBPCCTs in that area of medicine, and the interests of patients.

First, any person making choices about treatment should opt for the treatment that stands the best chance of returning him or her to health. There may, however, be specific reasons why some particular intervention is not acceptable to a person; for instance, a Jehovah's Witness patient may, on the strength of the sect's idiosyncratic interpretation of the Old Testament, refuse a blood transfusion. We could imagine a person with extreme racist views not wanting an organ transplant from someone of a different race—a decision that might be abandoned when the patient is in extremis.

Second, it is rational for patients to accept the best available treatment according to the current state of knowledge at the time of their illness and what contemporary clinical care, particularly in academic hospitals, recognizes as the prevailing standard of treatment. It is quite possible, however, that an ideally informed clinician would be in a state of equipoise between the currently accepted standard treatment and a suggested modification or innovation. In such a case, the doctor does not know whether the treatment proposed for a given patient at a given time *is* the best thing to do. Therefore, patients have no more (rationally grounded) interest in any particular one of a range of possible treatments than any other of the possibilities on offer. In fact, patients, considering that they may require further treatment at a later date, have a definite interest in their doctors getting to know as much as possible about their conditions and making well-considered judgments about their management as patients undergo ICU treatment. This is most likely to happen in the context of a well-designed scientific trial.

A treatment in ICU is trialed only if equipoise exists as to whether it or an alternative treatment is actually more beneficial. It follows, therefore, that it is a matter of ethical indifference, objectively speaking, which of the two arms of a clinical trial (the *treatment arm*—where something new is tried, or the *control arm*—where standard treatment is used) any given patient is assigned to. For this reason, it is rational, on the grounds of self-interest, for an ICU patient to be enrolled in a trial of treatment where significant uncertainty exists about how he best ought to be treated.

Third, it would be in accordance with self-interest, more broadly conceived, for people to want to contribute to medical knowledge in conditions of uncertainty. This is almost self-evident, and the justification is to gain more complete knowledge about the patient and his problem—but there is an added factor: the benefit to a patient of being cared for by a medical system in which active clinical research is going on and clinical knowledge is being extended. Indeed, given that there is a certain amount of community feeling and parochialism in all of us, we should all want for the members of our community to benefit from lessons learnt when misfortune befalls anyone, given that gaining that knowledge will not increase any of the known risks of clinical treatment. In retrospect, of course, it may turn out that patients enrolled in one or other arm of a study (sometimes the opposite one to that intuitively expected) have been disadvantaged by the clinical trial, but that outcome cannot be known at the time of enrollment, and the dangers continue to exist until the relevant facts are discovered. Therefore, we must conclude that clinical research trials of treatment in ICU exposes no patient to any extra risk over and above those that exist for them by virtue of their eligibility for the trial and that the cessation of that research means that they and their fellow citizens will probably be exposed to unnecessary risks in the future.

Fourth, it is reasonable to assume that every person has a modicum of altruism, however limited in scope, and that altruism should be encouraged by anyone interested in ethics. This attitude is rational for the following reasons.

1. Most people are members of a community and have a positive interest in the well-being of the fellow members of their community. Where this well-being is affected by a medical crisis, most people therefore have an interest in the best evidentially grounded treatment being used in the care of those in the community to which they belong (another way of stating the principle of broadened self-interest).

2. Where a person stands to gain by a community practice, it is morally unsustainable to abstain from participating in that practice. Best ICU care and the research that supports it is such a practice and therefore

(for reasons parallel to those about moral freeloading in the clinical management of AIDS) ethical arguments favor participating in it.

3. We all recognize that a degree of altruism is virtuous, and therefore it is something to which, in our best moments, we ought to aspire. It does no harm to make the charitable assumption that people should be treated in the way they would be if they always acted in accordance with the decisions that reflect their values (unless that decision involves heroic self-sacrifice by forgoing one's own objective best interests). Therefore, they should be enrolled in properly conducted trials of ICU research. In fact, it seems that most people are indeed glad to have contributed to public good research even without their consent. (Davidson, Dawson, and Moore 2001)

Fifth, relatives are often badly placed to make life-and-death decisions for any person. This has been objectively demonstrated (Coppolino and Ackerson 2001), and it is easy to understand. When patients are admitted to ICU, all the uncertainties associated with life-and-death decisions cluster around every conversation between the ICU team and the patients' relatives. In addition to this informational turmoil, there is an emotional cauldron. Some family members feel shocked, others guilty, yet others protective. Some will not want to agree to anything that puts their relative at risk and will hear words such as *experimental* and *trial* only in a way that creates confusion about equipoise and the clinical uncertainties that abound in this area of medicine (and, as we have seen, in every other). Consider the situation that provokes surrogate consent: a mortal decision must be made; the context is heavily overlaid by technology, the power of the medical establishment, and urgency, and there are often conflicted feelings that cluster around one's role as surrogate. It seems neither rational nor realistic to believe that anything like informed surrogate consent can prevail. In reality, many such decisions miss the mark in one way or another (Coppolino and Ackerson 2001), although we should still share clinical information and updated assessments of the patient's condition with those who are in attendance as sensitively and supportively as we can. This is part of the partnership between the clinical team and the patient's whanau.

Sixth, clinical staff are most likely to make the best decisions for any given patient, provided only that they are suitably sensitive to the realistic interests, concerns, fears, and expectations of ordinary folk (and not laboring under undue influence from distorting factors such as extreme right-to-life or euthanasia views, fear of litigation, or financial gain). This solution seems obvious given the arguments to date and is definitely most likely to offer us all the best chance of getting soundly researched clinical care in an area of medicine where intuitions and theory-based reasoning can mislead even the best of well-intentioned clinicians.

It emerges that, in general, it is best for the clinical team looking after you to make a plan for your management if you are incompetent and in dire or mortal threat from a debilitating influence. In fact, in most countries, the clinicians make recommendations, and the support people for the patient give their assent. It is clear that in ethical terms, this should be the default position with disputed cases being arbitrated by some suitably impartial body such as an ethics committee. The extreme remedy of litigation should be used only when, here as elsewhere in medical care, things cannot be managed in a more rationally defensible way.

What is more, we can commend, in ethical terms, the general practice of doing ICU research under the condition that the clinical team, acting in good conscience, can enter their patients into the trial, even where informed consent prior to entry into the trial cannot be obtained.

Elective Ventilation

Elective ventilation (EV) is ventilation initiated not in the interest of the patient but in the interest of somebody else. This may occur if a relative has not arrived in time to see the patient alive or needs a few hours to come to grips with a sudden and unexpected catastrophe. It may also occur to facilitate organ donation. In that case, it poses special questions that are not answered by the kinds of arguments in support of ICU research without prior informed consent (Browne, Gillett, and Tweeddale 2000).

There is one use of EV in which the person is dead according to brain death criteria, and EV is used to keep the organs perfused because of the patient's wish to be an organ donor. There is also a more problematic application of EV after a medical catastrophe when it is expected that the patient will proceed to brain death.

The former type of elective ventilation is justified according to a broad construal of what is fitting in terms of the patient's life and values. People who are concerned enough to offer their organs for postmortem donation would be unlikely to object were their official "moment of death" to be delayed or certain steps taken while they are dying to ensure that their wishes are carried out. A similar argument, based on the best interests of the patient and respect for the patient's values, supports a sensitive decision made to delay the declaration of death and withdrawal from treatment for reasons to do with the well-being of someone the patient clearly loved.

However, we cannot begin to justify such a practice if the patient has indicated that he or she would not want to be an organ donor. The real issues bite when it is a reasonable presumption that the patient would find postmortem organ donation an acceptable or preferred option. The pressing questions in such cases concern the risks of EV to the patient and the burdens imposed on those working in ICU settings. To assess these questions, we need to evaluate the seemingly tortuous arguments for and against the practice of EV in the relevant circumstances.

Arguments for and against EV

I will assume that the patient has not explicitly consented to the practice of EV after a clear outline of the advantages and pitfalls in the practice. Given that, we must rely on the general arguments in favor of unconsented interventions or proxy consent to measures that are of no benefit to the patient and, arguably, pose certain risks.

Arguments for:

F1. Consent to be an organ donor implies consent to the procedures necessary to become one and, hence, to EV whatever the circumstances.

F2. EV can increase the supply of transplantable organs by making available organs that would otherwise be lost. This may save a life, remove an incapacity, or ease the family's burden from the loss of a loved one.

F3. Families can give best effect to the wishes of the patient. Some patients are willing to undergo EV to become organ donors, and families are in the best position to know about such wishes.

Arguments against:

A1. The RUB. Patients undergoing EV may not die but instead (and as a result of EV) proceed to a persistent vegetative state (PVS) or some similar condition. The risk of surviving in such a state, even where it is followed by death as a result of the withdrawal of life-sustaining treatments (with consequent distress to relatives and loved ones), is a risk that many would regard as unacceptably bad.

A2. EV imposes a burden on ICU staff coping with the conflicting intentions to preserve organs in the best possible condition but not to treat the patient's brain injury. The conflicts touch many decisions about interventions to maintain life while allowing brain death to occur (e.g., should patients on EV be resuscitated in the event of cardiopulmonary collapse, treated with antibiotics if they develop infections, and so on). Families are also put under stresses; the decision about EV may be forced on them under difficult circumstances, and yet they must try to be level-headed about the risk of their loved ones surviving in a PVS or other unacceptable condition.

A3. The practice of EV in ambiguous circumstances might decrease the supply of transplantable organs by deterring people from volunteering for transplant programs. This might happen if it were ever suspected that physicians in transplant-related hospitals sometimes modified their intention to do the best for their patient in order to increase the number of organs available for transplant. This, as they say, is not a good look.

A4. Third parties cannot ever validly consent to procedures not done in the patient's interest and that may be contrary to the patient's interest.

These arguments should be assessed not only on their own merits but also against the background of a sensitive appreciation of the dilemmas involved in caring for and making decisions about a patient who has suffered a life-threatening catastrophe.

The Utility of EV

We can first examine the consequential arguments about EV (F2, A2, and A3).

The strains put on health care providers and families by the practice of EV are not a decisive argument because both negative and positive features of such a policy must be weighed before the overall utility can be assessed. The possibility of an increased supply of transplantable organs would offset the negative effect of the burdens on ICU staff and families if F2—it will increase organ supply—is more plausible than A3—aggressive organ harvest in ambiguous circumstances would be a sufficiently bad look to put people off EV. It is clearly disastrous for a program that relies on goodwill and altruism (as the transplant program does) to be smeared with the ghoulish taint of "organ snatching" or anything similar. Furthermore, the argument concerning the unenviable conflict imposed on ICU staff is consequentially relevant in that EV could make such staff disenchanted with the whole transplant program and therefore affect their cooperation.

Perhaps I ought to set the consequential arguments aside for a moment and then see what is left.

Giving Effect to the Patient's Wishes

I have argued that it is important to respect the patient's values even when the clinical staff would rather follow their own treatment plan, so the stresses on the ICU team should not be allowed to outweigh the patient's wish to be an organ donor. But in order to get support for EV from the simpler premise about patient's wishes, we now need the argument that consent to be an organ donor entails consent to EV.

Consent to x entails consent to y in only two circumstances. The first is where the person can be presumed to understand that consent to x entails consent to y (as in surgery and anesthesia). Thus, it is plausible that consent to being an organ donor entails consent to surgery to retrieve the organs, despite the mutilation of the body that is involved. Yet we cannot similarly presume that persons who have consented to be organ donors thereby consent to EV in problematic circumstances, for the simple reason that most people have never heard of EV. There are added risks in terms of the fittingness of the ending of the patient's life which are not immediately obvious (unlike the damage caused by a postmortem organ harvest). Therefore, mere consent to be a donor does not plausibly constitute consent to EV.

The second circumstance is where the person may not understand that consent to x entails consent to y, but y is necessary for x, and y does not carry any added risk that the person might reasonably find significant. Thus, it is plausible that consent to being an organ donor entails consent to the unproblematic EV when death is inevitable. However, this condition is not satisfied in precisely the problematic cases of EV. EV in the problematic or uncertain circumstances raises the question posed in A1—the RUB—the patient may survive in a PVS, which many people would find unacceptable.

Third-Party Consent

Failing implied consent based on the patient's wish to be a donor, the acceptability of EV rests on whether third parties can validly consent to it on behalf of patients. The first obstacle to third-party consent for EV is A4, according to which health care providers can never initiate any procedures on patients which are not performed in their interest and which are potentially harmful to them. The relationship between health care providers and patients should be one of trust, and this (it may be claimed) requires that A4 be strictly observed.

But the possibility of third-party consent does not fall over quite this easily. For if EV will increase the supply of transplantable organs, as F2 urges, one may reasonably ask why that should be trumped by the importance of maintaining trust. Perhaps respect for the trust shown by the dead is not a significant consideration. If that is so, then the debate turns on F2 and F3 (increased supply and respecting donor wishes).

F2 and F3 favor the use of EV, but they do not clinch it because the good results of EV may be offset by the even worse things that it produces. Thus, the argument requires that the good produced for transplant recipients outweighs the harm to health care providers and families specified in A2. It also requires that A3 is false, that is, that EV will not result in a net loss of transplantable organs from the practice. Whether these conditions can be satisfied is quite unclear.

If EV posed no risks for the patient, and we waived A2 and A3, there would be no difficulty in seeking third-party consent to organ donation when EV was required, but, as A1 claims, there is a risk. It is clear that EV would be a good thing if we could accept that the risks involved were not horrendous and that a great deal of good would come and could come only if EV were accepted. Otherwise, there is a difficult moral problem. Given the risk to the person undergoing EV—that his or her life will have an unfitting end and that he or she is exposed to the RUB—the procedure falls into the class of the supererogatory. A third party should not consent to a heroic act on my behalf that I might well not consent to myself.

Now, some have claimed that EV poses no threat of harm at all to patients (Kluge 2000). The argument is that there can be harm to patients only if they experience distress. This condition does not apply to patients in a coma being cared for in an ICU or patients who are in PVS; because they are insentient, they cannot experience distress. Thus, some claim, EV does not pose a risk of harm to patients.

The fault lies in the assumption that patients can be harmed only if they can currently and consciously experience distress. A narrative approach to ethics implies that persons are harmed if their interests are damaged. Interests are what persons care about, and we can care about things that lie beyond the possible bounds of our experience. For instance, persons can care about their reputations or memories of themselves surviving intact, or a dignified funeral, or their lives having a certain "shape" that is incompatible with their falling into a deep dementia, or (to speak to the point) surviving in a PVS, or a PVS followed by an engineered death, or a state very similar to PVS. If this is so, persons can be faced with the possibility of harm when there is no possibility of their suffering distress. What is more, we have ample reason to be skeptical that families can be sure about such things (i.e., that the person would be willing to accept the RUB and go with EV).

Therefore, EV carries significant risks of ambivalent treatment in which one's likelihood of living or dying is subject to certain uncertainties and also "narrative" risks associated with the final chapter of one's life having a shape that one finds abhorrent. I can imagine saying that I would not run the risk of EV, even though I am in favor of being an organ donor. Now if I, who have thought a lot about such things, cannot know whether I would want EV, my whanau could not be confident about their decision. On the other hand, even if individuals know they would want EV, we must question whether a whanau should be asked to take on this choice absent an explicit discussion (given that they cannot infer it from the consent to be an organ donor, nor can they infer it from a demonstrated willingness to help others at some cost to oneself). One must conclude that unless the person and their whanau quite explicitly have embraced EV, then we should not assume it is OK to do it. These problems by themselves give us sufficient reason for not approaching families about EV, but there are also dangers in the approach itself.

First, there is evidence that donating the organs of a loved one eases the burden on the family, and it is plausible that families take guidance from what doctors suggest, let alone recommend. Thus, a family asked about EV has a conflict of interest: it may coincide with their attitudes and dispositions to consent to something that puts the patient at a risk which is far more than minimal. In this situation, it is all too easy for the family to rationalize (unconsciously, of course) and say that the patient would have wanted to run the risk, even though there is, in most cases, insufficient evidence for that view and later they may regret it (particularly if the patient ends up in PVS).

Second, there is the question of whether the circumstances in which the family are approached about transplant ever allow for adequately considered consent sufficient to safeguard donors and relatives in this specially problematic situation. Grief, anger, gratitude, guilt, despair, and a desire to have some good come out of a tragedy, together with the social awkwardness of refusing an earnest humanitarian request from a physician, certainly make a request difficult to refuse. Many of us who doubt our ability to make a substituted judgment are even more uneasy in the light of these subtle pressures. Any clinician who has "walked the walk" with a family facing decisions about a loved one in PVS and near-PVS conditions knows that the reality is almost impossible to convey prior to the event and that the emotional strain is intense. Thus, we should not seek family consent to EV because it is invalid, and we know that there is a good chance of getting it despite the unpleasant reality it may cause.

There is a huge difference between family involvement in therapeutic decisions at the end of life or more normal organ donation cases, and the case of EV. In most cases, we can rely on a best-interest judgment, and the family can speak to this as well as can health care professionals. In relation to organ donation, there is a foreclosure of the patient's interests at the point where brain-death becomes inevitable. This, together with the fact that persons who do not wish to be organ donors have a realistic opportunity to make their wishes known, makes it reasonable for the family to be consulted. But these considerations do not apply to family consent to EV. It therefore seems that, absent explicit consent from the patient, EV is not permissible. The question remains whether EV should be initiated in those rare circumstances when health care providers have explicit consent from patients, and whether transplant programs should provide public education and consent mechanisms explicitly addressed to EV.

Giving Your All

Organ transplantation is an issue in which stereotypes abound. In general, it seems worthwhile to improve the lives of people A, B, and C by transplanting organs for which person D, unfortunately, has no further use. Therefore it seems wrong to have reservations about the donation and transplantation of organs on the basis of lingering mysticism about death and respect for the dead. However, ethical debate, in part, uses terms and concepts springing from our basic emotive and value commitments, so we cannot resort to a narrowly rational hatchet job in the face of serious concerns by sensitive and informed human beings. It is, after all, possible that some of our intuitive reservations may capture something that escapes our rational analysis of ethical issues.

Some folk worry that the possibility of organ donation means that we care less about saving the lives of those who might be donors than we would if they were our only focus of care. This theoretical worry raises its head in relation to the debate about EV and becomes pressing in any environment where medical care is being marketed and institutions may have greater incentives to perform good outcome, high-tech, transplant surgery than poor outcome, expensive, resuscitative care for victims of severe multiple trauma. The worry is allayed somewhat by the dedication of ICU doctors to high standards of excellence in critical care medicine. However, it does highlight the need for clear standards for the determination of death and for the ethical aspects of intensive care medicine. These are especially important in a health care system where there are other incentives potentially conflicting with the welfare of some patients.

The medical profession has, in fact, strict requirements for the determination of death and, in particular, brain death so as to safeguard potential donors against undesirable practices. I have laid out the arguments why issues about brain death can be treated on their own merits, without sidelong glances at such things as the need for donor organs, and in accordance with the principles that affirm the right of every patient to expect care directed primarily at his or her own benefit as far as justice permits.

Our ability to act for the benefit of any given individual may, however, be tempered by the requirements of justice, particularly when the benefits are marginal and obtaining them may be very expensive in terms of the level of health care provided by a given health system and the opportunity costs they impose on others. These factors apply *a fortiori* when there is competition for a scarce resource such as transplantable organs.

It is tempting to believe that there must be some ethical way of regulating such competition; surely people can be ranked in terms of some measure of ethical entitlement, just as medical triage can tell us which patients are most likely to benefit from a given intervention. However attractive this idea, it is difficult to formulate in useful terms. If we suggest that some individuals are more worthy or deserving than others, we find ourselves making value judgments about human lives which smack of a kind of elitism based in a narrow idea of the ideal society. (For instance, were we to leave this question to somebody with management-based ideals, we would end up with pushy, commerce-speak, entrepreneurial, new-broomers being valued over and above salt-of-the-earth traditionalists and romantic or artistic types.) We are therefore cast back on the utilitarian maxim that "every individual should count for one and nobody for more than one." This implies the waiting list, modified only by medical indications relevant to the likely outcome of the procedure. The more one debates the issue, the more it seems that waiting lists are the only fair way to determine how to distribute scarce resources. Thus, from a narrowly rational point of view, the ethical issues that dominate discussions of transplantation from dead donors revolve around issues of justice.

Live Donors

Here again, justice issues surface. Nobody chooses lightly to give away an organ and submit themselves to transplant donor surgery, and thus the issues raised by obtaining organs from live donors concern the level of coercion that a potential donor might feel either because of financial inducements or for other reasons. Both types of coercion are problematic, not the least because their ethical status is unclear.

Financial inducements to organ donation are usually rejected on the basis that it is wrong, without qualification, to trade in human bodies. Often this is linked to fundamental human rights; Justice Manohar remarks that "profiteering by procuring organs and inducing the poor and needy to violate their bodily integrity are violations of these rights" (1990). But it is not so simple. After all, if the donor is part of a family in which four children will have severely deprived lives with all the attendant risks unless one or two members run the (comparatively minor) risk of being organ donors, why should the donors concerned not be able to make that choice? The proponents of this argument claim that only those of us who have the resources to indulge our refined moral sensibilities oppose the option of a transplant market. They point to the fact that we are quite willing to let other relatively disadvantaged people do life-threatening things such as work in coal mines and clean skyscrapers for financial inducements. What is more, we should remember that heroism and self-sacrifice by members of a family to save each others' lives is a widely endorsed human phenomenon.

Against this, we could argue that the existence of systems in which such exploitation can occur because of highly disparate financial circumstances is, in itself, an evil and that we cannot condone an action merely because it is the least worst option taken in an evil context. We could make an analogy with the concentration camp guard who executes inmates because he "has no choice" given the circumstances and reasons that it is a kinder fate for some of them than that they would otherwise suffer. Neither his lack of real choice nor their unenviable fate make his action right, although it does spread the attribution of evil beyond him as an individual. There is, however, a fine line between a considered choice made by a family in response to difficult circumstances and a coercive situation where people are exploited by a corrupt society and a complicit organ-procuring organization. The problem reminds us that we need to be aware of the difficulties faced by disadvantaged groups for whom life is a series of unenviable choices and of the need for health care ethics to have a concern for social justice.

Charles Dickens was the master of narratives in which the correct moral response to many of the unenviable choices forced on his characters could only be to fight for social reforms that had little to do with the individual case and otherwise to bear up as best one might, doing what one could to bring about the least worst outcomes.

The problem of donor relatives is just as difficult. There is, of course, emotional coercion in any family with a severely ill member, but it is unclear that it is wrong in itself or that it is wrong for an individual to respond to such pulls. And we should not, as I have mentioned in relation to research, be too swayed by the illusion of autonomy and self-centered best interests that smack of Hobbesian egoism as the basis of rational behavior. There is a fine line between a sacrifice made out of commitments to people dear to oneself and coercion of a type that exploits an individual without regard for that individual's real wishes. Children are obviously very vulnerable here, but it would be wrong to adopt a blanket prohibition against organ donation by children. Such a donation might, plausibly, come about as a result of the child genuinely wanting, more than anything else, to help a sibling or relative or to save that person's life.

The issues are intensified by the trade in human organs, where the organs may be obtained in ways that do not meet ethical criteria for organ donation. We worry that the harvesting of organs for money does violate our respect for the human body and, therefore, our respect for human life. We worry that the sensitivities of relatives and loved ones of deceased persons will be callously overridden in the interest of a thriving trade. We also worry that the practices of obtaining donors might neglect some of the important safeguards about death and terminal care that have already been discussed. The general point to be drawn from these worries is that we should not let our concerns for transplant organ availability (or some even more abstract and unrealistic ideal like the free market) blind us to the dignity and importance of each human being and the need for fundamental fellow-feeling as the basis of our associations with each other.

Our fundamental commitments to and links with other human beings as individuals form a deep-rooted foundation for ethical debate reflecting that we do not and cannot submit all of our moral intuitions to narrow rational scrutiny. Thus, if they are problematic, the questions may have to be resolved other than by rational argument. Many of us share semimythical fears about the grafting into one person of a body part from another. This fear goes beyond rational considerations and embraces the deep, indeed symbolic, associations that underlie many of our value commitments. The thought that, when transplantation occurs, a person literally and symbolically takes into him or herself aspects of the donor person is able to be understood in illness and remedy terms at one level even though it seems to have far deeper connotations at another. Where such symbolic associations are at work, we often need strongly countervailing images to resolve our ethical worries in a satisfying way. Such images should not be thought of as propaganda or emotional manipulation any more than the idea that morning is a reclaiming of life from the darkness of night or that spring is a renewal of vitality after the cold and numbing grip of winter should be thought to be unfounded in fact. The long cold night of the soul is not just a poetic phrase but a state of being to be avoided. In this spirit, a key concept in transplantation is that of a gift.

Tom Murray argued that this concept is an underpinning for many of the aspects of collective human life that we most value and that it is fundamentally different from other types of social transaction (1987). The most powerful image associated with such giving of self is expressed in the familiar words, "Take, eat, this is my body broken for you." The images of the Eucharist transform the symbolism of organ donation so that our thoughts do not become absorbed by pictures of organ harvest and the cannibalizing of the dead by others (something of which the early Christians were accused) but, instead, focus on the gift that is made when one person is enabled to give life where there was previously no hope of life.

This concept so closely parallels the highest ideals of most moralities, be they religious or secular, that it is a fit image to inform our discussion of transplant issues in abstracto (in ethical discussion) and in concreto (at the bedside of the newly dead person). A dignified recognition that one human life has ended and the sensitive suggestion that this person may have wanted to give life to someone else has shades of meaning which take the discussion to a different place from that to which it tends in contemplating the paid procurement of organs.

Cardiac transplantation in particular inherits a burden of imagery and association that has deep roots in our fundamental feelings about ourselves and other human beings. I have noted that where our thoughts and responses are engaged in this way, an ethical problem is not susceptible to purely rational resolution, and the deeper aspects of our being need to be recognized and respected. I have suggested that the concept of a gift, particularly as exemplified in the Christian Eucharist, is eminently suited to inform our ethics in this area. The symbolic giving of self to benefit another is so central to our highest moral ideals that it can serve outside of the particular faith and doctrine in which it has its home. The idea that a donated heart is a precious gift given by a fellow human being who has died can restore the felt "rightness" that transplantation may otherwise lack. This felt rightness is a vital part of our moral (and mortal) lives together. Similar styles of thinking are, I believe, important in considering the issues surrounding euthanasia.

CHAPTER TWELVE

Euthanasia, the Pause, and the Last Rights

> I will not give a fatal draught to anyone if I am asked, nor will I suggest such a thing. —THE OATH

"It's a helluva thing, killing a man. You take away everything he's got and every-thing he's gonna have." So Will Munny (Clint Eastwood) in the film *Unforgiven*, remarks to a young wannabe gunslinger who is vomiting his heart out after his first kill. Will voices a common intuition often translated into the sanctity of life principle (it loses something in translation). It can, I think, be truly said that we do have strong feeling that *there is an intrinsic value in human life, quite apart from whether it is currently thought to be valuable by the person concerned or indeed by anyone else.*

This is the principle we appeal to when an individual attempts suicide and we prevent it. The conviction that each human life is of unique value and ought to be protected and cherished on that basis alone seems to have been part of the ethos of medicine since the time of Hippocrates. The commitment is moderated by other considerations when our treatment becomes too burdensome and a person wants to let nature take its course, but even here many of us are con-flicted. The *pause* is a phenomenological marker of this conflict and the depth of the commitments that go into it (Gillett 1988, 1994).

The Pause

The pause is the hesitation or doubt you experience when, as a doctor, you decide that death is the right option for your patient, even where you have carefully considered the situation and feel that you are deciding (for instance, to withdraw treatment) on the basis of very good moral reasons. Think, for instance, of the problem of a newborn child with severe hydrocephalus, a large encephalocele containing a nub of poorly formed brain tissue emerging from above its eyes, and areas of perinatal brain injury evident on a postnatal scan. Imagine that the tests we have done—brain scans and EEGs, for instance—in the context of the history show that it is unlikely that the child will ever recover to a point where it can respond to those around it or develop purposive behavior. But looking at the child's face, one sees a cherubic visage (with a bandage hiding the deformity in the forehead). Even in such an extreme case, at the moment of recommending that no further intensive efforts be made to keep the child alive, one might experience, as I have, the *pause*. The pause may be almost unbearably intensified if, as one examines the child, some fleeting, primitive, and reflexive expressions play around the tiny mouth and remind you of your own children at a comparable age.

Such decisions make us delve deep into our characters as moral agents, and rightly so. The ability to heed such complex inner voices is arguably fundamental to the caring professions. In light of my discussion of clinical intuition, perhaps such moments confront us with the mismatch between informed and astute judgment backed up by careful attention to evidence and sound reasoning, and certainty in the face of diverse imagined futures. The pause alerts one to the seriousness of the decision being made, the dimensions of which are expressed by Will Munny's remark, and asks that one reflect on any lingering misgivings or unresolved questions that have perhaps been jostled to the back of one's mind in coming to that decision. In this way, the pause can indicate that the apparently clear-cut reasons leading to an apparently straightforward ethical decision may not have done justice to everything that is at stake in a particular decision (at least for creatures of our moral stripe).

Euthanasia is used here in the restricted sense that is the focus of discussion in the Netherlands, where it denotes "ending a patient's life at the patient's explicit request" (van Delden, Pijnenborg, and van der Maas 1993). The practice of actively ending the lives of patients has, in the Dutch setting, been extended to other categories where an explicit request is not made. This occurs at about half the rate, when surveyed, as those fitting the criteria laid down for active voluntary euthanasia (van Delden, Pijnenborg, and van der Maas 1993). As such, it takes one step further the kind of management I have recommended for PVS (and related states) by making the termination of such states an active decision to intervene with a lethal technique.

The intuitions that feed the pause are generally stacked heavily against the active killing of persons, and at this point they touch the roots of our moral sensitivity in general but also, and particularly, our moral sense as health care professionals. What is more, that "touch" is like all the things that touch any one of us at a personal level—elusive, evocative, and with inchoate but disturbingly resonant effects on one's psyche. We shall see that it is exactly the kind of thing that engages with "a sense of life," particularly when that is awakened by an imagination schooled to exhibit a narrative sense of the values in which life trades.

First, I ought to be clear that, by appealing to the pause, I am not arguing that a gut-level reaction is adequate to establish the morality or immorality of active euthanasia; rather, I am trying to deepen our focus on the unique and complex nature of human death. Parker comments that "we need to look closely at our intuitions, in order to rationally conclude about best courses of action, since without any such examination, it is just my intuition against yours, or perhaps mine against the patient's" (1990, 2). He argues that when we are deciding about such an event, our intuitions can be sensitive guides to the right choice of action in the situation, but there is nothing in the pause itself that tells uniformly against active voluntary euthanasia.

He also notes that arguments claiming that the inadequacy of palliative care induces requests for euthanasia neglect that, in his experience, "well informed and compassionately cared for patients will continue to make such requests" (3). He therefore concludes that neither the ethical considerations based on autonomy, nor those based on a fiduciary relationship between doctor and patient, nor those based on the values guiding medicine tell definitively against active euthanasia. It is a step taken at the patient's request, by a doctor who is keeping faith with a duty to care and who is influenced by the important value of relieving suffering by whatever means we can even where that is inconsistent with preserving life. This seems like a well-rounded and persuasive case for admitting the permissibility of euthanasia. It remains to be seen whether an inquiry into euthanasia, couched in terms that pay philosophical attention to the pause and conducted in the light of the narrative approach of this book, tends toward a slightly more traditional conclusion.

Narratives, Lives, and Deaths

Human beings, as Kübler-Ross notes, "create and live a unique biography and weave ourselves into the fabric of human history" (1969, 102). Therefore, a human death is unique with respect to all of those things that make a human being what he or she essentially is. There are many meanings, aspects of relationships, and unspoken words that may be disrupted by a technological hijack of this area of human life in terms of a range of techniques designed to be wheeled in when life becomes too painful (for whatever reason) and death becomes the preferred option. For this reason, a viewpoint reacting to extreme contingencies of pain and perceived worthlessness may not evince the requisite sensitivity if and when the "final solution" is waiting in the wings and can be fairly readily produced. Active euthanasia is almost too clean and rational to engage with the dying person because the decisions here are not as simple as they are in the case of nonhuman animals (Mullen 1995). To appreciate this, we need to stray, once again, into the nature of narrative and the sensibilities it enhances.

Martha Nussbaum discusses the moral perceptions that inform our sensibilities at intense and conflicted moments of our moral journeys by discussing Henry James's novel *The Ambassadors*. She explores the territory of moral reflection and moral perception in complex human situations, unashamedly espousing an Aristotelian stance that "speaks about us, about our lives and choices and emotions, about our social existence and the totality of our connections" (1990, 171). These explorations, she argues, give rise to "the vigilant and responsive imagination that cares for everyone in the situation and refuses . . . to 'simplify' for the sake of purity and safety in the midst of wonderful puzzling mysteries" (184–85). To be sure, she is discussing a nuanced novel that deals with the discovery of a richer, fuller life by a limited young man with previously narrow horizons and a very conventional and functional background in terms of life, love, marriage, and career, but the lessons are meant to be general. The sensibility and imaginative capacities that she explores lead to a somewhat messy sketch of the moral landscape that is not likely to be satisfying to those with a penchant for clearly premised arguments leading to rationally coherent and apparently incontestable moral conclusions. For myself, I can only conjecture about a moral life that can see itself in those more clear-cut terms (although I always feel guilty that I cannot). Yet Nussbaum's recommendation for reflective equilibrium, suitably sensitized to human particularity and the subtle guidance of practical wisdom or virtue, does tend to bolster one's precarious confidence in the evident rightness of proceeding in a different vein. One can even take comfort from the fact that the ethical (or even the ethically informed) life was never meant to be easy.

What seems particularly hard, from a long way off—amid, as it were, the Apollonian heights of reason and argument—is attentiveness to the situation as it looks from up close. From up close we can hold the situations we are engaged in up "against our own experience and our intuitions" (Nussbaum 1990, 174). Thus, in this sort of close proximity, amid the smell of the clinic, one's neural networks can sniff out those nuances and styles of interaction and conversation that tell one how one ought to behave so that things are resolved in a way that all of us will be able to live with now and hereafter (Churchland 1996). This is the stuff of Aristotelian moral competence: the ability to do what is fitting in a complex situation that does not reduce itself neatly to a set of propositions on which one can perform a moral calculus.

A Unique Challenge

Death is a problem that we will all face, some suddenly and others of us after a period of preparation (for instance, because one knows one has a terminal illness). Although each of us "crosses over" as an individual, most of us need others to help in that uncertain (and literally awful) journey. All sorts of small kindnesses are needed to ease the way, and conversations need to be had; things need to be said that have often been left unsaid. Some loose ends need to be tied up and others untied and retied so that those left behind have something with which they can carry on. Sometimes old wounds need to be forgiven and healed and sometimes acknowledged for what they really are. For these things to happen, the dying person must both anticipate death and be in a sufficiently clear-minded condition to attend to any remaining questions. But a person is also a body that needs to be cared for. The desire to have a good dying makes many people fear the worst scenario of all, where one is reduced by illness to an impaired and pathetic condition and is left alone with nobody to care or to create a place of being that can be departed from in a way that is fitting.

Death also raises other, less-defined fears because it is and will remain the great unknown. At the moment of death a person quits all that is familiar, some say for another kind of life, some say for oblivion. Although different beliefs abound, there is no knowledge in the ordinary sense to be had this side of death. Frances Dominica writes, "Two things are clear to me. One is that mystery and a sense of awe surround death and whatever lies beyond it. The second is that an effect of love and grief exposed, the soul laid bare, is to bring forth reverence in the beholder. Here we find ourselves beyond the realm of reason crossing all barriers of different faiths" (1987, 109).

Death is a final break with the relationships and everyday familiar things that fill the hours and days of human life. In the face of this unknown, many people need support and reassurance that they are not being abandoned. It seems that the feeling of being no longer of any worth is one of the worst aspects of dying for many patients. Yet it is not necessary for people to feel this way. Indeed, for many people, the time before death has much greater meaning and intensity than any other time of their lives. I recall that the wife of a young man (and father of three children) who was going to die of a brain tumor said, "The last three months have been the happiest of our lives together." Often only the threat of loss impresses on us the true value of what we have got.

The reassessment of life's values which we see here is a common experience in serious sickness in general and in the time before death. Many of our beliefs about what is worthwhile in life do not stand up under the personal challenge of a serious illness. For this reason it is important that the health care professionals dealing with a patient help to create an atmosphere in which such questions can be raised and worked through. This kind of thing, rather than just "pills and potions" or, even worse, surgical interventions, can make a time of tragedy into a time of intense personal worth.

Although doctors are often pivotal figures in this type of situation, medical training, at least in its scientific and technical aspects, does little to provide them with the resources that are most needed in dealing with death and dying. It is hard to say what prepares us apart from reflection on human life and what makes it go well. Exactly what is needed can become clear only as we spend time with those who are dying and seek to help them through the last days and weeks of their lives with as much dignity and patience as possible. Even then the most experienced of us can sometimes fail abjectly those who most need us.

The dying experience can, however, become a nightmare. The knowledge that someone has a terminal disease may cause other people to avoid him and can lead to a strange fabric of evasion and deceit which surrounds that person and isolates him from those whom he most needs. Guilt, embarrassment, or awkwardness can threaten to cut a person off from all his normal supports. This can sometimes be the case with AIDS patients, who can be rejected by many of those to whom they ought to be reconciled before they die, such as family or estranged "straight" friends. Only by realizing that our attitudes and actions can convey rejection and worthlessness to a dying patient, even when we do not realize what we are doing, can we ensure that dying is no more painful and desolate than it need be for those who must somehow find within themselves the resources to face it and conduct themselves in a manner that is fitting in the light of the life story they have written and inhabit.

There is, unfortunately, nothing we can do for some people but not usually because of uncontrollable pain. Some will never be able to approach death with any peace. We can do what is done for others and minimize pain, offer respect, and preserve the person's dignity as much as possible, but there will always be a small group for whom the prospect of death induces frantic searches for some way out. In this tragic situation, one can offer only commitment rather than abandonment and, by so doing, try to provide the sense of worth and reassurance that alone has a chance of allowing the person something like a good death. In such an atmosphere, one can come to be reassured that what lies ahead can be faced. Wittgenstein remarks, somewhat judgmentally, "Fear in the face of death is the best sign of a false, i.e. a bad life" (1969, 75). Despite the thought that this pronouncement cannot be the whole story, one is struck that there is something in it and in the related thought that the anxiety and fear that drive a person to want an early death must signal something bad, some need for healing, but perhaps a healing or wholeness of a kind about which medical textbooks do not have a lot to tell us.

It is abundantly clear that in the face of death we meet as person to person and that medical and health care techniques per se have a limited role. For this reason, some of us are deeply suspicious of the "technological hijacking" of death. It sometimes happens that a person can be rushed off to a hospital, admitted to an intensive or acute care bed, and treated with drips and drugs before anybody takes stock as to where it is all heading. This is worse in some countries than in others, but it is particularly cruel when it is demanded in the misguided name of not denying older people the best medical care. For each of us, medical care is good only when it offers what is fitting and realistic at that point in life's journey. It is clear that many people who suffer a really serious illness late in life want peace and comfort care rather than futile (but state-of-the-art) medical techniques. Here we cannot evade the real need for the understanding, wisdom, and sensitivity that are part of the art of medicine and that reveal to us what would be of substantial benefit to a given patient.

Suicide and Its Relevance to Euthanasia

Suicide is a growing problem in many Western societies, and much has been written to try to illuminate the issue. Only one or two points carry over to the euthanasia debate. The first is the well-known association between suicide and depression, and the second is the phasic nature of the desire for suicide. So closely are these phasic aspects of mood, attitude, and cognition linked that Boldt remarks "with rare exceptions, suicide is constrained by an urgent and intense need to relieve an intolerable life situation. This renders the notion of an autonomous, voluntary, or free choice in regard to suicide, inappropriate" (1989).

There can be a number of reasons for believing that death is more attractive (or less unattractive) than going on living. It may be that the person concerned feels that nobody loves or values him or her; life may seem to be of no value at all, or anything may seem better than some state of physical or emotional suffering; the person may feel cut off and afraid of the future; or a state of grief or impending loss may seem too much to bear so that the person just wants to "get it over with." No doubt there are many other stories of hopelessness and despair. In every case, we have to try and understand the person concerned and see why he or she wanted life to be cut short. That challenge is captured by the questions "How did we fail you?" and "Why did you not want to live out your time among us?"

These thoughts should give us pause when we find that terminal illness is associated with a high rate of clinical depression, which in many cases responds well to directed therapy (Block 2000). In fact, clinical depression does seem to be a significant factor among patients with terminal illness who desire an early death (Brown et al. 1986). For instance, a patient thinking about "getting it all over with" may have poorly controlled pain and real fears that it is going to get worse. Here it is relevant that up to 98 percent of patients who fail pain treatment in other institutions can be well controlled in an experienced hospice setting where pain, as an affliction of the whole person, is well understood and expertly handled (British Medical Association 1988, 12). Many of these patients will leave the hospice on lower doses of pain relief medication than those with which they were admitted but with better control of their pain. Thus, perhaps not always just the pain itself but the fear of what is happening and is going to happen may push a person toward a certain type of choice. This fear, the anxiety with which one faces unknown future prospects, and pain itself all enhance one another and contribute to a malignant psychic cocktail that the hospice ethos seeks to recognize and address. The hospice attitude—that death should neither be hastened nor delayed—provides the kind of framework within which patients and staff can be given time to take care of the pain, fear, and anxiety of dying without the background pressure of having to make a decision about a possible intervention such as euthanasia.

It is understandable that patients with a terminal illness who know they are going to die might feel unsure whether others still want them around. Even a passing brush with disability can make vivid the idea that one may feel worthless when severely debilitated, and, for this reason alone, it seems wise to encourage the attitude that death must take its own time and that we can only ease it and make it as "gentle" as possible. If a doctor were to inquire whether you wanted to be helped to die or to offer to help you to die (or actually to hasten your death), then that doctor, perhaps unwittingly, is conveying something about whether your still being around is worthwhile.

This last worry has drawn our attention to the fact that any patient, and particularly one who is seriously ill, is vulnerable to a number of subtle coercions. When you are admitted to a hospital for a procedure you feel a definite obligation to go through with the course of treatment as planned. Many patients will say something like, "Well, I've come this far. I can't really back out now." This may reflect genuine uncertainty or a rough-and-ready way of preventing anybody from revisiting a painful topic once some kind of decision has been reached. For most patients and most decisions about health care, there are, in fact, good reasons to stay on track, and we hope that in most health care these have been adequately discussed (to the patients satisfaction) before a decision is made so there is no real reason why the discussion should be reopened.

However, a decision about death is much less clear in that what is at stake is a deep human mystery, however painful it is to think about. We should worry that the tendency to not "want to go over all that again" or burden other people with doing so might make some vulnerable patients just go along with what is planned or what they think might be expected of them, even if nobody is saying so. Most people want to do the right thing, and in a climate of legalized euthanasia "the right thing" can be quite threatening if you feel you don't want to be a burden or cause too much fuss for others—which is a very common feeling.

The complex, conflicting, and often unclear ideas that surround decisions about death and dying further affect discussions in this area. On the one hand, there are really obvious things to consider, such as the fact that a person is dying, the fact that he or she suffers pain, disability, and so on, and the possibility of it just ending without further ado. Anybody can see and appreciate these, so they can be thought of as the only *real* features of the decision being made. On the other hand, there are more subtle and complex considerations that are usually better appreciated by those who have to care for people through the process of death and dying. These caregivers often are alerted to their misgivings by the pause, but then, when they turn their minds to the problem, they try to make sense of these less clear factors by saying they feel hesitant about helping a person to die, which sounds very weak and is, in those terms, indistinguishable from a gut reaction.

The ill-defined and poorly articulated feelings and perceptions that contribute to that felt hesitancy are difficult to capture and lay out in any cogent, logically argued form. Faced with such readily understandable arguments on the one side and merely a fuzzy discomfort on the other, those who support the traditional "respect for the sanctity of life" can feel somewhat overwhelmed. That is why euthanasia is a really difficult ethical challenge. Almost everything that is easily stated supports it in the right kind of circumstances, and it is often hard to put words to why some people feel so set against it (except where there are clear reasons, based in a code of beliefs, why some people do not agree with the idea). But, at least to someone sensitive to the idea of narrative, that imbalance suggests the possibility that we have not got our minds around all that matters here and that some traditional stances may have more going for them than just history.

The clear and desperate remedy on which the suicide victim seizes has exactly this same cognitive quality—a plethora of seemingly compelling reasons why it is the only thing to do which rationally overpower the misgivings of the spirit that speaks for life. Of course, we should reason about what life has in store for us, but we should also listen to the voices and the silences that alert us to the defects inherent in a rational approach to things. We have, after all, a powerful cultural precedent for the good voice being not in the howling wind of public opinion, nor the earthquake of existentialist iconoclasm, nor in the consuming fire of rational argument but in the still small voice heard within that confirms what it says by resonating with one's sense of life.

Care and Intervention

One of the impulses we serve by the practice of euthanasia is to do something for a suffering person. Yet it is not always true that doing something is the right thing to do, and even if it is right to do something, we need to be very clear about what is needed to be done (or perhaps more accurately, exhibited). Cicely Saunders and Frances Dominica are both highly experienced in the care of the dying, and their comments are illuminating.

Saunders remarks on the patient who asks a team just to "let me die."

> The team needs to discover what it is that makes continued life so grievous . . . Reassurance and explanation about the likely nature of the final coming of death may well be needed if anxious fears are to be eased. (Saunders 1994)

> "I want to die" expresses anguish that demands attentive and experienced listening . . . It often arises when past treatment for distress has been inept and listening cursory. (777)

> The specific request "Kill me" . . . is still extremely uncommon in spite of all the (often confusing) attention of the media to this subject . . . We need to give a clear answer, and a definite stance of this kind gives its own security. (778)

Saunders goes on to discuss the need for a caring and supportive atmosphere in which the patient's value as a person is affirmed and unresolved problems surrounding his or her life and relationships can be addressed. She counsels judicious use of pain-relieving drugs as these are often used to compensate for what is really inadequate listening and support. In her wide-ranging and sympathetic work, we see the narrative steal into the picture as the patient has words that need to be heard and that need therefore to appear in the text of his life. She notes of one patient who suffered from a widespread inoperable cancer that she needed "open and frank discussion and patience as she found her own way helped to a final peace that at one time seemed unlikely" (782).

Frances Dominica, from a similar tradition, writes on death in childhood and notices our impatience with tragedy and our tendency to try and get an expert to step in and handle it (1987). She remarks, "I condemn a society which prefers to have such things dealt with at a safe distance clinically and antiseptically, and seems to absolve itself from the responsibility for making itself available to be alongside and to stay alongside and to take on board some of the suffering and grief of others" (109).

Here is the guide, the one who does not abandon even though the pressure of life and one's sometimes irresistible desires to be up and doing intrude and displace the best intentions. She observes, in relation to her dying patients, "despite society's fear of death and ineptitude in the face of death, I believe that every individual has the potential to meet death with a severe beauty which in no way denies grief" (110).

These revealing glimpses into the experience of the seriously ill or dying patient and the insights of those who care for them and share the hyphenated experience of care-in-dying are highly relevant to a discussion of active euthanasia. The feeling one gets from both writers is that events surrounding death are subject to a different rhythm from the interventionist mode that prevails elsewhere in medicine and in a have-a-problem-fix-it society.

When a patient is killed—or helped to die at a given time and place—by a doctor, the mode and moment of death depend on an irreversible choice made as a result of a set of reasons. This finality places a great weight on those reasons and how adequate they are to deal with all that is important in human death and dying. It is not quite the same with the withdrawal of life-prolonging treatment because our actions have a different dynamic. The description "appropriate treatment for the dying or terminally ill" (Reichenbach 1987) captures this dynamic and allows one to hold together the universal tragedy of death and the limitation of human action in the face of it. The rhythm of mortality is varied and can, no doubt, accommodate the assistance that some find themselves able to give. Whether it should and how accommodating it can be before we find that we are changed into technologists who control life, birth, and death in a way that centrally or peripherally colors every human narrative is a question that seems to demand a wisdom beyond the reason of philosophers. The Hippocratic answer was clear.

When we intervene to alter a process that is at work in the patient's body, we intrude in what could be regarded as a *natural* change inherent in human life. Of course, medicine does this all the time. Defining what is natural is very hard, but people usually seek active medical help so that they might enjoy continued life as far as possible and be rescued from suffering or danger to their health. Some patients, however, get to the point where they say, "I have had enough" or

"I don't want to fight it anymore" or "Is that really going to do me any good, Doctor?" These conversations reflect a sense of the *fittingness* or *naturalness* of certain bodily changes that indicate that death is coming and should not be treated as an enemy any more. This is congenial to the Aristotelian position that acknowledges the fact that each of our lives has a natural form (see Appendix C).

At these points the patient and the wise health professional tend to "listen to the wisdom of the body" rather than wheeling in yet more technology to try and fix things. This may mean that the moral discussion of medical situations needs to find room for phrases like "allowing to die," "letting nature take its course," or "not prolonging the dying process." Such phrases are sympathetic to the feelings of the patient and somewhat respectful of the rhythms of mortality. They call into question the assumption that in life-and-death situations we are required to act as autonomous agents with clearly formulated reasons for our actions and that we need and should have a wide range of choices. Those in hospice practice argue that a lethal, fix-it solution to the problem of death and dying, especially where that involves major human suffering and distress, is a poor second best to careful attention to the needs of the suffering body and the patience that takes away any desperation induced by those needs. Stepping in "to end it all" is usually not what is needed. Perhaps if we answer the real needs rather than do away with them by killing the patient, we shall come to see that "technology rules" is not always the best way to serve the calling of the good life.

Law, Culture, Morality, and Death

There remains only one case where the law has specifically sanctioned a nationwide practice of active voluntary euthanasia, so it is useful to turn our attention to that setting in discussing the implications of these somewhat unclear ethical reflections for lawmakers thinking about this area of our clinical life.

The situation in the Netherlands has been developing since 1973 as case law has gradually crystallized a conception of what is permissible. It as accepted that a doctor is under conflicting duties when faced with a patient who is suffering intolerably. In this situation the doctor is held to have a duty to relieve suffering (as the patient's caregiver) and also a duty (as a citizen) to obey the law and not commit murder (van der Maas, van Delden, and Pijnenborg 1992). The former duty was thought to create a defense of force majeure, or necessity, whereby the doctor found that he was bound by the greater demand to do his duty as a care-giver and, acting under that necessity, ended the patient's life so as to relieve suffering even though that required him to fail in his duty as a citizen to not take the life of another citizen.

This kind of defense could be sustained if the euthanasia was performed under the following conditions:

1. there was a request by the patient;
2. the patient was properly informed about his or her condition;
3. the patient's wish was sustained or durable;
4. the doctor considered the patient's condition to involve intolerable suffering without hope of relief;
5. a colleague agrees with the doctor concerned. (Leenan 1987)

The crucial conditions clearly involved a free and informed request from the patient, thereby ruling out other forms of end-of-life decisions apart from that involved in active voluntary euthanasia. However, the assurance that this was the general case was dispelled by the Remmelink report of 1991 (summarized in van Delden, Pijnenborg, and van der Maas 1993).

In this report it became obvious that, in addition to voluntary euthanasia, cases of involuntary and nonvoluntary euthanasia were occurring and that assisted suicide was also widely being used as a means of helping patients to die. The contents of the Remmelink report have fueled the already existing worries about abuse of the provisions in the Dutch legislation (Keown 1992). This showed that, all in all, about 3 percent of deaths occurred as a result of euthanasia, assisted suicide, or "life terminating acts without specific request" (24). It therefore seems clear that the original very stringent guidelines have loosened slightly as the practice has spread. A recently publicized case raises further issues.

The Chabot case concerned a fifty-year-old woman, Mrs. B, who was supplied, at her request, with lethal drugs, which she consumed in the presence of her doctor; she died within half an hour (Griffiths 1995). Mrs. B had a particularly complex psychosocial history. She had had an unhappy marriage and had separated from her husband three years previously. She had lost both her sons; the older son had committed suicide in the army two years before her separation, and she had lost her second son to cancer four months before her death. She was diagnosed as having no major psychiatric illness but was judged by her psychiatrist, who gave her the lethal drugs, as suffering "intense, long-term psychic suffering that, for her, was unbearable and without prospect of improvement" (Griffiths 1995, 235). The case was heard in the district court, the court of appeals, and the Dutch Supreme Court. The first two hearings concluded that the doctor acted under the necessity to relieve the patient's suffering, but the highest court reversed that decision. It discharged the doctor who prescribed the drugs without penalty or any other measure. Although this case provoked censure, it also provoked a change in guidelines so that "11 of the 15 pending prosecutions (involving nonsomatic suffering or patients not in the 'terminal phase') were dropped" (Griffiths 1995, 247). This was seen as a fundamental step away from the approach to euthanasia which took as its basis the Hippocratic ethos toward a standard that gave primary weight to the wishes of the patient.

The result is therefore to release the profession from an atmosphere of careful respect for life into an atmosphere where we are to be seen as the technical adjutants of patients who have made their own significant health care decisions. Whether this accurately reflects the way in which Dr. Chabot and Mrs. B came to their decision, I am in no position to judge, but the worry is there that we are being asked to go "naked" out from under the canopy of sanctity of life into a world where what counts as good medicine will sometimes include acceding to a wish to actively end a patient's life. Most of us recognize that the worst equipment, morally speaking, that one could avail oneself of in this situation is a thick skin and that the most distressing will be an acute sensibility to the intricacies of terminal (or perhaps nonterminal suffering).

A nurse who recently visited some elderly relatives in the Netherlands mentioned to me that her elderly relatives living there have deep misgivings about going into hospital. They fear, in the light of the Remmelink report, that they may be victims of euthanasia with or without their consent. It matters little how widespread this apprehension is or how ill founded in the light of the attitudes and ethics of the medical profession in the Netherlands; it is an attitude not conducive to the kind of atmosphere we need to allay the widespread alienation of the public from the profession.

Hippocratic practice is founded on trust and reverence for life; these orientations keep one going when, for instance, one's "intestinal fortitude" fails at 2 A.M. with an eighteen-month-old infant bleeding badly on the operating table who could die from the neurosurgical operation one is performing (even if one's practice would still fall well within the acceptable mortality for operations of that type in such a case). But they can also drive us to *persist* when we should *desist* in the name of humanity and a realistic eye to the outcome of what we are doing. Despite these mixed blessings, the Hippocratic commitment to life and the well-being of our patients has delivered to us medicine as we know it and the safeguards that we have bred into us with our training. I think that is something we should not lightly abandon.

The Dutch experience with euthanasia should at least make us worry about the reality of slippery slopes and the possible climate of change that is created by legalization of euthanasia and assisted suicide. It may be that what we see in the Netherlands is a progressive move allowing us to clarify and refine the desirable safeguards and conditions under which decisions at the end of life can be taken. Some philosophers and lawyers are less optimistic and see genuine reasons for concern in the Dutch practice although they acknowledge that the issue is far from simple (de Wachter 1992).

Personal Morality and Legal Reform

At this point it is important to notice that the law does not merely reflect the moral standards of a society but, in fact, has a profound influence on them. If the law permits a certain type of action, then we as a society are swayed in our attitudes toward that action. This inevitably means that when an act crosses the line from being unlawful to being lawful it finds a new level of social acceptance. We have already seen that happen with abortion, which has gone from being a stigmatized, backroom activity (with all the attendant risks to women) to being an acceptable alternative in the face of what might be a terrible moral conflict for a young woman who finds her life and health or her life story, as she has composed and crafted it, threatened by an unwanted pregnancy.

It is clear that, as this last possibility indicates, the acceptable reasons for abortion have loosened somewhat from the initial very cautious legislation that focused on a serious threat either of death or to the continued health of the mother. I will, in due course, come to the importance of our attitudes to young human lives and will not visit the issue here, but what has happened in the area of abortion illustrates that once we have allowed some practice, the conditions under which it is allowed and the ways in which we form moral opinions about it change. With abortion this has led to a much more widespread performance of abortion and it looks as if, in the Netherlands, there have been similar trends with euthanasia.

Legislation allowing active voluntary euthanasia would affect the whole context of terminal and palliative care. The choice as to whether or not to ask for euthanasia would be there in the background for everyone. We would all, if suffering a terminal illness, be wondering what is expected of us. The realization that a request is purely voluntary does not close the issue as to whether acceding to that request might or might not be the right thing to do.

I have discussed the many ways in which dying people can be vulnerable, isolated, and distressed by what they perceive to be happening. Many of these reactions are, as Kübler-Ross has so eloquently shown, completely natural, but they may well lead a person to question the worth of their going on to live out their "natural span." The fact that the question of euthanasia is in the background and the implication that our society regards it as an OK thing to do would plausibly interact, in ways we do not feel comfortable about, with those uncertainties. Thus, legislative change creates a changed moral framework for terminal illness. It is a subtle change but, if viewed through the lens of the moral imagination, a real one. The words of *Evangelium Vitae* (John Paul II, 1995) are sharply relevant here. "The commandment 'You shall not kill' establishes only the point of departure of a journey to true freedom, a journey which must lead to the active promotion of life, the development of attitudes and modes of behaviour which serve life" (730).

There is clearly a difference between the arguments that bear on the morality of an individual act of euthanasia and the arguments that should be heeded at a social or legislative level. At the personal level there is a need for a sense of what is fitting in the context of the life that is coming to an end. My personal practice has always been to see the journey through to its end and neither hasten nor delay that end (in accordance with the hospice orientation). I find this in accord with my own sense of life, which is informed by those many texts that the lives of patients offer, that I find in the literature of our cultures and others, and that the experiences of hospice and other caregivers interpret for us. I find this body of knowledge deeply satisfying and fundamentally sound in its guidance and the help it gives me in dealing with my dying patients.

Those who exhibit the phronesis that incorporates schooled intuitions evident in the most experienced caregivers for the dying among us deserve to be listened to. I find that they as individuals exude a kind of calm and peaceful demeanor that makes me feel somewhat inept in the face of death and the grief of losing a loved character in the story of one's life. When I have to communicate to my patient that he or she is dying and that I have no magic answers, I find I have a need for imagination and identification with the living person who confronts me and whose face traces his or her reaction to what I am saying.

When contact is made and the hyphen in our relationship indicates a joining of consciousness on the ugly thing laid on the table between us, it rarely emerges that an intervention is up for debate; far more often it is a sense of traveling with, albeit at a distance, the person as he or she leaves my immediate care. If the contact is made, then it is made. When we meet, we share that time of contact and the understanding that it brought. As the death becomes closer there is a sense in which the shared understanding creates a kind of companionship that is at once personal and professional.

The need for a companion, someone who will be sad to see me leave and who does not want to hasten that ending, seems to me to be the most profound need of the dying person. I do not think I will want my companions to cling too much, but I also do not think I will want to be released too readily. I cannot think that the release of a negotiated arrangement at a given point in time is the kind of release that brings a good death, but then, I have not passed that way, and we all know that extrapolation is a dangerous game.

So What Do I Think?

In 1987 I wrote the following conclusion to an article on this topic: "Our official ethic, enshrined in our statutes as firmly as it is graven in our character, and thus proclaimed with all the gravity which justice can lend to any moral conviction must be, and must be seen to be, that human life is inviolate. Any doctor who feels bound by conscience to contravene this sanction must, I think, be prepared to submit his action to the deepest scrutiny that society can undertake and be vindicated by the overwhelming humanity of his act, and that alone" (Gillett 1987).

Maurice de Wachter makes the telling remark, "When euthanasia is negotiable and the end of life no longer a topic to be hushed up patients may find acceptance, tranquillity, even peace and happiness" (1992, 25). We ought also to notice that when the practice is met by unsympathetic attitudes from prosecutors and police, the notification rate goes down and the ends of regulation are not well served (van Delden, Pijnenborg, and van der Maas 1993, 25).

I have not really departed from my stance of 1987, although these days I would probably not express it with the same gravitas. My own clinical experience and the arguments inspired by the pause have kept me to that view.

Medical intuition and tradition is against active euthanasia despite that neither doctors nor nurses, according to various polls, are absolutely and universally opposed, nor are groups of individuals who have worked extensively with dying patients. I thus find myself in agreement with Philippa Foot, when she remarks, "Apart from the special repugnance doctors feel towards the idea of a lethal injection, it may be of the very greatest importance to keep a psychological barrier up against killing" (1978, 59). "But this is not to deny that there could be acts of voluntary euthanasia both passive and active against which neither justice nor charity would speak" (55).

Death is unique and its actuality something whose mystery somewhat escapes us. "Death is not an event in life. It is not a fact of the world" (Wittgenstein 1969, 75). Frances Dominica talks about a mystery and Will Munny talks about a "helluva thing"; each in their own way attest to the specialness of death. I have suggested that there is a Thanatos that is *Eu-thanatos* or a fitting, harmonious death in keeping with the rhythm that the life and story of the person impart to it. Our task in caring for the dying is to respond to and work with that rhythm whether in life or death.

I believe we all need to be needed, and we need to know that others are not dismissing us with any sense of untimeliness. I remember the patient with a severe spinal condition (syringomyelia) for whom I had intermittently cared for many years who sent her daughter to see me in the hospital where she had been admitted under another team's care. She was in a terminal condition with severe respiratory disease and yet had not agreed to start the morphine regime that was needed to ease her respiratory distress until she had seen me. I finally visited, after procrastinating for a day or so because I did not know what to say and had made myself busy as a clinician can always do. She greeted me and said, breathless and wheezing, "You know I have fought as hard as I can, don't you?" I said that I did, and then she said "It's OK now." The team looking after her started her regimen, and she died, quite peacefully, in the early hours of the morning of that night.

There is an Australian saying, "Nobody misses a slice off a cut loaf," which, although it is normally used in other contexts, is quite apposite here. Richard Hare observes that we have a tendency in our moral lives to find good general rules that will stand by us when decisions are personally demanding and that we ought to stick with them. He notes, like Philippa Foot, that there are some genuine cases that seem very hard and to call for a departure from tried and tested principles of practice, but he gives the following caution.

But since it is so easy to deceive oneself, and since in actual cases we never know enough and never have enough time to think about it, it is very hard to be sure that this is a case in which we ought to depart from the principle. Maybe it is; but maybe on the other hand, the case actually before us, is not really so peculiar after all; we are only trying to persuade ourselves that it is peculiar because we want to get away for the weekend. But even if it is peculiar—even if in this general case we ought to break the good general principle—we shall do so with the greatest misgiving, because it goes against our whole upbringing as doctors; and the occurrence of this general case does not in the least mean that the good general principles are no good. They still ought to be our main standby as doctors, and we ought not to do anything to weaken them. (1993, 14)

The debate around active euthanasia is beset with unbalanced arguments. On the side of the Hippocratic tradition there are indeterminate considerations that are difficult to state and summarize but that, when articulated as best they can be, cohere with one's sense of life and what is good and worth striving for to serve it and live it well. On the other hand, there are clear-cut reasons that tend to a decision that can be enunciated and acted on and that brings a problematic and sometimes painful situation to closure. However, closure is not that great, unless you are an accountant. I find I need to retain a kind of openness to experience which is attentive to the things that are not so easy to summarize in arguments but that emerge as one considers stories and incidents that illuminate clinical ethics in ways that have an effect on me. For this reason, I am suspicious of the apparently conclusive arguments, although I have the utmost respect for those whose humanity and care for their patients leads them, in the face of what could be potentially harsh judgments, to walk near the boundaries of medicine where the signs on all the old maps say, "Here be dragons."

I do worry about what medical killers do to medicine as a whole. I know that my own practice rests on the solid foundation of a commitment, where there is doubt about outcomes, to saving life and that this sustains me when I would be tempted to settle for an easier solution. Death and dying are problematic, emotionally, spiritually, ethically, and personally. I therefore worry about our acceptance of a technology or technological and interventionist mind-set that relieves us of our discomfort in this area. I am somewhat heartened by the voices of those such as Dr. H. S. Cohen, in the Netherlands, who, as a person who has helped a number of patients to die, remarks, "It is not easier to kill than to care" (de Wachter 1992, 24).

I have never found myself faced by the need to intervene lethally to end a patient's life, even though I have managed a number of dying patients with various conditions and I have been asked to do so. I have been involved in a number of deaths where life-sustaining treatment was withdrawn, sometimes at the patient's request. I cannot, as things stand, envisage myself needing to be the means of active euthanasia for any patient, but I have a great deal of respect for those whose humanity and care for their patient leaves them, they feel, no alternative. I do not envy them.

Part IV / The Beginnings of Human Lives

CHAPTER THIRTEEN

Ethics, Embryos, and Stem Cell Research

By now the foetus is formed. This stage is reached, in the female foetus, in forty-two days at maximum, and for the male in thirty days at maximum. This is the period for articulation in most cases give or take a little . . . The cause is that the female embryo coagulates and is differentiated later, since the female seed is weaker and more fluid than the male.

—THE NATURE OF THE CHILD

In this passage, cited by both Aristotle and St. Thomas Aquinas, Hippocrates attempts to define when the human organism achieves its characteristic form. This form was thought to be the basis of the functions comprising the human soul (or psyche). Given that the Hippocratic ethos fosters and encourages medical knowledge based on intelligent and informed experience, the Hippocratics studied miscarriages and fetuses in their attempt to understand human origins. The continuation of that course of inquiry has produced many of the most pressing problems for contemporary bioethics because knowledge of our own origins and the building blocks of human life makes us trustees of a power demanding responsibility and care in its exercise.

The enduring values informing our lives together as human beings (and therefore medical practice) give a central place to the uniqueness of each human being as a never to-be-repeated creation. What is more, each of us needs a place to stand and a story to tell which affirms that unique value.

We are now (or shortly will be) able artificially to produce human beings and have some control over their characteristics. Some of us (perhaps only those who can pay) may also, in future, have a tissue bank of our own stem cell–generated tissue for use to replace body parts and organs. Cloning may also give us the capacity to reproduce whole persons. These powers must be guided in their use by the values defining the place of human beings in the biosphere. We therefore need to consider how our attitudes toward young human beings, such as embryos and fetuses, interact with our moral thinking in general. In fact, we have distinct ethical intuitions about children and their place among us, related to thoughts about our origins and the ethical relevance of them to our autobiographies and our place in the world.

The Use of Embryos

How should we regard embryos? On the one hand, they are small scraps of biological matter (*coagula*—to use the Hippocratic term) and almost indistinguishable from collections of sperm and eggs or other bits of human tissue. On the other hand, some regard them as sacred beings, made in the image of God, and see embryos as children whom we must nurture. Our attitude to embryos is, therefore, an interesting study at the interface between ethics, social attitudes, cultural symbolism, metaphysics, and theology.

I think we can best understand our diverse moral intuitions about embryos if we adopt a view based on Aristotle's distinction between form and matter. Aristotle remarks, "soul is substance as the form of a natural body which potentially has life" (1986, 412a). His use of the term *substance* indicates a thing with a particular configuration (as distinct from undifferentiated matter), and he compares a substance to an imprinted wax seal where the wax is the matter and the imprint (creating the seal) is the form. The soul, we could say, is the living configuration of a type of thing. (For instance, the soul of a fox is the form making that animal a fox.) He remarks that the human soul has "nutritive, perceptive, and intellective faculties and movement [or activity]" (413b) and speaks of it as "the cause and principle of the living body" (415b). The soul forms the internal dynamic (that from which the movement itself arises), the purpose (that for whose sake it is), and the pattern (the formal substance), of an ensouled body. I have argued (Poplawski and Gillett 1991) that the form of a human being, as for any living thing, is one that changes over time while yet being part of the one unfolding reality (hence the narrative shape to life). In this view, an embryo is an early phase of a human person and should be seen in the context of human growth and development. Thus, the embryo is human but not quite in the same sense as an adult member of the human community.

The moral value of a fully developed person depends on his or her nature as a rational and social being, and Aristotle's treatise on ethics claims that ethics is a branch of politics because human beings necessarily, as part of their nature, live in collectives within which each person develops individual attributes (as a unique narrative project). The value of human life arises in this context and is then logically attached to the individual who is the actual and potential person bearing that person's name. The nature of a person, we could say, is to have a longitudinally extended form in which characteristically human features are progressively developed and then cease to be. The moral value of the human being attaches to all phases of human life as phases of a single being in whom the specific actuality of being human takes shape. I have called this the holistic longitudinal form (HLF) view of a human life, and it can be represented graphically.

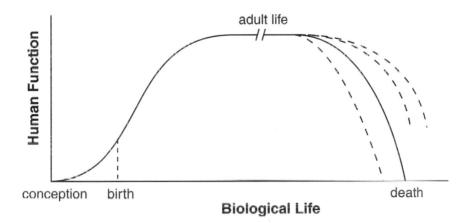

The HLF view underpins certain ethical intuitions (whether they are grounded in secular humanism or religious belief). Embryos (who later become adult human beings) have a special place in Christian writing even while they are being formed in the womb, but Mosaic law and Judeo-Christian writings do not regard the death of a child in the womb as equivalent to the death of a person (see Exodus 21.22; Psalm 139.13; Jeremiah 1.5). Taken together, these passages leave it unclear just what Judeo-Christian morality should say about embryos. Our ethical attitudes toward reproductive technology, controls on infertility treatments, and the use of embryos reflect this ambivalence. (The Aristotelian/Thomist view of the soul is widely accepted among those inclined toward natural law as the basis for morality and rational discussion between the faithful and heathen.)

In defining limits on the use of human embryos, the Human Fertilization and Embryology Authority in Britain recognized the widespread intuition (in accordance with the HLF view) that human life of whatever stage has moral significance. "The fact that the zygote [embryo] is a living being from conception onwards is a sufficient reason for many to recognise that it must be treated and protected not as a property but as a member of the human family" (Iglesias 1984). The same intuition is evident in recent Norwegian and European legislation (Holm 1988; Byk 1997), but these intuitions are not universally shared.

At the opposite pole of the debate, some argue that there are no rational grounds for an embryonic right to life and that human embryos therefore can be used as required for scientific research. They argue that embryos, though human in one sense, do not have characteristics of personhood such as reason, consciousness, and personality (Singer 1992). It is tempting to compromise and adopt the moderate view that embryos are entitled to respect but not the full rights of human beings per se. If this is to be more than a pragmatic compromise, we need some grounding for the moderate view in our general thinking about the beginnings of human life and the moral attitudes it should engender. Is there a basis for embryos and the early phases of human life having some but not all of the moral status associated with more developed human beings? Some thinkers explore this question by focusing on potential or on the idea of biological essence (Brody 1978).

Is there a metaphysical underpinning such as potentiality for human identity (Brody 1978; Lockwood 1985)? Rival accounts of the metaphysical basis for identity include the primitive streak as a distinguishing biological mark that determines that there is one and only one individual being formed, a more advanced level of nervous system structure and function, and the first dawnings of sentience or awareness of stimuli as the beginning of a continuous mental life (though not a fully Lockean consciousness and memory). These accounts have in common a commitment to the idea that the metaphysical underpinning unifies and provides a foundation for the moral treatment of a being. Some thinkers would, however, argue that metaphysical underpinnings themselves are rooted in our discourse and reflect our ways of dealing with each other. Such a discursive or postmodern conception holds that metaphysical underpinnings are no more than broadly and intricately interconnected patterns of thinking which inform many of our praxes and attitudes because they have the kind of stability and generality in our cognition that is characteristic of the roots of our understanding. Metaphysics, in this (post-Kantian or Wittgensteinian) interpretation, reflects nonnegotiable features of our thinking that are part of the fabric of our being as rational creatures. But which of our attitudes to the embryo have this deep-rooted and intrinsically compelling quality to them?

Arguing that embryos have the potential to grow into human beings who have moral rights is a promising start but only the beginning of this cognitive task. It is difficult to find a sense of potential that coheres with our general thinking about things in the world and that rationally grounds our moral intuitions about embryos.

In the view accepted by consequentialists like Singer, any mixture of sperm and ova have the potential to become one or more human beings, and yet it is ridiculous to treat such a mixture as a human being. Such views rely on a reductive account of potentiality such that what physically makes up and then follows from a situation encompasses all of its important properties. Potential is therefore a complex of possible future events expected to result from a current state of affairs through the operation of a causal chain. Thus, any state of affairs has the potential to be an X provided only that nature will produce an X from it. However, this does not quite catch our intuition that there is a potential or capacity that is properly intrinsic or belongs to things of certain types.

Aristotle argues for this intrinsic conception of potentiality when he remarks that the soul is present in a living person whether that person is sleeping or waking, but that its characteristic activity is evident only in the waking state (1986, 412a). Indeed, it seems natural to think that such a capacity as intelligence or liveliness is an enduring feature of an individual even if an intoxicated or somnolent state obscures the actuality at the time in question. There is a closely related sense in which the seedling has the potential to be a tree or the human organism increasingly gains and manifests the nature of a person. On that basis, we could say that the capacity for becoming a fully developed human being is an intrinsic capacity of the embryo in a way that it is not of a collection of sperm and eggs because such capacities (or potentialities) go along with an identifiable being to which we can attribute them.

I see no reason to prefer the kind of metaphysical thinking central to the reductive or consequentialist views over this latter Aristotelian view, which seems more holistic and better grounded in our experience of nature, and to reflect more accurately our intuitive understanding of natural kinds (Lockwood 1985). In general, the more reductive, snapshot, or "time slice" accounts of human life (Parfit 1976) seem less suited than philosophical conceptions that take serious account of the narrative aspect of life.

There are other challenges to meet in arguing about the nature and moral status of embryos. First, some thinkers (Singer 1979) argue that special consideration for human beings as distinct from other similar higher animals evinces "speciesism," a sin comparable to racism (a justification of grossly unfair treatment of beings who are racially different but, on any morally relevant ground, alike). The claim that human beings have a special status just because they are human and that killing a human being is different from killing animals, looks similar but is one that most people accept and would justify, if pressed, in the following general way:

1. by showing that human beings have a special moral status—different, in terms of conscious appreciation, interactions, and behavior, from that which reflects the functioning (or soul) of other forms of life (Thomson 2000); and

2. by showing that these things or the potentiality for them are the kinds of things that entitle any being to special moral regard.

The problem is that, even if we could show that certain features (to do with the intellective and social aspects of the soul) make human beings worthy of special moral consideration over and above animals, embryos (and other human organisms, including fetuses, anencephalic infants, and severely brain damaged adults) do not have those crucial features (consciousness, "relational potential," or whatever). A sound metaphysical concept of potential would help meet this challenge because it would distinguish those whose form implies they will develop such features from those who could never do so.

A second challenge arises because we seem to be caught between two arguments.

A. If an embryo is just a bit of tissue attached to the mother, then she should be able to do what she likes to it.

B. If an embryo is a person in its own right, then the mother cannot say what will happen to it.

Some people opt for A, arguing that the mother should have sole and final say about what happens to an embryo. Others opt for B arguing that the fate of an embryo cannot depend on the wishes of any other person. Neither option solves the problem, and between them they divide the moral universe into warring factions. Yet the choice is not that stark.

Even if the embryo is a person, we may still not have a right to limit a mother's choices about it, as is shown by Thomson's scenario—the famous violinist (1971). In this scenario, a woman is, through no choice of her own, abducted and connected to the life support system of a famous violinist who has a self-limiting but potentially fatal disease and requires nine months of life support. The analogy with pregnancy is obvious as is the fact that the violinist and those who campaign for his life have no claim on the liberty of the woman concerned. Thus, if we were to regard an embryo (or fetus) as a fully morally entitled human person, we could not, on that account, force a mother to nurture it. This holds even when her decision entails that it die. Therefore, a decision about the embryo's being a person seems irrelevant to the question of the mother's right not to carry it to birth.

However, this case can be given an interesting twist. Imagine that the individual at risk is a three-month-old child and that the father of that child is the one "hooked up." In this altered case, our moral intuitions are not so clear-cut. To be sure, a born child has some moral claim on the parent's love and concern, and it is arguably closer to the situation of abortion than the case of the famous but unrelated violinist and the woman. We should also notice that, whereas the father may not be legally bound to support the life of his infant daughter (which would be analogous to forbidding abortion under most circumstances), we might recognize, as the law does, some kind of parental duty in the paternal case. In any event, it is obvious that our moral intuitions crucially depend on factors such as relatedness and stewardship or duties of care. (I explore these in greater depth when I discuss young human lives and our ethical attitudes to infants.)

I therefore return to considering embryos, noting that we need to look deeply at our values with regard to human beings and their relatedness if we are to understand our moral intuitions about the use of embryos.

Grounding Our Attitudes to Embryos

I have already given reasons to set aside the idea, supported by one side and attacked by the other, that being a human organism (however defined) is equivalent to being a person with full moral status. That they are not the same has emerged in discussing end-of-life issues where it seems clear that some human beings are alive in some sense but have ceased living as persons. PVS was a case in point, and similar arguments touch on the status of anencephalic infants but have an added dimension. Most of us do not believe that anencephalic children should be treated the same as other neonates (either in terms of health care resources, or because of the emotional costs to parents of going through a series of futile efforts that will never result in a life worth living). However, most of us, despite arguments about current capacities, distinguish other neonates from anencephalics and reject infanticide as a permissible way of treating human infants (Tooley 1972).

Our thinking is explained when we accept that anencephalic infants differ from normal neonates in lacking the actuality of those properties that ground our moral being as well as the potential to develop them. Our moral responses are therefore based not merely on the fact that we are dealing with a biologically living human body but on the idea that it is a body capable of developing a certain level of functioning—a soul of a certain type (crucially related to the integrity of the brain)—a "person in the process of becoming." Therefore, our shared intuitions support the Aristotelian (HLF) view I have outlined.

Aristotle's claim that every type of thing has its own specific form, allied with the view that the human form essentially involves the activity of a rational, social being, has been taken to license a definition of personhood based on cognitive attributes. I would argue, in accordance with my overall position, that the pervasive moral judgments that inform our treatment of one another are based in the reciprocity implied by the fact that we are all beings to whom certain things matter. This claim is grounded in (actual or hypothetical) empathy for each other as beings in relation to one another. The fellow feeling that enables this empathy arises when we recognize in other people lively activity, relationships, sensitivities, satisfactions, vulnerabilities, and so on, and it takes us into the realm of discourse and relationships. Within that milieu we all develop unique life stories. Young human beings are, in that respect, no different from the rest of us. Embryos, fetuses, and infants are all examples of the type of being—human beings in the process of becoming—with whom we feel an intuitive commonality. One hears and understands the mother who has lost her baby and says, years later, "You know, it's times like this that I remember she would have been starting college this year." If, then, this human commonality, this involvement in each others' life stories, is what engages our mutual feeling and grounds our values, when does it begin? Does it begin only when relationships are developed, or does it come into play before there is any reciprocity at the level of animate, intellective, and social functions? I believe that we are attuned to the potential that will give rise to the actuality.

The HLF (or neo-Aristotelian) view I have outlined suggests that it is natural and reasonable to extend our moral concern to early stages of human life because it accurately captures a feature of our ordinary thinking. In general, the way we think of a thing takes a broad view of that thing. Imagine that my wife uses my ticket to the Boxing Day test (or the World Series finals) to start the fire. Imagine that I regain my self-control and that she, having avoided homicide or at the very least wife-beating, says, "But what are you so upset about? It was only a little bit of paper." Now, excluding the possibility of intentional malice, she does not comprehend what she has done. My ticket is just a piece of paper, but it has a value "not dreamed of in her philosophy." Here another image—that of a painting—is useful. A painting takes shape gradually, and its value increases as it develops. Thus, to destroy it when the painting is only a few brush strokes on the canvas, is a lesser thing than to do so when it is complete. Similar points inform our thinking about embryos and support a kind of gradualism that acknowledges the unique production that is a human being.

The ticket story bears directly on the reductive view of the embryo which equates the human embryo to the embryo of any other creature—such as a frog, a sheep, or a monkey—from which it might appear physically indistinguishable (in its manifest properties). Seeing my ticket as no more than a piece of paper is analogous to seeing the embryo in this light; it leaves out almost everything that makes the thing concerned important to us.

The painting story brings out a complementary point that tends to weaken the strong case for investing embryos with the moral attributes of developed personhood. Thomson argues for a conception of personhood based on "the suprarational capacity to discern right from wrong or at least the potential to develop this in due course" (2000, 35). This strong view of potentiality is, I would argue, parasitic on the Aristotelian view of potential and the human form but neglects the neo-Aristotelian considerations mitigating the application of moral properties (such as human dignity and human rights) to the embryo. Let us accept that interaction (or the capacity for such) in a human context (even if it is not fully reciprocal) places moral value on the life of the human being concerned. Like the painting, the human embryo develops from almost nothing (from a thing whose presence might not even be suspected) to the stage at which we have a living, loving, and loved child on our hands. This is true of any valued thing that it takes time to create. The gradualist position is that a human organism accrues value as it takes shape and appears among us so that at some point in the developmental process our responsibilities to nurture and protect each other come into full play. It is therefore highly congenial to the theological claim that the human soul is a feature of human beings that is truly developed through incarnate experience. The soul with its cognitive, emotional, and spiritual functions is, on this view, able to be fashioned only through mortal human life. The embryonic soul is therefore precious in a certain way but not in quite the same way as the soul of one who has truly come among us in a fully interactive sense. However, even here, things are not clear-cut.

Problems with the Relatives

For some parents, particularly prospective mothers in infertile couples or those who are hoping desperately for a child, the first missed period means that there is a baby on the way, and every subsequent period signals the loss of yet another potential child. Thus, a morally significant interaction with the potential child can occur much earlier in the gestational process than is usually recognized. Even though that interaction does not fit our normal conception of an interpersonal moral exchange, its role in a particular human story—the potential mother's—gives it a set of properties that are deeply morally relevant. This early (and perhaps unusual) maternal intuition is compatible with the metaphysical view that a distinct human being comes into existence at conception. The natural course of events for a thing of this type is for it to become a person whom we have a duty to love and nurture. This, we could say in the neo-Aristotelian view, is a potentiality or capacity that it possesses in itself, and departures from that course are to be thought of in terms of the total process that would normally occur. Thus, the embryo does not become a different thing as it develops into the child, and our moral attitudes to embryos should be continuous with those we hold toward children rather than totally different (as expressed in "a fortnight of my life is missing" [Holland 1990]). However, the analogy with the painting explains why for most of us the moral properties of the embryo are not the same as those of a child or adult. Yet what of the fact that abortion involves another person quite apart from the developing human being?

A Choice Too Bitter for Words

As I have not felt a child develop within me for nine months, I have not given birth, and I have not experienced a mother's closeness to her child, it is with great reluctance that I stray into the abortion debate. I have taken a view that precludes our treating abortion as the murder of one human being at the request of another. But these arguments do not touch the mother's experience of abortion, which is clearly a least worst choice for many women. Jing Bao Nie has given us an invaluable glimpse into the experience for mainland Chinese women, drawing his title "so bitter that no words can describe it" from the words of one of his interviewees.

> For Qianqian, like almost every other Chinese woman who has had an abortion, the experience can be characterized [as] having been engraved on one's bones and heart. (2001, 152)

> I watched the aborted fetus. It looked like a roll of fine air. I sighed, "Oh, my poor son, how miserable you are!" (152)

> Though I determined to do the deed, or get the "family physician" to do it, my womanly instincts, my reason, my conscience, my self-respect, my entire nature, revolted against my decision. My womanhood rose up in withering condemnation. (162)

These voices speak from a culture in which children have traditionally been welcomed and valued, but it is clear that even in China the experience varies widely. Women often write about this decision "not as a contest of rights but as a problem of relationships" and frame the discussion "based on a recognition of the continuing connection between the life of the mother and the life of the child" (Gilligan 1982). This connection repeatedly surfaces in feminist discussions, all of which tend to recognize that the mother and her fetus are intertwined in ways that no other two human beings ever can be and that this relationship should inform our thinking on the issue (Tong 1997). Warren defuses those arguments that dwell too heavily on the continuum between fetal and neonatal life by reminding us that "it is impossible to treat fetuses in utero as if they were persons without treating women as if they were something less than persons" (1992, 209).

It seems, then, that a complex tangle of conflicting moral pulls surrounds the issue of abortion, but it is the mother who is most likely to be drawn and quartered emotionally by their moral demands on her. The present view implies that the mother should be trusted and supported in making the decision that commends itself to her own moral sense, bearing in mind that she alone will live with the consequences of that decision because of her ongoing connection with her "little children" and the reminders of "how old they would now be if they had been born" (Nie 2001) that her life as a woman and perhaps a mother will constantly bring to her.

The present view implies that embryos are genuinely human and have an intrinsic worth but that their worth is not that of a child or an adult. We are bound together by our common humanity, and we are aware that the roots of that humanity are in small beings who come into existence in the midst of human communities. Embryos don't change into human beings; from their conception they are human beings with the potential that we value in human beings. That potentiality becomes actuality, and the corresponding (temporally changing) reality is a fact about our form as natural beings. By and large, except in unusual cases, embryos are inherently on the path toward being the kind of individuals who can be cared for, responded to, wondered about, grieved for, and so on. In an age of scientific investigation, though, we recognize increasingly that an embryo may not follow that path.

Assisted reproductive technologies bring these issues and uncertainties into sharp focus. In that arena, human embryos come into existence that will never develop beyond an early stage. We could say that their capacity or potentiality has no link to the actuality (or holistic longitudinal form) that is normally manifest. Nevertheless, the current argument implies that, as much as we can, we should not deal with embryos and fetuses in ways that neglect the inherent value that attaches to a human life from its earliest point.

We could say (at the risk of misleading ourselves) that an embryo has an interest in making it into the world, but the nature of the interest is not that different from the interests of any other biological organism until the embryo (and then fetus and then child) has come among us in a way that clothes it with the form of a person with whom we are morally engaged. The context that transforms an embryo into an organism with a potential life story is a discursive context and no less real for that. Thus, an embryo has a real nature that partakes of the world of meaning (or discourse) as much as the world of nature. This bipartite reality eventually exhibits itself as the capacity to participate in the public world where we recognize each other as persons and take some responsibility for each other, but in its earliest stages it is only an embryonic form of the unique production that is a human life, and, despite being precious in that sense, it is not a person.

It is a happy and highly appealing consequence of this view that the moral status of the embryo has only a slight connection with the stem cell debate.

The Stem Cell Debate

There are currently a range of variously realistic hopes and expectations that therapies using stem cells will radically transform our conceptions of incurable disease, severe tissue damage, and what insults to the human person can be healed. These hopes often fall foul of a debate about cloning and the use of embryos, but I will argue that they should not. We can use human tissue to provide stem cells without producing and destroying embryos. Therefore, my account defuses arguments that import issues about human embryos into the center of the stem cell debate.

I have argued that there is a natural trajectory and therefore an intrinsic potential attached to an embryo that comes into being within normal human relationships or even through high-tech processes aimed at producing a child. The events in this story are clearly related to our conception of the beginnings of a human life because that is their narrative context. But the events occurring in the production of stem cells are not necessarily the same because their narrative context is different. The argument depends to some extent on the idea that an event is identifiable by virtue of its narrative context or as a moment in a given story. This is a contentious metaphysical thesis that I cannot argue adequately in this context, but one or two remarks may help to make it plausible (see Appendix B).

Think of a range of events:

- Rutherford's splitting of the atom (to start with a New Zealand example);
- the beginning of World War II;
- the killing of John Lennon;
- the speciation of homo sapiens;
- the marriage of Charles and Diana.

In each case, there is a tract of time during which a number of things happen in a certain region of space (quantum energy changes occur; atoms jiggle about; chemical reactions progress; bodies move; words are spoken and written; people interact in certain ways; nations experience some meaningful moment). Yet exactly which of these things comprises the event to which we refer when we use these denoting expressions? A case that is readily understandable to bioethicists makes the inherent indeterminacy of the space-time specifications of an event evident. Consider the killing of John Lennon: does this happen when the gunman shoots the bullet, when the bullet enters his body, when his heart stops beating, or when his brain loses its functional integrity? Take his heart stopping: does this happen when the last beat happens, when the next beat does not happen, or at some objective point after the last recorded beat, or is this another case of "It ain't nothing 'til I call it!" It depends on the discourse in which one is engaged and the story one is telling. Events and the objects that they concern are, I would argue, able to be individuated only by the story in which they appear.

We tell all kinds of stories: quantum physical stories, causal stories, biological stories, biographical stories, political stories, historical stories, cosmological stories, and so on. For each one, we need a range of objects and events to refer to, and the story (or the discourse that furnishes the resources needed by that story) gives us the means of doing that semantic work. We could call this the *narrative theory of events* to capture the relevant insight, and it is sharply relevant to this discussion.

The narrative theory of events implies that the context of the production of a nucleated and living cell is crucial in determining what kind of thing that cell is. If the context is a reproductive story, then it is a pre-embryo and will, we all hope, go on to form an embryo and then develop in the normal way with the usual probabilities. If the context is not a story of that kind but rather a therapeutic story using stem cells for some experimental or clinical purpose, then the cluster of concepts that embed images and associations drawn from stories about the beginnings of lives are irrelevant. If we are telling a stem cell therapeutic story, it is just not apposite to import discourse with a totally different role in our general thinking and moral intuitions. The resemblance between what we are dealing with and an embryo is misleading and superficial or merely physical rather than metaphysical. I deal with the special issues associated with cloning below, but for now there are a range of issues peculiar to the therapeutic use of stem cells.

Stem cell–based technology does offer the hope that we will be able to reproduce tissues from a human being and potentially recreate that person's organs. If that becomes a reality, then the shortage of transplant organs will be readily addressed. Stem cells also offer the possibility of repairing such things as myocardial infarction or spinal cord damage, for which, at present, we can only support the person in coping with the problem and preventing the situation from becoming worse. The prospect of injecting cells into a damaged heart or spinal cord so as to initiate repair and restoration of function should silence the staunchest critic of such technology, but ethical problems lurk in the wings.

First, there is the *placebo effect,* which, as I have noted, is problematic when the gains are subjective in terms of improved cognitive ability, improved feeling in limbs or organs, and so on. I have discussed this to some extent in discussing surgical advances.

Second, there is a real problem with *therapeutic pressure* from patients and commercial interests. The latter are constantly on the lookout for surgical and other techniques and innovations that will make money in the lucrative medical technology market. It is not difficult to imagine that stem cell banks, accessible for a fee, will be well patronized by those hoping that the technology will come along to repair or regrow a liver, heart, kidney, or spinal cord should you need it. The prospect of "two-tier" medicine and serious injustice in these fringe areas looks to be not far off.

Third, there is a distinct prospect that some early attempts at stem cell therapy will have serious *long-term complications.* For instance, neural repair is a long haul, and neural complications such as neural stem cell tumors are quite slow growing, so they might not show up for some time after the stem cells have been injected or inserted into the site where they are supposed to do their thing.

There may well be other long-term dangers, the possibilities of which are suppressed or discounted in the vanguard of exciting new prospects for stem cell therapy. As well as these more detailed concerns, there are also metaphysical worries about our conceptions of ourselves and the nature of human life.

Human life has a mortal or finite span, and our conception of who we are is tied to that span. Heidegger, Sartre, and Kierkegaard all noted the special moral challenge and quality that goes with our humanity and mortality. If we harness the power of stem cells, perhaps the bodies of human beings as currently affected by the diseases of aging prevalent in Western society will be amenable to repair by cells conditioned to be eternally youthful. Does this mean that we ourselves will have hugely extended life spans? Some workers think so, and others think not. If it does, then our conception of the good life will need serious reflective scrutiny.

The use and investigation of stem cell biology is an intriguing way to look at this and other questions, but it is evident that as we set out on that journey, we should be aware that we are laying ourselves open to questions about our very being. In fact, the same questions are underlined by the ethical issues concerning young human beings, to which I now turn.

CHAPTER FOURTEEN

Save the Life of My Child

Come children, give me your hands, give your mother your hands to kiss them. Oh the dear hands, and O how dear these lips to me, and the generous eyes and the bearing of my children! I wish you happiness, but not here in this world. What is here your father took. Oh, how good to hold you! How delicate the skin, how sweet the breath of children! Go, go! I am no longer able, no longer to look upon you. I am overcome by sorrow.

—EURIPIDES, *THE MEDEA*

Medea speaks these words as she prepares to kill her sons. Because human infants invoke in us special concern and care, the act of infanticide is understandably condemned as unnatural and horrendous. Yet at least one major moral theory not only devalues these intuitions about human infants but actually suggests that they are radically mistaken (Singer 1979; Tooley 1972). The narrative approach, with its naturalistic grounding in human relationships, supports quite different conclusions that confirm our intuitions but allow us to moderate them when an infant lacks the human potential that was pivotal in the debate over embryos. In fact, the emphasis on narrative and virtues can fruitfully be contrasted with consequentialism (and its derivative, utilitarianism) by exploring life-and-death issues in childhood.

Consequentialism and Its Problems

Consequentialism is committed to the basic claim that the moral value of an action is determined by its consequences. What is more, consequentialists, undaunted by the fact that some of their conclusions are counterintuitive, insist that theirs is the only rational strategy in moral argumentation. Many consequentialists invoke a utilitarian calculus of some type to assess the relevant outcomes, but this is problematic because of the incalculability and even incommensurability of different types of outcome (Foot 1985). Glover attempts to alleviate this problem by arguing that utilitarianism is not a precise method of assigning relative values to outcomes but rather "an approximate guide to conduct" (1977, 62–63). However, we are surely entitled to a method suggesting an approximate weighting of different outcomes, and that usually entails that certain simplifications are needed.

The first simplification is that each human life should count as equal to every other. Thus, an outcome that produces five good-quality years of life for individual A should roughly equate to an outcome that produces five good-quality years of life for B (other things being equal). The problems occur when the consequences are of very different general types such as a year of pain-free life for A versus restoring the sight of B. There are even more difficulties once we opt for an acceptable way of assessing consequences and relate them to the preferences or satisfactions of the people concerned. I have already noted that any assessments of value should be completely general and therefore indifferent to which individual is benefited; we could call this the *indifference claim*. The indifference claim implies that nothing essentially individual, such as the death of a particular person (rather than the death of a person with features X, Y, and Z), should influence the moral values in a given situation (that is, apart from its contribution to the sum of general value or disvalue that is brought about). We can now derive two theses, which are important in certain arguments about the treatment of infants and other young human beings.

First, there is no direct wrongness in killing. This claim follows from the idea that the consequences of the killing are all that is important. Thus, provided that side effects such as the effect on other people and the loss of future positively valued states can be taken into account, the actual killing itself is not to be negatively assessed. This conclusion has immediate relevance for infanticide and the replacement of one child by another.

Second, animal lives are essentially equivalent to human lives, which presently realize the same general types of satisfaction (absent a nonconsequentialist reading of potential).

One further complicating factor will have to be admitted into any plausible moral reasoning about young human beings. Quite apart from bare comparisons of satisfactions across different lives, certain practices will cause widespread dis-affection. Thus, for instance, it might be counterproductive to merely sum the total of present satisfactions of an affected group of people because it is plausible that all human beings want the security of knowing that, in general, their own preferences will be respected unless some compelling justification can be given for overriding them. This provides a consequentialist justification for individual rights sufficient to avoid the disruptive effect of "warre where every man is Enemy to every man" (Hobbes). Glover, for instance, contemplates a policy of "euthanasia" for individuals whose lives are substandard to make space for more promising replacement lives. He remarks, "the side effects of such a policy would obviously be calamitous. The remaining population would feel grief, resentment and insecurity on an extreme scale" (1977, 72).

These consequences "show that it is not a policy a utilitarian would favour" (Glover 1977, 72–73). In fact, some utilitarians (such as Singer or Tooley) have a stronger case based in the *preference utility claim:* "an action contrary to the preference of any being is, unless this preference is outweighed by contrary preferences, wrong" (Singer 1979, 80–81). From this claim, it follows that the "kill and replace" policy for melancholics would be wrong. However, this underpinning of individual rights does not protect infants, who lack formed preferences or even ideas about the future.

There is a further problem when we take seriously the intrinsic generality of value that is supposed to guide right action. If my preferences to go on living (and the hypothetical social costs) were outweighed by a weighty set of preferences *out there* that I should die, then because my preferences are outweighed the right thing to do is kill me. But all is not yet lost. One way to save preference utility and avoid widespread social disruption (with its associated disutility) is to invoke a social contract whereby the preferences of each are, within certain limits, respected. Such a social contract might be justified by appeal to the "rule utilitarian" version of consequentialism, but another dilemma then arises.

The dilemma arises whenever my duties under the social contract conflict with my assessment of consequences in the particular case. Therefore, it is "fish or cut bait" time: either actual outcomes are decisive (rendering the social contract subject to so many exceptions that it may become worthless), or the social contract wins, and we have a duty-based morality, a theoretical inconsistency that should make us wary of accepting the underlying assumptions (Glover 1977, 62).

Things get even worse when we intensify our focus on young human beings.

Children and Utilitarianism

Young children are especially vulnerable to a consequentialist grounding of rights and the value of human life. A social contract or preference basis for moral behavior depends on the individuals concerned consciously valuing their own lives. Therefore, "no one capable of understanding what is happening when a newborn baby is killed could feel threatened by a policy which gave less protection to the newborn than to adults" (Singer 1979, 124). For instance, consider two three-week-old infants, both of whom need a neonatal intensive care bed. In the consequentialist view, the competing claims should be resolved in favor of the one who had the best chance of achieving higher net satisfaction in life. Thus, a child having any kind of defect is replaceable by a child not so affected. We might even go further and regard a particular attachment to any individual infant rather than a potential competitor (for instance, a possible future child) as irrational and indicative of deficient moral thinking. Singer claims that we are terribly prone to such thinking when children are being discussed (123).

The alleged mistake of attending too closely to our psychology and "natural attitudes" is generally regarded as unacceptable in philosophy because it substitutes psychologically attractive opinions for a critical evaluation of the conceptual claims being made. In logic or epistemology, this kind of psychologism substitutes persuasion of the many for a demonstration of validity. In moral theory, psychologism is more problematic because of the naturalistic view that there is an intrinsic connection between the psychology and responses of normal human beings and what is, in fact, good and bad. However, we should be able to defend some principled difference between what we feel about an issue and what we should think, where the latter is subject to argument or justification that goes beyond personal dispositions. Consequentialists claim that the relevant arguments turn on an impartial assessment of the outcomes of actions. I can illustrate this claim by returning to the problem of young human beings.

Recall that, in the search for a plausible and universal dimension to use in assessments of the moral value of different lives, we have mooted the idea of preference satisfaction. Such preferences include the desire to go on living, sometimes called future-directed interests or sense of continuing identity, and yield an argument for the right to life. As Tooley notes, such interests cannot plausibly be ascribed to newborn and young infants, and therefore there is no rationally defensible reason why such a right should be invoked when we make life-and-death decisions about such infants (1972). Singer concurs that "only a being which is capable of conceiving itself as a distinct entity existing over time—that is, only a person—could have this right to life" (1979, 82).

This approach effectively denies any such right to an infant, neonate, or fetus. "There are many beings who are conscious and capable of experiencing pleasure and pain, but are not rational and self-conscious and so not persons. Many non-human animals almost certainly fall into this category; so must newborn infants and some mental defectives" (Singer 1979, 84). He concludes, "No infant—defective or not—has as strong a claim to life as beings capable of seeing themselves as distinct entities, existing over time" (131). The conclusion applies, a fortiori, to the life of a fetus where the pregnancy is ended by an early termination. "We can look at the foetus for what it is—the actual characteristics it possesses—and can value its life on the same scale as the lives of beings with similar characteristics who are not members of our species" (117–18).

Having dismissed any special consideration for human beings, he then argues: "Taking the infant in itself, what we have is a sentient being that is neither rational nor self-conscious. Since its species is not relevant to its moral status, the principles that govern the wrongness of killing nonhuman animals who are sentient but not rational or self-conscious must apply here too. These principles are utilitarian. Hence the quality of life that the infant can be expected to have is important" (1979, 32).

That there is no defensible right to life for young human beings and that the essentially general quantum of (preference) satisfaction is the sole determinant of the worth of a life, taken together, yield the conclusion that any individual young human life (A) is disposable or replaceable by another (B) if certain conditions are met. The relevant condition is that life B is likely to exhibit more good experiences than life A. However, this conclusion is unsustainable in the light of a narrative approach, which puts special value on each individual life.

Before continuing, I ought to deal with the objection that the child does have a preference to go on living. This is usually argued on the basis that the child has a number of survival-enhancing dispositions, but, as Glover remarks, the existence of such dispositions implies nothing about any preference to avoid death or go on living. "A baby cannot want to escape from death any more than he can want to escape the fate of being a chartered accountant when he grows up. He has no idea of either" (Glover 1977, 158). He goes on, "The objection to infanticide is *at most* no stronger than the objection to frustrating a baby's current set of desires, say by leaving him to cry unattended for a longish period" (158).

If these conclusions seem callous, things only seem more so when we pursue this lack of intrinsic value even further. Given that children do not have future-directed self-regarding interests, their worth is largely determined by the moral evaluations of significant others. This is too bad for children who are killed by their supposed caregivers: such cases of infanticide then are seen as wrong only because parents and others find the death distressing but not because of the intrinsic moral value of the infant life itself (Singer 1979, 126). It follows that such "side effects" (Glover 1977) on others give only derivative value to the life of the infant, a line with unattractive (and counterintuitive) implications in cases of child abuse.

The theory implies that no special regard attaches to the lives of small infants, and they get moral value only from their parents' preferences. Thus, only if the parents value the infant's life is it valuable, and it is too bad for children whose parents abuse or reject them. If the child is resented and abused, then it follows that the child's life has minimal or even negative value, and we should be morally indifferent as to whether the child is killed or the parents are prosecuted. But it gets worse (or perhaps better if you have a limited child protection budget).

Given that we commonly override the preferences of abusive parents by punishing them and that there are no intrinsic moral goods associated with the life of the infant, then the right thing to do *is* to kill the (valueless) child. Perhaps, if the community in which the unwanted child lives is protein deficient, we should make unwanted children into delicatessen goods, as Swift suggested. According to consequentialists we should not shrink from the intuitive abhorrence of this conclusion merely on the basis of our intuitions.

There are four essential tenets of this objectionable view of the moral worth of children.

1. A life is of value because of features that are essentially generalizable rather than particular to any individual life.
2. A life is morally assessable in its own terms (allowing that ancillary factors such as parental preferences or social consequences must be factored in to some decisions).
3. The core features of any moral situations are essentially impartial so that our natural feelings should not sway our principled moral judgments.

4. Any act such as killing an infant can be adequately assessed in terms of predictable consequences rather than according to other aspects of it.

Metaphysical Reductions

There is a famous passage in moral philosophy in which Hume illustrates that moral judgments involve passion and not merely an appreciation of the facts. He denies that there is any factual difference between patricide and the case of an acorn that falls from an oak and, as it takes root and grows, eventually causes the death of its progenitor (1969, 518–19). Arguing that the facts in these two cases are the same, Hume claims that our moral response to patricide draws on passion and not on reason (call this the *Humean reduction*). However, the son has had a personal relationship with the father involving conversation (in its broadest sense), nurture, training, modeling of certain behavior, mutual understanding, and the many inarticulate things that pass between two people who are part of the same family. Thus, the whole character of the father-son relationship goes beyond anything that could be found in the plant kingdom. Moreover, when one recognizes that these distinctive facts are plausibly central to moral judgments, it becomes obvious that an informed moral judge cannot view the two cases as being the same (even if the natural case was an alligator eating its offspring).

Now we can concede that any moral judge, for instance, in the case of Oedipus, might not be able to come to a clear-cut moral judgment of the patricidal son and might even endorse what he does, but moral indifference (plausibly appropriate in the other cases) is a sign of insensitivity rather than rationality. The facts of the case, rightly considered, are central in our assessment of the moral issues even though the relationship between morals and metaphysics may be quite complex. I would argue that our moral judgments are inextricably interwoven with an interconnected web of ideas, including what Strawson calls "reactive attitudes" (1974).

Strawson notes that our beliefs in such things as the freedom of the individual and responsibility for one's own actions are inseparable from a range of reactive (including moral) attitudes such as resentment, indignation, praise, blame, entitlement, compassion, and so on. He argues that these (reactive) attitudes are part of a way of thinking that is integral to our everyday life together as human beings. This way of thinking is, however, quite distinct from a scheme portraying human beings as biological entities caused by impersonal forces and internal mechanisms to behave in certain ways (although that might also be true of us in the terms of a certain kind of discourse). What is more, he argues that our reactive attitudes are part of what we call rationality or reasonableness, in that they are indispensable to the cognitive world in which we deal with each other as meaningful individuals. By contrast, the "objective or reductive scheme" concerned with purely physical descriptions of objects, mechanisms, and impersonal forces, if uncritically applied to human behavior, undermines the interpersonal attributes that structure our discursive and moral universe.

In thinking about very young human lives, we are obviously torn between wanting to regard them as human beings and acknowledging that they are not the kind of human beings who are part of our moral discourse. If we then extend our reflection to things such as human embryos, we find ourselves in a place where our moral judgments no longer have clear implications. Reflection on the moral thought of either Aristotle or Wittgenstein tells us that we are plagued by moral uncertainty in our life-and-death decisions about embryos and fetuses because these are not part of the normal fabric of our moral experience.

However, consequentialist ideas are worse than useless in this area. I have already made use of potentiality to illuminate the debates surrounding embryos in the face of enjoinders to look at the very young human life only in terms of "the actual characteristics it possesses" (Singer 1979, 117). "Actual characteristics," read too narrowly, makes us overlook important morally relevant characteristics of the object or event being discussed. Without suitably sharpened sensitivities, when we are faced with the ambiguities I have already canvassed and the threat of the Humean reduction, our thinking can be deflected away from the intuitions that are essential to moral reasoning and that draw on our life among other human beings with whom we are in a myriad of emotionally and psychologically significant relationships.

Anticonsequentialist Thoughts about Young Human Lives

I can deepen and articulate certain features of this dilemma by considering the central questions that are problematic for consequentialist writing about young human beings.

Does the moral worth of a human life depend essentially on general features that a life currently realizes or is likely to realize? I argue that the case of children suggests that this is not true to our moral thinking and that therefore this tenet, basic to most types of consequentialism, should be rejected. It is tenable only if a selective Humean reduction is allowed to color the metaphysics of young human lives and the assessment of their moral value.

Is each life separable from each other and individually assessable for its intrinsic moral value? This reductive methodological individualism about human lives and their value is central to many theories, including many varieties of social contract theory, but it is questionable when looking at issues in infancy and childhood.

Can we justify the exclusion of significant and directed emotional attachments and commitments from rational moral deliberation? I do not think we can, and to do so exposes us to rationalistic bullying (of which consequentialism is the most obvious type) in ethics.

Are acts properly evaluated according to consequential assessments of them so that, for instance, contraception = abortion = infanticide? I think not.

In What Does the Worth of a Young Human Life Consist?

Why do human lives matter morally? A utilitarian would say that they matter because each person's life has the consequence of adding to the (indeterminate) sum of preferences and satisfactions in the universe and also because they matter to the human being concerned. Yet this gives us no basis for claiming that any particular individual matters, all things being equal. To be sure, we can say that the early death of someone like Mozart matters on three counts: (1) he is deprived of a future life with its satisfactions; (2) these near to him are deprived of his company in which they find pleasure; and (3) he might have significantly added to the pleasures of many others through the music he would have composed had he gone on living. For lesser mortals, the first two of these apply, but for *young* lesser mortals only (2) applies.

Thus, when asked why children matter and why, in particular, it should matter to a parent that a particular child should die from cot death (SIDS, or sudden infant death syndrome), we are struck dumb by the strong consequentialist line. Given that the child might be replaced by another, that the parents might find equal satisfactions in raising that other child, and that the replacement child is likely to achieve similar states of well-being, it seems irrational to regard the loss of that particular child as anything special. It follows that, for a consequentialist, health care resources devoted to saving particular infant lives, through, for instance, a cot death prevention program, are not to be valued because they save the lives of particular children. Any value would seem to come from relieving irrational parental distress. The irrational attachment that seems to form between parents and particular children is, of course, problematic, but there may be other more general reasons for tolerating it.

However, most of us believe that each individual child does matter and that the way in which each one matters is quite independent of any attitudes of their parents. In fact, rather than making parental attitudes definitive of the moral worth of children, we look askance at parents who do not form a caring and individually directed attachment to each of their children. But can we defend this belief?

A child, from birth at least, and some would claim from conception, can truly be perceived as having a unique relational and discursive place among us. I am reminded of a little boy whose infant brother died when a few weeks old. Some weeks before he died, the boy had said, when holding the baby on his knee, "I am your older brother." Now, this boy had already embraced that infant, as had the whole family, as a unique human being with his own name and history (albeit short), his own time of coming into the world, and any number of other features that, subtly but unambiguously, made that infant one of us and also different from any other individual.

These aspects of our thinking are an inherent part of our rationally articulated interpersonal and moral lives, hence the importance of an individual infant. For this reason, the individuality, and indeed irreplaceability, of each infant is a basic feature of our thinking about them. In the account of metaphysics that I have sketched, Singer's sparse view of "actual characteristics," couched in general terms, does not capture the metaphysics of young human beings and therefore fails to reveal the things that are directly relevant to our moral thinking about them.

We could say that a being is intrinsically of value if, even potentially, it is a being who is one of us in a morally reciprocal sense (Thomson 2000). It has this value in that the only basis on which we can understand and relate to an infant as a metaphysical type takes origin in the complex reactive and interpersonal attitudes that cause us to respect and value each other as individuals and the infant as one who belongs among us.

Is Methodological Individualism Sustainable in Ethics?

I have sketched a relational basis for our moral attitudes and traced it to the essentially reactive milieu in which infant lives are located and in which our thinking about them makes sense. In this milieu, an infant engages me and offers me an opportunity to care for him or her as an individual. I cannot prize the individual loose from his or her discursive location so as to define his or her "actual characteristics." Therefore, only if the consequentialist bestiary of essentially general and impersonal metaphysical properties is uncritically accepted can we regard young human lives as of diminished worth and therefore disposable or replaceable. When we consider the uniquely instantiated set of relations we have with any particular young human being who is among us, related to us, and vulnerable to each of us in terms of its very survival, then the infant is seen to be unique and can be replaced only in an attenuated sense. Another individual child who will make the same kind of demand for my nurture and care might come into my life, but this "replacement" does not compensate for our loss (and carries its own moral and psychological hazards). Any infant or young human being not only has a place of belonging ("a place in our hearts") but also inspires nurture in the rest of us for that very reason.

Another fact relevant to our moral thought about young human lives is that they are, as I have noted, subject to noncontractual attitudes (because they cannot form reciprocal contracts of consideration and respect). Therefore, our moral responses to them reflect the value we place on human life in itself as distinct from the value we place on the lives of those whom we have self-directed interests to respect. It follows that our answers to moral questions about young human lives evince our commitment to the values of being-with in contrast to attitudes based on individualistic conceptions of good. I have argued that attitudes of the relational or being-with type are inherently more virtuous than individualistic attitudes. We might go so far as to say that a moral system truly counts as such only insofar as it is built on attitudes of the former sort and, as a result, pays special regard to the vulnerable and powerless.

Making Visible the Sources of Moral Judgment

These speculations about what counts as a moral attitude lead naturally to reflection on the sources of moral judgment. I have suggested that the fundamental bases of moral reasoning arise within relationships and include relational facts such as dependence and attachment. On this richer basis we might be able to locate intuitions that lie deep in our ethical reasoning and focus on the inherently intersubjective nature of human well-being. Intersubjectivity then appears to be not incidental to but formative of human identity, and it produces a range of implicit demands and commitments operating between human individuals. Consider the child who is held by his father and thereby becomes *this little child whom I have held, who needs me, and in whose life I have a nurturing role.* That father cannot regard this child with indifference because it does not have the cognitive life that he has. And if he could do so, he would not be rational and morally intelligent but rather evince an impaired personality and character. A psychopath, for instance, might act this way. The kind of moral sensitivity involved when I engage with or open myself to a little child does, of course, make me keenly aware of any consequence of my actions on that child, but that feature of my moral attitudes is not at all like the objective considerations that figure in consequentialist writing about such situations.

Actions, Consequences, and Moral Value

I have attacked a strong consequentialist position, and yet consequences have an obvious role in our assessments of actions. Does this mean that I am a closet "weak consequentialist" who is reluctant to "come out" as such?

I have already noted that certain kinds of social contract or rule utilitarianism veer close to alternative metaethical theories such as deontology, or duty theory. I might similarly challenge a consequentialist justification appealing to such things as the general undesirability or inherent disvalue of a society in which people are disposed to act in nasty ways. This latter view comes so close to virtue ethics that its distinctively consequentialist character dies the death of a thousand qualifications.

Any view that commends certain actions because we are essentially beings-in-relation with certain types of dispositions is not really a kind of consequentialism. For instance, a view in which we ought to treat certain beings in certain ways just because they are of a given ontological type should be grouped with deontological theories. Similarly, the idea that we ought to act in certain situations as guided by the caring relationships in which we find ourselves should be placed within the ethics of care. In any or all of these approaches, we might consider the consequences of our actions, but this does not group those theories, in any interesting way, with the more full-blooded kinds of consequentialism.

Looking only at consequences does not allow us to make visible the differences between the destruction of embryos, abortion, and infanticide. But these actions are different. In my view, the young human lives involved instantiate different chapters of the human story that is an individual life. The embryo is so early that the human form is not really evident, and it is also a phase of development where there is a high rate of natural attrition. Our attitudes toward an embryo are, as a result, much more remote from our attitudes to children and our peers than are our attitudes to formed fetuses at later developmental stages. The fetus changes from something barely human to something with an instantly recognizable human form, and our attitudes shift accordingly. The reactions we have to the loss or sacrifice of such a thing also change. Here on the horizon of life (albeit nonsentient and inaccessible to empathy) is one who was coming among us but whose journey has failed. Then, after birth, "the mewling puking infant" is there with his or her demands on us, a small and sacred charge for whom we feel responsible. This being calls forth in us empathic and caring responses that are unambiguous. He engages us as an individual, and we give him a name. He is unique. His loss will be felt as a small void in the human universe that can never quite be filled by any other. That is the reality of the thing, and that is what makes ethics so nonnegotiable for all of us, even though if a book contained the whole description of the world it might not capture that remarkable fact (Wittgenstein 1965, 6). It falls to ethics to bring out what is valuable and really important here, which are things connected with the meaning of life and "what makes life worth living" in the right kind of way (5). I think that our moral thoughts and attitudes regarding children are genuinely instructive in that respect, and it seems to me remarkable that so widely prevalent a set of ethical theories should get them so spectacularly wrong.

Our attitudes to children and to our origins as human individuals are sharply relevant to the fraught topic of cloning, which will bring this volume to its close.

CHAPTER FIFTEEN

Joanna May Revisited

The Cloning Debate

> Sperm is a product which comes from the whole body of each parent, weak
> sperm coming from the weak parts, and strong sperm from the strong
> parts. The child must necessarily correspond. If from any part of the
> father's body a greater quantity of sperm is derived than from the corre-
> sponding part of the mother's body the child will, in that part, bear a closer
> resemblance to its father; and vice versa. The following cases are impossi-
> ble: (a) the child resembles the mother in all respects, and its father in
> none; (b) the child resembles its father in all respects, and its mother in
> none; (c) the child resembles neither parent in any respect. No: it must
> inevitably resemble each parent in some respect, since it is from both par-
> ents that the sperm comes to form the child.   —THE SEED

The age-old wisdom captured by the Hippocratic writers (and explained according to their own ideas—which seem remarkably accurate if one substitutes either
the term *DNA* or *genetic material* for *sperm*) no longer holds in an age of cloning.
Reproductive cloning allows us to recreate the genetic template of a human individual. When it was first mooted, it drew almost universal condemnation (Brock
1998, 141) but it has proved difficult to enunciate just what is wrong with reproductive cloning and why we have such strong intuitions about it. Is this a case
where our intuitions stand in need of schooling by reasoned debate? We ought
first to survey those moral intuitions and see why they do not survive reflective
scrutiny.

There are arguments that condemn our interference in fundamental decisions about life and death. Perhaps it is wrong for us to manipulate fundamental natural givens that God (in her infinite wisdom) or nature (after years of slow
evolutionary change) has decreed. But this argument seems to ignore the evident fact that much of what we do in contemporary medicine is aimed precisely
at human intervention in and manipulation of birth, life, and death.

There are a set of ideas about the identification of clones as duplicate human beings (genetic reductionism) and the justifications and harms attached to being a replacement child.

Three areas of significant debate concern our socioculturally entrenched beliefs about reproduction and its significance, the idea of parenting, and the intention to make copies of existing human beings. These debates engage us with human individuality in a way that links metaphysics and cultural signification. I argue that something lurks at the root of these latter issues that is the real source of our moral discontent about cloning and also forms an important and semistable basis for intuitions about human beings and their value.

What Is the Problem?

In Fay Weldon's *The Cloning of Joanna May*, Joanna May's ovaries, at her husband's request and without her knowledge, are stimulated. Four ova are taken and cloned, and the resulting human individuals are implanted into four different women, each of whom comes to believe she has been enabled to give birth to her own child. These four women raise their clones of Joanna May in ignorance of the existence of the others and as individuals.

This is hardly a model of ethical practice in reproductive medicine, and Joanna May's treatment would undoubtedly be condemned throughout the ethics community in the Western world. The reasons given would surely include that Joanna May did not give consent to being reproduced in this way. The general public, judging by the widespread reactions to cloning, would go further and argue that even if an individual did want to be reproduced by cloning, it should not be a permissible choice. Why is this?

Cloning produces a genetic replica of an already living human being. This could be achieved by a number of means: by taking a cell from an existing person, causing it to dedifferentiate and form a pre-embryo, and then regrowing it into a new human being; or by taking genetic material from one person and inserting it into the cytoplasm of a cell, which would then be grown into a human embryo; and so on through a range of techniques currently being devised.

Yet we ought to question the motives for cloning. In the Joanna May story the husband wanted to have replacement "Joanna Mays" available in case he lost his wife. His motive seems to violate something basic about Joanna May herself and the kinds of relations that ought to prevail between men and women and that may well serve as a clue to the moral disquiet that inchoately clusters around these issues.

I therefore look at the following arguments:

1. It is not right for human beings to meddle in basic matters of life and death ([Danish Council of Ethics 2002]—already looking flimsy).
2. We should not copy existing human beings (Danish Council; Brock 1998; Thomson 2000).
3. No child should be a replacement child (Danish Council; Brock).
4. Cloning treats children as commodities (Thomson; Brock; Danish Council).
5. Cloning exposes children to unknown risks (Brock).
6. The right to reproduce is insufficient to justify cloning (Thomson).

I explore these arguments and the ethics of cloning through three hypothetical scenarios.

Bob and Alison and the Argument about Intervention in Nature

Bob and Alison are devastated because they have learned, from an intensivist, that their three-year-old son, James, has suffered severe brain damage in a road accident and will almost certainly be dead within twenty-four hours. However, they have read that doctors in the United Kingdom can take a few cells from a child and form new embryos. The technique involves extracting the nucleus from the child's cell and introducing it into an enucleated cell of the mother to form a new single-celled pre-embryo. They envisage cloning a new James, having the embryo implanted in Alison's womb, and getting James back again in nine months time. They approach James's physician with their request.

Most of us, faced by this increasingly possible situation, feel that there is something wrong with Bob and Alison's request. Some answers, though, do not wash. We could not, for instance, say that we should not decide about life and death because we have allowed James to be admitted to the intensive care unit so as to try to save his life.

Hume makes a similar response when he addresses the argument that human life is not ours to give or take in relation to the wrongness of suicide ([1776] 1980, 100). He observes that the claim that our lives belong to God and that he is sovereign over their endings (and beginnings) does not ring true in practice. For instance, we would not dream of standing by and watching a brick fall onto a person's head and kill her just because we felt that it might be God's time to take her. The fact is that we do "give" and "take" human lives in a number of different circumstances including:

1. the use of artificial reproductive technologies when people cannot have children without help;
2. refusal of medical treatment in conditions where we feel it is wrong to prolong life;
3. strenuous attempts, particularly in neonatal care, to save children whom nature (or God) would otherwise take from us.

We therefore need an ethical justification for objections to cloning other than a reluctance to deliver mortal responsibilities into human hands.

In the case of Joanna May, there was no informed consent to the embryo donation nor to the embryos being implanted. What is more, we were suspicious about the motives being served by the cloning. Are there any parallels in the present case? If there are, they concern the ethical status of the parents' wishes and the best interests of the to-be-cloned child.

Although parents would normally give consent to procedures on behalf of a child of three (indeed, that seems inescapable when the child is comatose), we should always ask ourselves whose needs are being met and whether the planned intervention is *in the best interests of the child.* This is crucial, for instance, when we do not allow Jehovah's Witness parents to refuse a blood transfusion for their child. Thus, when asking parents about a procedure on a child, we consider whether the intervention is justified from the child's perspective. In the present case we should therefore ask whether James should be cloned to produce James II (or, in terms of the parents' fantasy) whether James should be resurrected. If they are going to think that way, then we might be concerned about whether they are well placed to consent to this procedure. The idea of James's "coming back to life" raises both a metaphysical issue and a concern about the consequences for James II of being born as the quintessential replacement child.

Who Is James II?

The metaphysical issue raised by the cloning of James is best approached through a question. Bob and Alison might well ask, "What is the difference between restoring a baby to life through neonatal intensive care and restoring our James through this cloning technique?" The most persuasive response here is that the individual that results from the cloning procedure, whoever it is, would not be James. However, it is not quite so clear that this is correct because the new individual would have James's genetic constitution and be gestated by the same mother, within the same family setting. If we were to accept a view of identity according to which my identity is jointly determined by my derivation from a pair of gametes (Parfit 1986; McMahan 1998) and accept that the same gametes yield the same human individual, then it follows that James II is James reborn. However, if individuality goes with some sort of historically indexed Aristotelian form claim then, arguably, James II is a different individual because his life trajectory starts at a different point in time, comprises different events, and does not conform to the kind of trajectory normally counted as one life. I have opted for the latter view and therefore am inclined to think that Bob and Alison are making a metaphysical mistake, but the problems and the arguments are sharpened by exploring two other, closely related, scenarios.

Consider, to make vivid the hope implicit in Bob and Alison's request, a different case.

> Carrie and Dave have a three-year-old son, Karl, who, like James, is expected to die within twenty-four hours. They are told of a new and experimental treatment that promotes reconstruction of injured nerve pathways. The patient spends weeks or up to a year recovering but, if successful, the recovery is miraculous. The fact that the method is reconstructive causes psychological differences between the individual that emerges and the one that was injured. For instance, cognitive skills must be relearned, most of the person's memories (crucially dependent on the integrity of the whole system) are lost, and some aspects of temperament may be altered. However, the technique has produced good results and, if it does, the doctors expect Karl to emerge, amnesic but recognizably the same as before the accident. Carrie and Dave are very keen to go ahead.

I have described Karl postreconstruction as recognizably the same as before his injury. Notice that Karl has never been declared dead and then buried. These crucial facts are evidently discursive, but then so are other important aspects of our lives. Death and burial would presumably happen in James's case and are important cultural ways of marking the end of a human life (just as a ceremony marks the beginning of a marriage). Now, if we are attentive to our moral intuitions, it is hard to dispute Carrie and Dave's decision because it offers them the hope that Karl will be restored to them. Before the choice was offered, they had no hope, and it seems little different from a course of neurological care producing recovery from head injury not altogether different in its effects from current intensive care and neurorehabilitation. It seems hard to advance ethical objections to this type of technique.

There are similarities between the stories of James and Karl, but a third hypothetical case sharpens the need for an analysis that underlines significant moral differences between them.

> Evan and Fiona's son, Luke, has a severe brain injury and is predicted to die, but they receive new hope when a "neuroreconstructionist" tells them about a technique whereby a combination of enzymes, growth factors, and microelectrical stimulation according to a three-dimensional graphics program could restore John's brain. The process takes about eight months (i.e., the same as fetal growth and differentiation of the brain). Luke will lose all his memories, may have a different temperament, and will require reeducation as for a newborn baby (he will catch up with his peers three or four years after his reconstruction). Evan and Fiona realize that they are facing an enormous task but are so overjoyed at the prospect of not losing Luke that they are more than willing to go ahead.

Those philosophically inclined to accept a "mind/brain life" or Lockean view of personal identity (as outlined in chapter 10) would regard Luke's case as almost identical to the cloning of James in that it is a rebirth, at least of the brain. How similar are these two cases?

If genetic and biological factors are all important, and if rebirth is possible within numerical identity, then James II could be James reborn. But there may be a difference between James and James II if human identity is not just a function of genetics and narrow biology such that the neo-Lockean (mental life) view should not be construed purely biologically. I believe that an account of individual identity in which each of us is a narratively defined individual within a network of relationships is a more adequate basis for dealing with our moral intuitions.

Locke and his followers, as we have seen, link individuality to the "mind," conceived of as an inner component of the person which is, in some sense, like an object and could be transferred from one individual to another (Locke [1689] 1975, 336). This idea is central to Locke's thought experiment about the prince and the pauper. But a better conception of whatever underlies personal identity would be the functioning of an individual who has the form of a rational and social being and has a unique discursive place among others. Such an Aristotelian conception focuses on a process or "dynamic" rather than a type of object (albeit of an odd metaphysical kind—mental, spiritual, or nonphysical in some other way).

The discursive view is that individuation takes place in a set of formative relationships, subtly different for each numerical individual. In this account each individual is a "node" of significant human interactions that affect and mold that human being so that he or she develops self-understanding and a conception of his or her own identity (Harre 1983; Hacking 1995). These thoughts are incorporated into the discursive view of human identity. "The discursive view of individuality and personality does not need to find a distinct constellation of inner processes to explain the uniqueness of each human being because every human being is given as unique in ways directly relevant to psychological explanation. Each human being stands at a unique intersection point of human discourses and relationships" (Harre and Gillett 1994, 132–33).

The discursive view implies that the difference between James on the one hand, and Karl and Luke on the other is significant. Being declared dead and being buried in a funeral ceremony (or whatever is done in that individual's culture) are significant moral moments in the history of an individual in a community. They mark the fact that that individual's narrative is closed, however tragically short it might have been, and they give a narrative or discursive expression to the reality of death. James II is discursively marked as a different person from James. Whereas Karl and Luke (pre- and postreconstruction) both have bodily continuity and can continue their lives after recovery from a near-tragic episode, the same does not apply to James. Imagine that Bob and Alison have James's body cremated, thinking of this as discarding a body that James has left behind while he is waiting to be reborn. Now perhaps there are cultural settings in which that view might prevail, but it is not ours. In a Western cultural setting, we would expect Bob and Alison to declare James's life ended when his body is destroyed so that any subsequent events would be predicated in that ideological framework.

According to Western culture, James dies, his body is destroyed, and in Alison's womb a new human life begins. This new person has a unique (in the simple scenario) relationship to James, but there is a break that prevents us thinking of him as James. One might posit many aspects of the newness and difference of that life (biological differences between James and James II, such as that Alison is older and her hormonal state has changed, perhaps in part because of James's death), but none of them encompasses the discursive reality that, applied to an embodied being living among us, forms the individual as a person.

And there are other influences structuring the situation into which James II is born:

1. Alison will feel differently about this pregnancy than she felt about James' pregnancy;
2. James II will have a different place in the family from James—he will be a child who has been born following a devastating accident to an older child;
3. James II will at some stage have the knowledge that he has a dead older brother;
4. James II will, perhaps, note a wistful déjà vu quality to some of the ways in which his parents regard him although he may not be able to name that (Nussbaum 1998).

These and many other significant psychological, relational, and therefore moral, differences will tend to make James II different from James. Therefore, we can say that we should not think that James is resuming his life, or coming back to life, or even "entering into his mother's womb and being born again." James II *is* a replacement child a fortiori, and we must deal with the ethics of creating replacement children if we want to look out for his best interests.

Replacement Children

James II will be born as a replacement child, even more so than in the currently possible scenarios in which children can be called that. He will almost certainly be compared with James throughout his developing life and contrasted with the ideal and unrealistic image that is the legacy of the dead. This set of expectations and parental responses can be a major and often quite destructive burden for such a child. The Danish Council of Ethics remarks that "it may be negative for children to be born or adopted either as surrogate children for dead siblings or to come into the world under parents who, for other reasons, have an overt desire to shape their personality in the image of another (2002, 21). However, we must also recognize that something similar can happen when a family loses a child through cot death and is encouraged to have another child. Although this advice may seem harsh and even to embody the view that children are replaceable commodities, it need not. Yet is the disvalue of James II being regarded as a replacement sufficient to entail that he should not be born? Prima facie one could argue that to be born at all is good rather than bad (McMahan

1998), and Brock argues that "these psychological burdens, hard though they might be, are not so bad as to make the twin's [clone's] life, all things considered, not worth living" (1998, 156). Thomson counters: "every child should be valued in his or her own right, and not seen as a replacement for an earlier sibling" (2000, 36). However, often the "have another child" policy is an eminently sensible response to the grief and guilt of a mother who, whatever we say, tends to believe that she has failed when a cot death occurs. The new child is a new chance to nurture and care for a child and for her mothering story to end quite differently than it otherwise would. A child dies, and a new child comes to birth; most families are not under the illusion that the new child is the old one recovered. Unlike the cot death case, however, Bob and Alison are choosing to have "another James," whom they expect to be like James. It would therefore be hard to deny that James II would live with a magnified version of whatever burdens replacement children suffer. However, even if all that is true, is James II likely to suffer to the extent that he should not be born?

This proscription seems a bit excessive because, even though it is hard to talk about the best interests of a child who is not yet conceived, it is an argument against his parents thinking of him as being another James and not an argument against their having him at all. Also, when we consider arguments for having a replacement child and weigh them against the burdens that might accrue to the child as a result, we are still prepared to recommend it after a cot death. Thus, we do not seem to have a good enough reason in the "replacement child" argument to oppose cloning. We could just as well stipulate that Bob and Alison have some counseling about treating the clone as another James. Yet if we do persuade them that the clone will not be another James, then their principal motivation for cloning is gone.

Images of and Reasons for Reproduction

Joanna May's husband cloned her because he wanted to retrieve, own, or control a "Joanna May" that would be his in the way that she was when they were younger. What is more, he would have four copies that he knew about, could locate, and regain power over because they would be versions of her that had not undergone what he regarded as adverse changes. But the four clones were not "Joanna Mays"; they had their own names and identities, which resembled Joanna May in some respects and differed from her in others. Fay Weldon describes five very different women, all genetically identical, none of which could replace any of the others except in the sense that one person can take another's place. If Weldon is right, then Joanna May's husband has made a serious mistake. Joanna May is not a property that he can duplicate at will, and she does not develop only in predictable ways that make her authorship of her own life irrelevant. Joanna May is her own person and not a doll to be kept in a doll's house life. These misgivings apply to any person who will not accept that another human being is to some extent a "self-maker," and would be equally true if a woman used cloning to try to produce a tame or dependent version of her lover (perhaps as a child copy).

These transactions and relationships, like all moral exchanges, take place in a cultural setting overlaid by the cultural symbols and images surrounding procreation: bloodline, *whakapapa* (genealogy), lineage, continuity of ourselves through time in our offspring, and so on. The cultural significances of human birth, life, and death are not mere illusions associated with the real facts of the matter (revealed by biology), they are the fons et origo of moral thinking. Their power is evident when we hear of aging bachelors wanting to "sire" a son and being ready to pay someone to act as "dam." Imagine that the desire is focused and includes a readiness to support the child but no further demands for relationship apart from the knowledge that the son exists and "lives on." A number of intuitively suspect meanings combine to set up such a scenario. Not least among these are the many patriarchal stereotypes about women as fetus producers necessary to perpetuate the male blood lineage. Further images of "potency," "planting of seed," and "getting with child" also spring to mind, with similarly uncomfortable moral overtones. The power of the procreative images that pervade our thinking about human origins and the need to take them seriously when we consider technological interventions in human origins is demonstrated in another area of our thinking about children.

Adoptees seem to have problems in constructing self-narratives; the most major seems to be a deep sense of abandonment that motivates the concept of "the primal wound" (Verrier 1991). "Genetic bewilderment" is another issue affecting such children, and both concepts are obliquely relevant to cloning, as can be seen when we pursue the phrase "a place to stand."

We all seem to need some idea of where we fit and of how we came to be born with a particular identity and name that determine just who we are. This need is recognized when we grasp the wrongness of an adopted child being raised in complete ignorance of his or her origins and siblings. Children have a "Who am I?" or "Where do I really belong?" reaction when they learn of their adoption.

Many try to find their biological origins and to recover some relatedness to the parents and siblings with whom they might otherwise have been raised. A sense of personal self-location seems, therefore, to be important to children. The idea of genetic bewilderment is also common in ethical debates about the interests of children produced by assisted human reproductive techniques. Such unease or bewilderment could arise from either uncertainty about lineage or perceived differences between oneself and one's peers. Only the latter would apply in cloning, but concepts like the primal wound emphasize the deeply relational nature of the identities of children and therefore reinforce the significance of origins that deviate from the sociocultural norm. The Danish Council for Ethics argues that cloning violates an important kind of intuitive knowledge about our own origins (also expressed in the Hippocratic writings): "That new human life is formed by the union of a sperm cell and an egg cell from two different people of different sexes, thereby having both a biological father and a biological mother and simultaneously coming into existence as a unique individual that is not a replica of another person who has already lived" (2002, 18–19).

Again we must ask whether these worries are sufficient reason to proscribe human cloning. What if we could strip these images and symbols from our reproductive lives? Would cloning then be acceptable? What if the intuitions clustering around genetics were jettisoned?

These suggestions are clearly on the wrong tack. To think that we could jettison such deep-rooted intuitions and attitudes is to betray an almost staggering naïvety about human thought and meaning. A number of literary works, albeit influenced by the science of their day, demonstrate that these intuitions are firmly rooted within us, planted and nurtured by biology and culture, which jointly form, for human beings, their natural and evolutionary history (as postmodernism reminds us). They are not detachable from our conception of the kind of beings we are, which is, at least in part, a cultural production. I have claimed that any sensitive account of the metaphysics of human lives does not clearly separate cultural conceptions of humanity and the metaphysics of personal identity. Therefore, James II cannot easily be released from his fate as a clone of James, and that may not be a healthy fate. There are also reasons to believe that at least some of the wishes and choices that go into the making of James II or the clones of Joanna May are themselves sufficiently misguided for us not to encourage them. These have to do, among other things, with images of parenting.

Parenting

In discussing the ethics of parenting and arguments about whose interests are served by bringing a child into the world, we might, at first pass, think of Kant's dictum that every person should be treated as an end in himself and not purely as a means to anyone else's ends. Yet this dictum is hard to apply in any straightforward way to parenting.

First, the reason for creating James II no more makes him a means to the parents' ends than the creation of any child whose parents desire to have a child (for whatever reasons). We surely cannot accept a blanket condemnation of procreation in general (although one might not favor evolutionary ethics, surely antisurvival ethics is a nonstarter). The counterargument that reproduction is acceptable provided that it is done for reasons of duty alone and not because of the desires of parents (a kind of "close your eyes and think of England" view of marital relations) also fails. It fails because then the child would not be produced for the sake of the child but because of the parents' urge to fulfil their duties to procreate. Kavka (1981) speaks of a modified categorical imperative according to which we are not to treat rational beings or their creation as a means to an end, but it is not clear that his idea solves any of these problems.

Second, if the child is born not because parents deliberately decide to have a child (for its own sake or for the sake of duty), then the child is a mere side effect of the means to another end entirely, that of sexual gratification. This, of course, does not harm the child, but it does make the production of the child an accident that may or may not be welcome. Even though it is common, the inadvertent creation of a human individual does seem somewhat careless and therefore mildly irresponsible if not downright vicious. This argument is not applicable to cloning, but it does affect our moral assessment of the virtuous reasons for parenting (to which I shall return). In most cases, the serendipity of conception and the creation of life are both absorbed in the open-endedness of a good life and the goods arising from a child coming into a loving family.

There are, however, circumstances in which we might be worried that the clone or clones were being regarded as commodities. Imagine, for instance, that Bob and Alison are both intelligent but poor (philosophy graduates perhaps) and that James was a good-looking, normal-to-advanced child with predictions that he would be above average on most indicators. Bob and Alison ask if not one but five clones can be made so that the other four can be sold to give James

II the financial security that they, despite their intelligence and good looks, cannot be sure they will be able to provide (they are utilitarians). Here the other four clones, apart from the one they keep, are clearly commodities, and, although there might be four couples made very happy by each having one of the clones, we might balk at the prospect. What is more, even though Bob and Alison are making the other clones for the sake of James II and his future, it is a matter of chance which of them is chosen as James II and therefore they are all tarred with the same (market-oriented) brush.

For many people, the whole idea of commodification damages our image of children and renders the motives in such a case vicious *sans phrase* (Danish Council of Ethics 2002, 19). But I have noted (as has Dan Brock) the many, albeit consequentialist, arguments about the prospective benefits to everybody involved (to Bob and Alison, James II, and the four other clones), which seem to undermine our moral scruples about commodification or a modified categorical imperative (four of the clones were clearly created as means to ends). One might wonder, however, if there is a conceptualization of parenting that makes it come out as virtuous rather than vicious and that redeems the inadvertent conception case.

Tom Murray offers an argument about eugenic attitudes and practices and nondirective genetic counseling that seems relevant to human clones. He identifies an understanding of parenthood that is intrinsically wrong because it "grants to prospective parents the right to seek a child as near perfect as possible, leaving it to those prospective parents to make their own definition of 'perfection'" (Murray 1996, 133). Now, Murray does not object to measures that parents might take to correct genetic problems in a potential child where the correction is aimed at a widely recognized severe genetic defect that produces significant suffering. Yet Murray's antieugenic stand in favor of nonjudgmental (or nonselective and nonperfectionist) parenting is relevant to the cloning case envisaged because Bob and Alice conceive of the clone as being the same as James and they would be less than satisfied with any other child. This does not evince what Murray calls the "unconditional acceptance" that is an important part of parental love for children and that we ought to value. The Danish Council of Ethics takes a similar stance, arguing "that each of us comes into the world as something new and something special" (2002, 19). Even if we accept this, though, we must ask whether psychological harm is significant compared with nonexistence (Brock 1998).

The unconditional acceptance of the carelessly created child can be seen as a morally redeeming feature common to much everyday parenting and so receives further support from its role in that discussion, but it is hard to assess the moral weight it should be given. It is also unclear whether these "eugenic" (or conditional acceptance) worries apply if the only reproductive choice available to provide a couple with a genetically related child is to clone one of the parents.

Something important is being asserted here, and it is clear that the glib face-off between nonexistence and the elusive psychological harms of being a replacement do not quite capture it. In fact, there is a suspicious move made in setting up the debate in that way because, on reflection, it is far from obvious that there is any such thing as "the harm of nonexistence." For a start, there is no one to be harmed. Therefore, this has meaning only if we assess harm as accruing when some metaphysical or utilitarian sum of states of happiness is diminished because some of the possible subjective loci of happiness are not in existence. I have questioned every facet of that conception of goodness and suggested that it "dies the death of a thousand qualifications."

One Person, One Life

If we regard James II as James reborn, we might argue that each person should have one life and that we should not use medical technology to pander to the abnormal desire of some individuals that someone (perhaps themselves) should have two. Nevertheless, there are a large number of people who believe that human beings do not have only one life. If, as some believe, a reincarnated life allows you to improve on your first effort and come closer to the ideal, why not have two or even more lives in which to become perfected as a human individual? This (possibly vulgar) interpretation of a widespread belief implies that the stark claim that we should have only one life does not have any privileged status as one of our basic intuitions.

However, it is not that simple. Reincarnation emerges from a tradition with a different symbolism and foundational set of images than Western individualistic views of human identity. For instance, Christians might see a person's reincarnated fate as the outcome of some judgment or choice by a divine being, but Hinduism sees that as an inevitable karmic outcome of the evolution of spirituality within a given mortal life, and it is not clear that anything like the named self-conscious person or individual (as conceived of in the West) returns to live among us in any form whatsoever. Thus, we have to face the cultural embeddedness of our moral convictions and, in the light of that realization, turn to the nagging thought that some regard as an unquestionable moral intuition that each human person should be regarded as a unique creation and not a copy of anyone else (National Bioethics Advisory Commission 1997).

In discussing this thought, I should note that it does not apply to twins or n-tuplets of any other kind (apart from the so-called GIDA—genetically identical different aged—twins that cloning produces [Thomson 2000]). The situation of ordinary identical twins is similar to that of clones (or GIDA twins) in that they are genetic duplicates, but I have already argued that genetics alone are not enough to secure identity of the person. Identical twins are formed from the same pre-embryo, which splits at a certain point, and from that point they develop separately and are born at more or less the same time. They are raised as contemporaries and usually in the same interpersonal, social, and cultural setting, and yet, even with all these similarities, the existence of each is not thought to diminish in any way the life of the other. So what is the difference between twins and clones?

The first difference seems to be that twins are coequal in priority. They are also two numerically distinct bearers of the personal descriptors that we use to address and distinguish each other, and each twin participates in relationships simultaneously and independently without any thought that "this path of life has been walked before" (however mistaken that might be). Because there are two numerically different individuals, there come to be two qualitatively different individuals, no matter what fundamental or biological similarities may link them. They have different names and individual life stories, and they have their own designated places in the discursive contexts in which they develop. Also, and importantly, twins raised together can adapt to each other's presence and construct their personalities and life history in light of each other's existence. Each is part of the completeness of the other in a way that can be woven into their personal narrative and thereby accommodated in the process of becoming a person with a certain identity. Neither is a copy of the other even though their genetic template is identical. They are not clones, they are twins, and, as we all know, "Everything is what it is and nothing else."

That n-tuplets, particularly nonidentical n-tuplets, are not the same as clones somewhat weakens a possible comparison between cloning and the deliberate production of n-tuplets. If, for instance, we found a drug (we could call it Quintrisium) that helped us produce successful pregnancies as a result of assisted human reproduction but always resulted in quintuplets, the considerations for the quints would be the same as (ordinary) twins. Again, we are not copying, although we might quasideliberately produce multiple instances of the same genetic constitution.

These considerations leave us struggling to find a good reason why cloning should be regarded as wrong, as has every group that has considered the issues. There remains, however, a seemingly unsupported intuition indicated by the use of the word *copy*.

No person should have a copy made of him or her, and no person should be made as a copy of another human being. This principle seems to be robust after reflection and seems to have something to do with human dignity and the uniqueness of each human being. Some thinkers have tried to capture it in the idea of a right to an open future, thereby linking it to intuitions that favor the freedom of children to become who they are and not merely to fulfil somebody else's expectations (vividly portrayed in films like *Dead Poets Society*). James II could be thought of as a copy in this sense because James has died and the parents have set out to make as a copy. I have identified "metaphysical" reasons (to do with the importance of individual discursive history and in particular interpersonal relationships in the formation of a person) to believe that Bob and Alison are misguided because no person will ever duplicate a predecessor (but their metaphysical mistake does not alter the wrongness of their intention). A rehabilitated Karl or Luke, or a set of twins are not copies nor are they thought of that way. I have argued that it is impossible to make exact copies or replicas of persons because of the nature of our human ontogeny. There are also reasons in biology to believe that the idea that genes completely determine phenotype is a naive view of the complex relationships between genes, organisms, and the expression of those genes.

The case of James can be extrapolated to pose an even more delicately poised ethical dilemma, in which a couple after a long period of infertility treatment finally manages to conceive a child, who tragically threatens to miscarry early in the pregnancy because of some transient disorder. What would we say if they wanted to clone their developing fetus so that after the miscarriage they could still have their own genetic child (which had cost them, in every way, so much to produce)? In such a case the gradualist view helps a great deal because, even if there is an existing human life to be copied, there is not an existing person who has started his or her engagement with us as an identifiable individual. We might, in such a case, think of what has happened as involving a false start and then a true beginning. In this case I cannot identify any clear and cogent moral objection to their plan.

I have similar intuitions in the case of a couple who, for whatever reason, cannot have genetic offspring by the normal methods and who could use a cloning technique to produce a child who is a nuclear genetic clone of one of them with some contribution from the other.

Cloning is problematic and leads us to reflect deeply on our basic conceptions of individual identity and the roots of our moral understanding of human beings in the traditional (Hippocratic) view that two people are required to produce an offspring. These reflections do not give us a knock-down, drag-out argument against the cloning of any human being in any circumstances but suggest that a policy that embraces cloning as a way of duplicating human beings may have a significant impact on our beliefs about the worth of each individual human life. I would argue that a society in which human beings are seen as the kinds of things that can be copied (even if that is a deeply false belief) is an undesirable society.

So, as I draw near to the end of this intellectual journey, I arrive at the beginning and know the place anew. Human life has a certain significance and moral value from the start. That is grounded in the idea that each of us has a place of origin and belonging and an individual story to tell because the like has never been seen before. Thus it is appropriate to regard us as being akin to works of art or unique creations rather than precious commodities of some generally valuable metaphysical type. If bioethical reflection on such things as cloning can deliver and make meaningful that single thought, then, on that basis alone, it seems to deserve a place in civilized discourse.

Epilogue
Mildly Philosophical Remarks

This book has been a lot of fun to write, even though it has taken a lot of hard work. Several characterizations of bioethics emerge from it and express where my thinking has arrived in the subject that took me on as a young brash surgeon, brimming with answers and certain that they were right. I now see bioethics in several guises:

- bioethics as bric-a-brac;
- bioethics as making vivid the human reality of the clinic; and
- bioethics as subversive and ironic;

Bioethics as Bric-a-Brac

It should be evident from this book that I am an unprincipled magpie in terms of argumentation and the "wheeling in" of this or that style of analysis, or source of insight as and when it seems helpful. This method is usefully seen as a *bric-a-brac* approach to bioethics in which no source of illumination is ignored in negotiating the complex labyrinth that is the human, political, and scientific world of the clinic. Different approaches—virtue oriented, consequentialist, duty or code based, legal, narrative, and postmodern—all offer glimpses that enrich our understanding of the whole situation at various points and therefore all have their part to play. Some approaches I am precluded from using by biological accidents of my birth, and where they are important I have tried to indicate my inadequacies. When it comes to real-life clinical bioethics, theoretical purity is gained only at the expense of phenomenological distortion, and that is a price I will not pay.

Bioethics as Making Vivid the Human Reality of the Clinic

The aim of the exercise, as I see it, is to make vivid the human reality behind sanitized medical accounts and the well-ordered ethical analyses that offer neat pigeonholes for messy clinical problems and sometimes difficult conversations. Our personae as doctors and our professional interventions in the lives of others are many and varied and draw on various strengths while also reflecting our various weaknesses. This multiplicity makes us increasingly aware of the need for our professional and personal lives to be illuminated by the kinds of reflection available through the humanities. It is a real source of encouragement for those of us who have taken this aspect of medicine seriously to now see fruits in those contexts where we encounter our younger siblings in the Hippocratic family. Despite all the pressures of modern medicine, the humanizing of the profession has enhanced our ability to realize in our lives as doctors those ideals of practice that are our legacy. This result is far better than finding those ideals abandoned in the skins we have been forced to shed so as to grow that glistening, shiny, and tough chameleon coat that seems prototypical of the successful physician.

Bioethics as Subversive and Ironic

Because it undermines the generalizations and pretensions of medicine's Olympian self-image, bioethics has a subversive effect. Medicine as seen by bioethics should be like Freud as seen by Wittgenstein—a figure for which one has immense respect but in relation to which one maintains a critical attitude. Medicine and its protagonists deserve our support and respect, but they also need our criticism, humor, and ironic realism. In this respect, and also in the spirit of Wittgenstein, bioethics should propound no theories and doctrines but rather offer itself as a trustworthy companion who reserves judgment until that judgment is properly informed. Yet this approach often leaves us with a question that is much more complex than it might first appear.

What Is Ethical Expertise?

Ethical expertise is phronesis. It is practical wisdom developed in the context of the clinic and informed by a thoroughgoing reflection on science and the human condition. Philosophy contributes to such expertise not in terms of schools or dogmata but more as an attitude. The philosophical attitude is to investigate and question, to seek clarification, to bracket the assumptions that often polarize or obscure an issue, and to be attentive to experience. It is also a scholarly discipline, attentive to its roots and able to trace the genealogy of its great debates. When we take these orientations into our study of bioethics, the intellectual rigor of Aristotle can be brought into fruitful engagement with the clinical dedication and moral certainty of the Hippocratics to provide what others have called "a more natural science." That science will, as good science tends to, leave us with more questions than answers, but then, even in our questioning, others will find help with problems that could never have come from neatly packaged answers. What is more, I have often found that the help we can give is intensely practical, as any truly Hippocratic enterprise should be.

The phronesis required for bioethics is bought at a price. The price includes one's clear and forthright beliefs, one's self-assured analyses, and—transiently—one's comfort with oneself as a person. At every point on the journey these are interrogated by experience so that, one hopes, what emerges is a little more worthy of commitment than its forebears. Wittgenstein seems to characterize this kind of intellectual journey in relation to more mainstream philosophy. "You see, I know that it's difficult to think well about 'certainty,' 'probability,' 'perception,' etc. But it is, if possible, still more difficult to think, or try to think, really honestly about your life and other people's lives. And the trouble is that thinking about these things is not thrilling, but often downright nasty" (Malcolm 1958, 39).

Thinking about oneself can turn up downright nasty results, but I guess that the response of an ethicist, as for a reflective practitioner of medicine, is not to reject the truth about those things but to incorporate them and transform the tendencies in oneself that lead to the nasty material appearing in one's auto-biography.

I might finally express a somewhat naive hope that I will see something like the "looping effect" of a book like this. The concept is due to Ian Hacking, and the hope is that reading this kind of thing enables individuals to form them-selves in a Hippocratic likeness within which they can find satisfaction and a measure of joy.

Appendix A. On Metaethics

When I was young, moral questions had a generality that ranked them among the most basic questions facing mankind (the gender is important). But then came the fall. I now see in the detail and particularity of moral challenges that which makes ethics a vital inquiry for all of us.

A discussion of metaethics often concerns moral realism, but I now have great problems with philosophical realism (although for most of us being realistic is thinking about the world as it really is). My allegiance to Aristotle and Wittgenstein prompts me to follow Philippa Foot (2001) and Sabina Lovibond (1983) in exploring links between natural history, moral perception, the grounding of meaning in human life as it is lived, and the centrality of reflection in ethics. This is close to the narrative approach to ethics derived largely from the work of Martha Nussbaum.

Aristotle and Naturalism in Ethics

Plato asked, "How should a man live?" and then answered by examining the intuitions attributable to wealthy young Athenians whom he educated.

Aristotle, more naturalistic in orientation, examined what made for a good human life. His answer, to those obsessed with the is-ought distinction, equivocates between a description and a prescription. I think that the fundamental ethical imperative finds expression in Wittgenstein's final words when he remarked that he had had a wonderful life (Malcolm 1958, 100). Clearly he exemplified a kind of human excellence even though his personal life seemed deeply troubled and unhappy. Wittgenstein, in fact, offers us a way out of the fact value dichotomy by reflecting on the everyday use of language. This stance embraces a kind of realism (particularly in the lay sense) even though the emphasis on *use* suggests a pragmatism in philosophical epistemology and metaphysics that is often opposed to realism. Lovibond unpacks Wittgenstein's approach in her *Realism and Imagination in Ethics* (1983). She argues that the realism debate in philosophy focuses on moral statements and their relation to matters of fact: "judgments of intrinsic value are held to be warranted not by the actual obtaining of a certain state of affairs which they declare to obtain, but by some phenomenon which, pending a better use for the word, can be called 'subjective'" (2).

The thought in question is the empiricist claim that there are two distinct kinds of statements: *propositions,* representations of the world; and *pseudopropositions,* which may look like statements about the world but are actually expressions of some attitude in the speaker, such as "It is wrong to betray a person who loves you." This statement cannot be true or false but rather means "I (We) disapprove of people who betray those that love them." Given that, you can say "It's not so bad" and not disagree about any state of affairs but rather express a different attitude toward human relationships. This position in metaethics is called subjectivism, expressivism, or noncognitivism (the boo!-hurrah! theory) and implies that statements about facts and statements about what one *ought* to think are different in kind, the latter reflecting an evaluative attitude.

Wittgenstein locates all statements in forms of life where people are enabled to communicate and share their lives by using language grounded in judgments about basic things around them ("That is a dog," "That is my mother," "Dad takes care of me," "That is cruel," "People need to eat and drink," "Pain is not nice," and so on). These judgments are basic to a network of practices and also, looked at as a whole, "a 'totality of propositions'—the theoretical counterpart of a common way of acting" (Lovibond 1983, 172). This shared resource binds a group of human beings together, creating common expectations and patterns of interaction with each other. Factual propositions are taken to reflect the general thought <that is how things are around here> and moral propositions are a subset capturing <how we do things around here>. In the milieu of shared human activity pervaded by language of this type, one negotiates a way of conducting oneself. As I have argued elsewhere, one's own psychological constitution is to such an extent a production of membership within that group that there is something inauthentic or even unnatural about alienation from the prevailing norms of the group.

In effect, Wittgenstein's answer to a question about the reality of moral values is reminiscent of the old timer who was asked about marriage.

"Jed, do you believe in marriage?"

"Believe in it, Hell, I seen it!"

This brings me to the reason why ethicists of my metaethical stripe often talk about moral perception.

Moral Perception

The idea that we directly or indirectly perceive states of affairs that ground factual beliefs is fundamental to empiricist philosophy. On this basis, empiricists often argue that moral facts must be "queer" because they cannot be perceived in the same way as other facts, and facts alone are not intrinsically action guiding. However, virtue theorists often remark that we can directly pick up certain features of our shared human environment. Such features and their pickup depend, like many perceptual capacities, on a skill resulting from a certain kind of training. Moral training sensitizes one to aspects of interpersonal situations which allow fine-grained and often subtle judgments about distress, cruelty, concern, kindness, manipulation, oppression, and so on. Detecting these things is useful, and there is every reason to believe that finely tuned neural networks such as those we possess might find them salient (Churchland 1996, 101). What is more, once noted, the relevant facts would be expected to move us in certain ways. Wittgenstein's later philosophy stresses the rules and techniques we learn in human forms of life and therefore welcomes this conception of perception and cognition. We can, in fact, find within it useful and interesting insights into certain kinds of mental disorder, for instance, autism and psychopathy, where interpersonal understanding is deficient in developmentally and morally relevant ways (Gillett 1999a).

Also, our perceptions and sensitivities can be enriched and refined by the kind of exposure to human situations that are explored in ancient and modern literature (Nussbaum 1990). This book's narrative approach to bioethics goes beyond relating ethical judgments to stories and uses the detailed exploration of human reactions and responses that are laid bare for us in great literature to inform our moral judgments about situations encountered in the clinic.

The idea that we are creatures who form relationships with each other, care for each other, react to others in morally relevant ways and shape each other as participants in communities is, as Kant noticed and as I have crystallized in one of my naturalistic axioms, fundamental to understanding ourselves as moral beings. It is ridiculous to argue that the realities that come into existence in that context are somehow less real than the sticks and stones that nature leaves around the world in which "we live and move and have our being" (to use Saint Paul's phrase). Thus, I am a moral realist, although not an absolutist in the accepted sense of that word (morality is based on absolute and inviolable principles or duties). For me, the absolute basis of morality, whether we correctly discern its implications for a situation or not, is in the quality of our relationships with each other and in the value each of us puts on him or herself as a unique individual in the human universe of life stories. This conception of morality implies that there are knowledge-transcendent truths even for inclusive human collectives, and that is about as strong a realist as, in the post-Wittgensteinian view I favor, one can be (Elliot 2001).

Narrative, Language, and Morality

Tom Murray asks, "What is narrative ethics?" (1997). The idea begins with writers like Howard Brody and Art Frank and centers on the narrative of the patient who is the central participant in the health care encounter. Frank has linked it to postmodernism and the multiplicity of stories and values that cluster around and in part constitute a clinical situation (1996). The link to postmodernism may be taken to imply that an inherent instability, intertextuality, attention to relations of power, and an essential partiality or incompleteness may characterize this way of doing ethics as distinct from the more traditional and coherent systems of metaethics, related as they are to mainstream Anglo-American philosophy. Attentiveness to experience and the perspectives of participants also links this approach to a pragmatic, Aristotelian position rooted in the Hippocratic approach I have tried to develop. Clearly, there is a central place for narratives in understanding the patient's illness and in reflective consideration of the professional's experience (as the traditional case study and casebook indicate). Just behind this attention to narratives or stories is the realization that all narratives are situated and emerge from a lived experience, a point that reinforces the Aristotelian and the postmodern links.

Murray considers four ways in which we might explicate the essential nature of narrative ethics (1997). First, we could claim, somewhat uncontroversially, that we learn our morality from stories told so as to confront us with the human heart of morally challenging situations. This claim I wholeheartedly endorse.

He then asks whether stories also have a role in ethical methodology and traces links between narrative ethics and casuistry—the discussion and resolution of cases. He considers this link not to exhaust the potential contribution of narrative to ethics. The third contribution that narratives bring to moral discussions is a richness of perception whereby the cultural and biographical context of a situation deepens our appreciation of the ways that varying interpretations may or may not do justice to what is at stake for the participants. There remains a fourth, substantive question about whether a narrative could ever provide justifications for conduct that cannot be conceptualized in other ways (for instance, by appeal to principles, duties, likenesses between cases, the exhibition of admirable character traits, and so on).

A telling example of the exact rightness of an action in its narrative context comes from Ferenc Molnar's book *The Paul Street Boys* (1998). Gereb, a young lad who has always been marginalized in one way or another, has betrayed the Paul Street boys and joined a rival gang, the Redshirts. He comes to regret his betrayal and asks to come back to the Paul Street boys because of the way that they have acted with courage and dignity in their dealings with the Redshirts and with his own father. He tries to redeem himself by undertaking a dangerous spying mission on the Redshirts and reporting to Boka what he has learnt. Boka, the leader of the Paul Street boys, takes a vote (which is inconclusive) and decides to readmit him, despite Gereb's betrayal and the inevitable suspicion of somebody who has changed sides at least twice. Boka speaks to the other Paul Street boys about the fact that Gereb has rejoined their gang, and he forbids any of the Paul Street boys to say anything about Gereb's treachery.

In the silence that follows, the boys think: "Boka is certainly a smart boy; he deserves to be our general" (137).

In the context of the story, bearing in mind Gereb's character and the reasons for his temporary shift of allegiance, the reader is struck by Boka's considerable sensitivity and wisdom in his handling of the situation. The general description of his action as one of *overlooking treachery and dissension* might, in another context, be exactly the wrong thing to do. In my view, however, Boka's action does not indicate a moral vacillation or inconstancy but rather tends to show what Nussbaum characterizes as "the ethical crudeness of moralities based exclusively on general rules and [a need] to demand for ethics a much finer responsiveness to the concrete" (1990, 37). Ethics is the critical scrutiny and development of what constitutes practical wisdom in the rich tapestry of human life (to use Tom Murray's metaphor). Virtue ethics concentrates on the virtues, those excellencies of human function that guide us and allow us to weave our small portion of that tapestry so that it brings harmony and completion to what is around it and has a particular beauty of its own.

Murray uses the metaphor of a tapestry to capture the idea of images, moments, and patterns in life that give meaning and depth to our goings-on and that can potentially create within themselves a kind of beauty or goodness that throws human activity into relief. Seen in this way, a sense of narrative offers glimpses of value in the midst of the complexity of life as it is lived where this value is not reducible to rankings or orderings derived from more abstract conceptualizations of moral problems. One might therefore say of an action, "That was the right thing to do" and mean that it was fitting in a way that implicitly contextualized the action to the situation, but it may not generalize to other moments of life along any recognizable or generally accepted evaluative dimensions (life-saving, lawful, respectful of autonomy, consensual, or whatever).

The sense of fittingness that goes into such a judgment is developed by experience and the intuitive adjustments one makes to one's behavior by using tools provided within a discourse in which some things are lauded and others condemned, and individuals are nurtured, educated, corrected, and sometimes rejected. This interpersonal or cultural arena is full of narratives, and they interact with each other in complex and demanding ways that often stretch our abilities to cope and maintain the social intercourse we all need to nourish our spirits and make life worth living. It may require subtle and well-honed discernment to be able to judge reliably whether an act is fitting in this sense. That skill inevitably affects one's reactions and responses in ethically demanding situations so that justifying how one has acted may need the relevant "sense of life" to be equally present in one's audience. Hilde Lindemann Nelson states: "Moral resolutions arrived at through this process of collaborative narrative construction are justified ultimately by the habitability and goodness of the common life to which they lead" (2000, 18 19).

It is clear that one can be under no illusion that one should emerge unscathed from this process. One cannot be an impartial moral observer of life if the relevant learning is to be done. That contrasts starkly with the stability and objectivity of principles or character dimensions that might form a pivotal point for moral judgment and action according to some moral theories.

The Moral Self and Reflective Equilibrium

In her discussion of narrative ethics, Nussbaum (1990) finds several points to commend in Rawls's conception of the moral life as involving a "reflective equilibrium" in which not only one's moral decisions but also one's intuitions, principles, and character are negotiable. This dialectic between self and situation considers a mixture of perceptions, reactions, responses, resolutions, and commitments and is part of the moral story. It is central in the participant narrative of moral development, and in clinical life it takes on an intensity that is seldom encountered elsewhere. It is no wonder that Toulmin concluded that bioethics had saved the life of moral philosophy. As one watches the kaleidoscope of reactions passing across the face of a mother whose child is pronounced brain dead, a man in the prime of life who learns he has an incurable malignancy, or a young woman who realizes that the operation she must have will mean that she is destined to be infertile, one cannot treat ethics as an abstract study of concepts informing practical reasoning in the way that a different set of concepts informs our theoretical reasoning.

Ethics is for creatures who sweat, bleed, love, and die and who live with uncertainty about who they are and what, if anything, is the point of it all. Ethical challenges make us confront these things armed with our vulnerabilities, needs, skills, and commitments to one another, and we become aware that there are a number of paths that any life could take, constrained but not determined by the natural endowments of the traveler. There is a map that helps one to walk these paths, but it cannot be surveyed from any privileged point of view. Therefore, there are no eternal propositions that reveal canonical truths about the moral domain. (Such truths are not to be found in any domain except those artificially constructed out of intellectual tools that are designed to be rigid in the face of a shifting world.)

For the later Wittgenstein, the idea of an objective map that accurately pictures the world in its entirety and includes within itself all the truths that will ever be known is an illusion. Therefore, for any follower of Wittgenstein, the very human creation that is a moral map, revealing as it does what in social and personal life counts as something, is just as true to the world as we live in it as any other map could ever be.

Appendix B. Narrative Metaphysics

Narrative metaphysics claims that objects and events cannot be individuated or specified independent of the narrative in which they appear. It is not just that things and events are named differently in different narratives; you cannot even determine the boundaries of their being unless you give the framework within which they can be meaningfully discussed. Here the term *narrative* is used in its broadest sense (as in postmodern critiques) to refer to a coherent account of phenomena or a localized history, as in the evolutionary narrative, the narrative about the splitting of the atom, the life story of Anna Pavlova, or whatever. Therefore the concept covers any coherent and organized body of knowledge and its way of understanding things.

Narratives use terms referring to objects, and it is generally assumed that those objects can be unambiguously identified for the purposes of constructing a coherent story. There are clear resonances between a critique of exclusive discourses and the objects they name and the evaluation of nonorthodox accounts of healing. One or two examples illustrate these ideas, but a carefully constructed argument for them would be out of place in the present context.

Stories are made up of events. Yet when we look more closely, it becomes problematic to say which conditions which. Take a typical event—my arriving home from work. Is it part of this event that a small pollen particle comes through the front door as I open it, even though that is neither known nor mentioned? That my daughter calls out, "Hi, Dad," is surely part of the event, but are the disturbances in air particles in the vicinity of her mouth? What about the movement of acetylcholine molecules in a million synapses in her brain or the influx of calcium ions into muscle cells in her diaphragm as she speaks? Clearly, if one tried to describe the event mentioning facts at this level, its identity as an event would be lost to view. Thus, we get into indeterminacy issues when we start asking questions about what is part of an event and what is not.

Imagine that one wanted a "topic-neutral" specification of my coming home. Would we include all the displacements of matter occurring in a certain region of space between T_1 and T_n? How do we specify the region of space, given that my daughter is two rooms away from the front door? Do we say that the event includes everything in the house? What if my cat, on the back lawn, hears the door and comes bounding around to the front of the house, and my daughter greets him more warmly than me? Was he part of the event while he was not in the house? But this is getting ridiculous. Other events on the back lawn include a bug eating a smaller bug under the beech tree; so how much of the bug's repast, occurring as it does within the favored region of time and space, is part of my homecoming?

A quasi-physical account of what goes on in the space concerned may mean nothing to any possible receiver of that information. (The event we are talking about is lost among all the molecular interactions, electrochemical forces, quantum changes, and so on.) What is more, a series of irrelevant matters get into the picture like the draft caused in the laundry (roughly the same magnitude as the disturbance of air around my daughter's face); the interaction of photons with the wallpaper opposite the front door; the lowering of mean kinetic energy in the water in the fishbowl due to the transient cooling that goes on, et cetera, et cetera, et cetera (to quote the king of Siam). The details of the physical story totally obscure what is happening, particularly if something about my daughter's tone of voice conveyed her displeasure that we had been on her back about her overdue assignments. Of course, the physics and chemistry of my homecoming is equally inaccessible in the human story.

Therefore, the meaningful human event that occurs at this point is not picked out—in its essential details that make it the event it is—from the myriad of happenings in the universe by anything other than the story that deals with my homecoming as a human event. There is no "topic-neutral" way of carving the world and its goings-on so as to clip out just what counts as my homecoming without having a grasp of the kinds of things that matter and the concepts that one might apply for this or that purpose to an event of that sort and that our participation in stories by doing this is foundational in our form of life. A physical, biochemical, meteorological, or political story carves up the whole mishmash in a way that makes a different kind of picture. Then we find that we can pick out a different set of events and objects which differentially come into relief. The general point is that there is a two-way relationship between stories and the events that make them up.

Events comprise objects and what happens to them, and therefore the story you are telling (which frame of reference you are in) affects the objects and their parts, which are also subject to certain kinds of indeterminacy.

Consider Ben Lomond and a piece of stone from the side of Loch Lomond lying half buried in the turf of the mountainside. Is this piece of stone a part of Ben Lomond or not? Imagine that the stone has in fact risen to the surface over time. Here one would say that it is a part of Ben Lomond. Now imagine that it was found on the lakeshore and carried up the mountain by a tramper. What if the stone is carried off and dropped into a concrete mixer in Glasgow. Is it still part of Ben Lomond? If so, then Ben Lomond becomes a scattered object. Now I can believe in an Irish diaspora but a Ben Lomond diaspora—that strains the brain too much. Similar indeterminacy affects the limit of the mountain in relation to the underlying geological formations—one is tempted to say that the roots of the mountain have a fuzzy boundary with respect to the rock beneath it. Now Ben Lomond becomes a vague object even though I seem to know exactly what I am talking about when I talk about it. Perhaps mountains are adequately identified only in geographic accounts rather than geological or geometrical accounts. Ben Lomond exists as an identifiable item primarily in a geographical description of Scotland and may not have any such existence in a quantum description of the universe or, for that matter, a cosmological one.

Even the president of the United States of America is a problematic object (that should come as no surprise). At any given time this is a human individual, but would that individual appear in the story of a water molecule or an ecological account of the impact of human beings on the environment?

Take the first case. Imagine that this water molecule is breathed in by the president but that it stays in his airway. Now, in the story of the water molecule, its time in the lungs or digestive tract of the president is nothing special except as a time when its mean kinetic energy corresponds to a temperature of about 37.4° C and it has certain chemical interactions. In fact, it is debatable whether it was really *in* the president at all compared with a water molecule bound to a protein molecule in one of the president's liver cells. Surely there is an answer as to whether or not our favored water molecule is part of the president of the United States! It depends what story you are telling. It depends on the story whether the president of the United States is an object of which the water molecule is a part.

In fact, where does the president begin and end? (Some might say, "Wherever he likes!" but that won't do for metaphysics.) Does the president include a molecule floating in the air in his airways or is it not part of him until the molecule has crossed the wall of an alveolus and entered the body? I can think of no reason why such a question would ever need to be answered—in that respect, the object that is the president of the United States can remain indeterminate. But let us say that the president sent you a letter apparently pardoning you for a fraud. Is this a pardon? It depends on exactly which body signed it. No chemical specification of the letter will decide the issue about what it actually is. Some complex story about the signature, the authorization for it, and so on determines whether this is an actual pardon or not. Thus, its nature is radically dependent on the story that surrounds it.

Explanation has the same indeterminacy. If I want to explain the extinction of a species of Amazonian bird or monkey, I might try and do it in purely biological terms, but I will not succeed. To understand it, I might have to say something about the president of the United States (qua leader of the most powerful economic and industrial nation in the world) and his attitude toward some critical agreements about sustainable use of the earth's resources. This political and economic fact and the objects involved (the U.S. legislature, multinational corporations, and so on) could be a vital part of explaining the extinction of the Amazonian animals even though many of the "objects" concerned come into view only in politicohistorical stories.

The underlying point is, I think, simple and familiar to all those acquainted with Frege's theory of sense and reference (1980) and its development in Wittgenstein's discussion of the fundamental components of reality (1953, 47). Any language game is a set of tools to carve up the world and what goes on in it so that according to our interests at the time certain things spring into relief as figures perceptible against a ground. The constitution of a figure depends on the concepts applied in that language game, and these are developed because they assist us to notice the things that engage with our interests and powers of action. Language provides us with tools that enable us to adapt our cognitive systems to the world around us. The stories we are acting out or participating in determine which of those tools will be employed on a given occasion, and the tools differentially make things visible and invisible (or more accurately cognizable or uncognizable—except that these are horrible words fit only for psychologized postmodern arguments).

Very similar points are made by Lyotard, Foucault, and Deleuze in the postmodern context.

Appendix C. The Idea of a Form

Aristotle's doctrine of form claims that a thing is essentially of a certain kind not just on account of what it is made of. For instance, the human body turns over all its molecules and a large number of its cells as the years roll by. Despite this, I remain the same person I was when I married, graduated from medical school, or enrolled at Oxford University. What is constant is my form as a person, despite changes in my appearance and other properties. Yet some subset of these properties makes me the person I am, and various people would opt for various subsets—my personality, my genetic composition, my narrative, my discursive or historical place in the human order—the detail does not matter. Form is whatever makes a thing essentially what it is, and it grounds the claim that I am encountering that thing when I do. Thus, something about me apart from molecules grounds my claim on my belongings after an interval of years. Aristotle does note that a given thing comprises both form and matter, so, for instance, a particular chair is bronze or wooden, but its general form is that of a chair, and its particular form is that which takes account of certain characteristic artistic and compositional features.

The form of a natural thing such as an animal also has a characteristic type of life—or psyche. This animal form comprises the characteristic functions that go into being a creature of that type, and there is a norm for creatures of the relevant kind. This norm not only is statistical but also has *normative* implications because any creature has certain adaptations that suit it to its mode of living and make life go well for one of its kind. For instance, a gazelle *should* be swift and vigilant, a beaver *should* be good at making lodges, a lion *should* have strength and sharp teeth and claws so as to kill its prey, and any creature *should* be fertile to enable procreation.

The sense of *normal* in play here has implications for what can be said to be good and what could be said to be defective for a creature of the type in question (Foot 2001). This gives us the linked Aristotelian doctrines about human form and human well-being (or eudaemonia).

The human form implicitly defines what it is to be excellent or deficient in function as a human being and is used by some philosophers to generate a definition of disease based on mental and physical defects or deficiencies in functioning (Boorse 1975; Megone 1998). In the broadest possible construal of this account, an organism has a disease where there is a functional change in that organism such that it becomes less than well suited to its natural environment. Narrower construals stipulate that the change must be in the intrinsic functioning of the organism, and broader, particularly postmodern, interpretations allow for relational breakdowns that problematize the notion of disease as a construct applied to individuals.

The human form implies that certain characteristics are required for a human being to function well in a typically human setting and allow us to reflect on what would constitute excellence in those functions. Given that the set of functions can be referred to as the *psyche* (or soul), then virtue becomes defined as excellence of soul, however realized in detail. Such a view can be interpreted to endorse a perfectionist morality or a more modest (as good as it gets) approach to life. My kind of Aristotelian naturalism recognizes many possible varieties of harmony that can be attained within the context of a particular human narrative with the result that the life concerned goes well (all thing considered). In fact, I opt for a relatively Dionysian version of that view.

One further point deserves mention. The human form operates as a formal cause of certain properties exhibited by a human being. Thus, the matter incorporated by the thing takes on, as part of its assimilation (and through metabolic work), the form it needs to contribute to the functioning of the human body. In answer to the question, "Why does the heart operate like that?" or "Why does the heart look like that?" one can properly reply, as Aristotle notes, "Well, that's what it is to be a human heart." The answer does not identify efficient or material causes—the things that explain the process of bringing something about and those that account for what it is made from—which are the normal terms in which we discuss causes in current philosophy. However, recent work in cell-to-cell and top-down effects in embryology, and the arrangement of body cells has given this ancient notion of formal cause a new lease on life.

References

The chapter epigraphs and other quotations from Hippocratic writings are taken from the Penguin translation by Geoffrey Lloyd.

LEGAL CASES

Airedale NHS Trust v. Bland (1993) AC 789
Auckland Area Health Board v. Attorney General (1993) 1NZLR 235
Re a Ward of Court (1995) 2ILRM 401
Re G (1996) NZFLR 362 also Judgement of Fraser J.
Rogers v. Whitaker (1992) 175 CLR 479
Sidaway v. Board of Governors of the Bethlem Royal Hospital and the Maudsley Hospital (1985) 2 WLR 480

BOOKS AND ARTICLES

Almond, B. 1988. AIDS and international ethics. *Ethics and International Affairs* 2:139–54.
———, ed. 1996. *AIDS: A Moral Issue.* 2d ed. London: Macmillan.
Angell, M. 1997. The ethics of clinical research in the third world. *New England Journal of Medicine* 337:847–49.
Angell, M., and J. Kassirer. 1998. Alternative medicine: The risks of untested and unregulated remedies. *New England Journal of Medicine* 339:839–41.
Aristotle. 1925. *Nicomachean Ethics,* tr. d. Ross. Oxford: Oxford University Press.
———. 1986. *De Anima.* Trans. H. Lawson Tancred. London: Penguin.
Balint, M. 1957. *The Doctor, His Patient, and the Illness.* London: Tavistock.
Beauchamp, T., and J. Childress. 1989. *The Principles of Biomedical Ethics.* 3d ed. Oxford: Oxford University Press.
Block, S. 2000. Assessing and managing depression in the terminally ill patient. *Annals of Internal Medicine* 132:209–18.
Boldt, M. 1989. Defining suicide. In *Suicide and Its Prevention,* ed. R. Diekstra, R. Maris, S. Platt, A. Scmidtke, and G. Sonnieck. Leiden: Brill.
Boorse, C. 1975. On the distinction between disease and illness. *Philosophy and Public Affairs* 5:49–68.
Boozang, K. 1998. Western medicine opens the door to alternative medicine. *American Journal of Law and Medicine* 24:185–212.
Bordo, S. 1985. Anorexia nervosa: Psychopathology as the crystallization of culture. *Philosophical Forum* 17, no. 2:73–103.

Brennan, T., et al. 1991. Incidence of adverse events and negligence in hospitalized patients: Results of the Harvard medical practice study 1. *New England Journal of Medicine* 324:377–84.

Brennan, T., C. Sox, and H. Burstin. 1996. Relation between negligent adverse events and the outcomes of medical-malpractice litigation. *New England Journal of Medicine* 335: 1963–67.

British Medical Association. 1988. *Euthanasia.* London: BMA Publications.

British Medical Journal. 1999. Editorial. 7212:717.

Brock, D. 1998. Cloning human beings: An assessment of the ethical issues pro and con. In *Clones and Clones,* ed. M. Nussbaum and C. Sunstein. New York: Norton & Co., 141–80.

Brody, B. 1978. On the humanity of the foetus. In *Contemporary Issues in Bioethics,* ed. T. Beauchamp and L. Walters. Belmont, Calif.: Wadsworth, 229–40.

Brody, H. 1987. *Stories of Sickness.* New Haven: Yale University Press.

Brown, J., P. Henteleff, L. Barakat, and C. Rowe. 1986. Is it normal for terminally ill patients to desire death? *American Journal of Psychiatry* 143, no. 2:208–11.

Browne, A., G. Gillett, and M. Tweeddale. 2000. The ethics of elective (non-therapeutic) ventilation. *Bioethics* 14, no. 1:42–57.

Byk, C. 1997. A proposed draft protocol for the European Convention on Biomedicine relating to research on the human embryo and fetus. *Journal of Medical Ethics* 23, no. 1:32–37.

Byrne, D., A. Napier, and A. Cushcieri. 1988. How informed is signed consent? *British Medical Journal* 296:839–40.

Campbell, A., G. Gillett, and D. Jones. 2001. *Medical Ethics.* 3d ed. Oxford: Oxford University Press.

Camus, A. 1971. The Myth of Sisyphus. In *The Existentialist Tradition,* ed. N. Languilli. Sussex: Harvester, 453–56.

Carson, R. 2002. The hyphenated space: Liminality in the doctor patient relationship. In *Stories Matter,* ed. R. Charon and M. Montello. New York: Routledge, 171–82.

Carson, R., and C. Burns, eds. 1997. *Philosophy of Medicine and Bioethics.* Dordrecht: Kluwer.

Cartwright, S. R. 1988. *Report of the committee of inquiry into allegations concerning the treatment of cervical cancer at National Women's Hospital and into other related matters.* Auckland: Government Printing Office.

Chin, A., K. Hedberg, G. Higginson, and D. Fleming. 1999. Legalized physician-assisted suicide: The first year's experience. *New England Journal of Medicine* 340, no. 7:577–83.

Churchland, P. 1996. The neural representation of the social world. In *Mind and Morals,* ed. L. May, M. Friedman, and A. Clark. Cambridge, Mass.: MIT Press, 91–108.

Clark-Grill, M. 2000. The languages of healing. Unpublished student essay.

Coates, J. 2000. "Report cards": The public's access to indicators of clinical performance. *New Zealand Medical Journal* 114:342–43.

Cochrane, A. L. 1972. *Effectiveness and Efficiency.* London: BMJ Publications.

Cochrane, J. 2000. Narrowing the gap: Access to HIV treatments in developing countries. *Journal of Medical Ethics* 26, no. 1:47–50.

Concato, J., N. Shah, and R. J. Horwitz. 2000. Randomized controlled trials, observational studies and the hierarchy of research designs. *New England Journal of Medicine* 342: 1878–86.

Coppolino, M., and L. Ackerson. 2001. Do surrogate decision makers provide accurate consent for intensive care research? *Chest* 119, no. 2:603–12.

Coulter, A. 1999. Paternalism or partnership. *British Medical Journal* 7212:719–20

Coxon, A. 1996. Coping with the threat of death. In *AIDS: A Moral Issue,* 2d ed., ed. B. Almond. London: Macmillan, 131–38.

Crisp, R. 1996a. Autonomy, welfare and the treatment of AIDS. In *AIDS: A Moral Issue,* 2d ed., ed. B. Almond. London: Macmillan, 56–70.

———. 1996b. Modern moral philosophy and the virtues. In *How Should One Live?* ed. R. Crisp. Oxford: Oxford University Press, 1–18.

Crombie, A. 1994. *Styles of Scientific Thinking in the European Tradition.* London: Duckworth.

Danish Council of Ethics. 2002. *Cloning.* Copenhagen: Danish Council of Ethics.

Davidson, A. 1996. Styles of reasoning, conceptual history, and the emergence of psychiatry. In *The Disunity of Science,* ed. P. Galison and D. Stump. Stanford: Stanford University Press, 75–100.

Davidson, H., J. Dawson, and A. Moore. 2001. Law ethics and epidemiology: The case of the cervical screening audit. *New Zealand Bioethics Journal* 2:8–26.

Davis, P., et al. 2001. Adverse events regional feasibility study: Indicative findings. *New Zealand Medical Journal* 114:203–5.

Deuchar, N. 1984. AIDS in New York city with particular reference to the psycho-social aspects. *British Journal of Psychiatry* 145:612–19

De Wachter, A. 1992. Euthanasia in the Netherlands. *Hastings Center Report* 22, no. 2: 23–29.

Dominica, Sister F. 1987. Reflections on death in childhood. *British Medical Journal* 294: 108–9.

Drury, M. 1984. Some notes on conversations with Wittgenstein. In *Recollections of Wittgenstein,* ed. R. Rhees, 76–171. Oxford: Oxford University Press.

Editors. 2000. *New Zealand Medical Journal* 113, no. 1116:345–46.

Edwards, S. J. L., R. J. Lilford, and J. Hewison, J. 1998. The ethics of randomized controlled trials from the perspectives of patients, the public and healthcare professionals. *British Medical Journal* 317:1209–12.

Elliot, C., ed. 2001. *Slow Cures and Bad Philosophers: Wittgenstein, Medicine and Bioethics.* Durham, N.C.: Duke University Press.

Ellis, J., I. Mulligan, I. Rower, and D. Sackett. 1995. Inpatient medicine is evidence based. *Lancet* 346:407–10.

Emanuel, E., D. Fairclough, F. Daniels, and B. Claridge. 1996. Euthanasia and physician-assisted suicide: Attitudes and experiences of oncology patients, oncologists, and the public. *Lancet* 347:1805.

Engelhardt, T. 1986. *The Foundations of Bioethics.* Oxford: Oxford University Press.

———. 1997. Bioethics and the philosophy of medicine reconsidered. In *Philosophy of Medicine and Bioethics,* ed. R. Carson and C. Burns. Dordrecht: Kluwer.

Evans, D., and M. Evans. 1996. *A Decent Proposal: Ethical review of clinical research.* Chichester: John Wiley & Sons.

Feyerabend, P. 1975. *Against Method.* London: Verso.

Fitzjohn, J., and D. Studdert. 2001. A compensation perspective on error prevention: Is the ACC medical misadventure scheme compensating the right sort of injury? *New Zealand Medical Journal* 114:432–34.

Foley, K., and H. Hendin. 1999. The Oregon Report: Don't ask, don't tell. *Hastings Center Report,* May-June, 37–42.

Foot, P. 1978. *Virtues and Vices.* Oxford: Blackwell.

———. 1985. Utilitarianism and the virtues. *Mind* 94:196–209.

———. 2001. *Natural Goodness.* Oxford: Oxford University Press.

Foucault, M. [1954] 1987. *Mental Illness and Psychology.* Trans. A. Sheridan. Berkeley: University of California Press.

———. 1965. *Madness and Civilization.* London: Tavistock.

———. 1977. *Discipline and Punish.* Middlesex: Penguin.

———. 1984. *The Foucault Reader.* Ed. P. Rabinow. London: Penguin.

———. 1994. Two lectures. In *Critique and Power,* ed. M. Kelly. Cambridge, Mass.: MIT Press.

Frank, A. 1996. *The Wounded Storyteller: Body, Illness and Ethics.* Chicago: University of Chicago Press.

Freedman, B. 1987. Equipoise and the ethics of clinical research. *New England Journal of Medicine* 317:141–45.

Freeman, T. B., et al. 1999. Use of placebo surgery in controlled trials of a cellular-based therapy for Parkinson's disease. *New England Journal of Medicine* 341:988–92.

Frege, G. 1980. *Translations from the Philosophical Writings of Gottlob Frege.* Ed. P. Geach and M. Black. Oxford: Blackwell.

Freud, S. 1940. An outline of psychoanalysis. *International Journal of Psychoanalysis* 21: 27–84.

Fulford, W. 1989. *Moral Theory and Medical Practice.* Cambridge: Cambridge University Press.

Gillam, L. 1998. The "more-abortions" objection to fetal tissue transplantation. *Journal of Medicine and Philosophy* 23:411–27.

Gillett, G. 1987. AIDS and confidentiality. *Journal of Applied Philosophy* 4, no. 1:15–20.

———. 1988. Euthanasia, letting die and the pause. *Journal of Medical Ethics* 14:61–68.

———. 1992. *Representation Meaning and Thought.* Oxford: Clarendon.

———. 1994. The pause and the principles. In *Principles of Health Care Ethics,* ed. R. Gillon and A. Lloyd. Chichester: John Wiley & Sons.

———. 1995. Virtue and truth in clinical science. *Journal of Medicine and Philosophy* 20: 285–98.

———. 1997. Is there anything wrong with Hitler these days? *Medical Humanities Review* 11:9–20.

———. 1998. Innovative treatments: Ethical requirements for evaluation. *Journal of Clinical Neuroscience* 5:378–81.

———. 1999a. *The Mind and Its Discontents.* Oxford: Oxford University Press.

———. 1999b. Consciousness and lesser states: The evolutionary foothills of the mind. *Philosophy* 74:331–60.

———. 1999c. How should we test and improve neurosurgical care? In *Ethical Dilemmas in Neurology,* ed. A. Zeman and L. Emanuel. Edinburgh: W. B. Saunders.

———. 2001. Wittgenstein's startling claim: Consciousness and the persistent vegetative state. In *Slow Cures and Bad Philosophers: Wittgenstein, Medicine and Bioethics,* ed. C. Elliot. Durham, N.C.: Duke University Press, 70–88.

Gillett, G., L. Goddard, and M. Webb. 1995. The case of Mr. L: A legal and ethical response to the court sanctioned withdrawal of life-support. *Journal of Law and Medicine* 3: 49–59.

Gillett, G., and J. McMillan. 2001. *Consciousness and Intentionality*. Amsterdam: John Benjamins.

Gilligan, C. 1982. *In a Different Voice*. Cambridge, Mass.: Harvard University Press.

Gillon, R., and A. Lloyd, eds. 1994. *Principles of Health Care Ethics*. Chichester: John Wiley & Sons.

Glover, J. 1977. *Causing Death and Saving Lives*. London: Penguin.

Griffiths, J. 1995. Assisted suicide in the Netherlands: The *Chabot* case. *Modern Law Review* 58:232–48.

Hacking, I. 1983. *Representing and Intervening*. Cambridge: Cambridge University Press.

——. 1995. *Rewriting the Soul*. Princeton: Princeton University Press.

——. 1996. The disunities of the sciences. In *The Disunity of Science*, ed. P. Galison and D. Stump. Stanford: Stanford University Press, 37–74.

Hahnemann, S. [1833] 1993. *Organon of Medicine*. Trans. W. Boericke. New Delhi: B. Jain.

Hamblin, J. 1994. HIV in the developing world: Lessons for health care in Australia. In *National Bioethics Conference Proceedings*. Sydney: Christian Centre for Bioethics.

Hare, R. 1981. *Moral Thinking: Levels Methods and Point*. Oxford: Clarendon.

——. 1983. *Personal Being*. Oxford: Blackwell.

——. 1993. *Essays on Bioethics*. Oxford: Clarendon.

Harre, R., and G. Gillett. 1994. *The Discursive Mind*. London: Sage.

Hebert, P., et al. 1999. A multicenter randomized controlled trial of transfusion requirements in critical care. *New England Journal of Medicine* 340, no. 6:409–17.

Heyssel, R., et al. Decentralised management in a teaching hospital. *New England Journal of Medicine* 310:1477–80.

Holland, A. 1990. A fortnight of my life is missing: A discussion of the human "preembryo." *Journal of Applied Philosophy* 7, no. 1:25–37.

Holm, S. 1988. New Danish law: Life begins at conception. *Journal of Medical Ethics* 14, no. 2:77–78.

Hudson, R. 2001. Discoveries, when and by whom? *British Journal of the Philosophy of Science* 52, no. 1:75–94.

Hull, D. 1982. The naked meme. In *Learning Development and Culture*, ed. H. Plotkin. London: John Wiley.

Hume, D. [1740] 1969. *A Treatise of Human Nature*. Ed. E. Mossner. London: Penguin.

——. [1776] 1980. *Dialogues Concerning Natural Religion and Posthumous Essays*. Ed. R. Popkin. Indianapolis: Hackett.

Hunter, K. M. 1991. *Doctor's Stories*. Princeton: Princeton University Press.

Husserl, E. 1962. *Ideas*. Trans. W. R. Boyce Gibson. New York: Collier.

Iglesias, T. 1984. In vitro fertilization: The major issues. *Journal of Medical Ethics* 10:32.

Jaffe, M. 2000. *Sleeping with Your Gynecologist*. Cleveland: West St. James Press.

Jay, M. 1986. In the empire of the gaze: Foucault and the denigration of vision in twentieth-century French thought. In *Foucault: A Critical Reader*, ed. D. Couzens-Hoy. Oxford: Blackwell.

Jennett, B. 1986. *High Technology Medicine*. Oxford: Oxford University Press.

John Paul II. 1995. *Evangelium Vitae: Encyclical Letter on the Value and Inviolability of Human Life."* 11th papal encyclical, March 25. Rome: Vatican Press.

Kant, I. [1789] 1929. *The Critique of Pure Reason*. Trans. N. Kemp Smith. London: Macmillan.

Kavka, G. 1981. The paradox of future individuals. *Philosophy and Public Affairs* 11, no. 2:93–112.

Kelly, M., ed. 1994. *Critique and Power.* Cambridge, Mass.: MIT Press.

Keown, J. 1992. The law and the practice of euthanasia in the Netherlands. *Law Quarterly Review* 108:51–78.

Kienle, G., and H. Kiene. 1997. The powerful placebo effect: Fact or fiction? *Clinical Epidemiology* 50, no. 12:1311–18.

Kluge, E. H. 2000. Elective, nontherapeutic ventilation: A reply to Browne et al., "The ethics of elective (nontherapeutic) ventilation." *Bioethics* 14, no. 3:240–47.

Komessaroff, P. 1995. Micro ethics. In *Troubled Bodies,* ed. P. Komesaroff. Melbourne: Melbourne University Press.

Kopelman, L. 1997. Medicine's challenge to relativism: The case of female genital mutilation. In *Philosophy of Medicine and Bioethics,* ed. R. Carson and C. Burns. Dordrecht: Kluwer, 221–38.

Kripke, S. 1980. *Naming and Necessity.* Cambridge, Mass.: Harvard University Press.

Kuhn, T. S. 1962. *The Structure of Scientific Revolutions.* Chicago: University of Chicago Press.

Kübler-Ross, E. 1969. *On Death and Dying.* London: Tavistock.

Lacan, J. 1977. *Ecrits.* New York: Norton & Co.

———. 1979. *The Four Fundamental Concepts of Psycho-analysis.* Trans. A Sheridan. London: Penguin.

Ladd, J. 1983. The internal morality of medicine: An essential dimension of the patient-physician relationship. In *The Clinical Encounter: The Mortal Fabric of the Patient-Physician Relationship,* ed. E. Shelp. Dordrecht: Reidel.

Leape, L., and D. Berwick. 2000. Safe health care: Are we up to it? *British Medical Journal* 320:725–26.

Leape, L., et al. 1991. The nature of adverse outcomes in hospitalized patients: Results of the Harvard medical practice study 2. *New England Journal of Medicine* 324:377–84.

Leenan, H. 1987. Euthanasia, assistance to suicide and the law: Developments in the Netherlands. *Health Policy* 8:197–206.

Lindley, R., and C. Warlow. 2000. Why and how should trials be conducted? In *Ethical Dilemmas in Neurology,* ed. A. Zeman and L. Emanuel. Edinburgh: W. B. Saunders.

Lloyd, G. 1973. *Greek Science after Aristotle.* London: Norton & Co.

———. 1978. *Hippocratic Writings.* London: Penguin.

Localio, A., et al. 1991. Relation between malpractice claims and adverse events due to negligence: Results of the Harvard medical practice study 3. *New England Journal of Medicine* 325:245–51.

Locke, J. [1689] 1975. *An Essay Concerning Human Understanding.* Ed. P. Nidditch. Oxford: Clarendon.

Lockwood, M. 1985. When does life begin? In *Moral Dilemmas in Modern Medicine,* ed. M. Lockwood. Oxford: Oxford University Press.

Lopez, B. 1990. *Crow and Weasel.* Toronto: Random House.

Lovibond, S. 1983. *Realism and Imagination in Ethics.* Oxford: Blackwell

Lurie, P., and S. Wolfe. 1997. Unethical trials of interventions to reduce perinatal transmission of the human immunodeficiency virus in developing countries. *New England Journal of Medicine* 337:853–56.

Macklin, R. 1999. The ethical problems with sham surgery in clinical research. *New England Journal of Medicine* 341:992–95.

McDowell, J. 1994. *Mind and World*. Cambridge, Mass.: Harvard University Press.

MacIntyre, A. 1984. *After Virtue*. Notre Dame, Ind.: University of Notre Dame Press.

———. 1988. *Whose Justice, Which Rationality*. Notre Dame, Ind.: University of Notre Dame Press.

McMahan, J. 1998. Wrongful life: Paradoxes in the morality of causing people to exist. In *Rational Commitment and Social Justice*, ed. J. Coleman and C. Morris. Cambridge: Cambridge University Press.

McNeill, P. 1993. *The Ethics and Politics of Human Experimentation*. Melbourne: Cambridge University Press.

Malcolm, L. 2000. The rise of clinical leadership in New Zealand: Towards clinical governance. *New Zealand Medical Journal* 113:177.

Malcolm, N. 1958. *Ludwig Wittgenstein: A memoir*. London: Oxford University Press.

Manohar, S. V. 1990. Medicolegal issues of the 1990s: An Indian perspective. In *Papers of the 9th Commonwealth Law Conference*. Auckland: Commerce Clearing House.

May, L., M. Friedman, and A. Clark. 1996. *Mind and Morals*. Cambridge, Mass.: MIT Press.

Megone, C. 1998. Aristotle's function argument and the concept of mental illness. *Philosophy Psychiatry and Psychology* 5:187–201.

Miller, F., et al. 1994. Regulating physician assisted suicide. *New England Journal of Medicine* 331, no. 2:119–22.

Mirkin, B. 1995. AIDS clinical trials: Why they have recruiting problems. *AIDS Treatment News* 217:1–4.

Molnar, Ferenc. 1998. *The Paul Street Boys*. Budapest: Corvina.

Monaco, G. P., and S. Green. 1993. Recognizing deception in the promotion of untested and unproven medical treatments. *New York State Journal of Medicine* 93: 88–91.

Moore, A., K. Hall, R. Hickling, and K. Sharples. In press. Critical care research ethics: Making the case for non-consensual research. *Journal of Clinical Ethics*.

Morris, D. 1998. *Illness and Culture*. Berkeley: University of California Press.

Mullen, P. 1995. Euthanasia. An impoverished construction of life and death. *Journal of Law and Medicine* 3, no. 2:121–28.

Murray, T. 1987. Gifts of the body and the needs of strangers. *Hastings Center Report* 17, no. 2:30–38.

———. 1996. *The Worth of a Child*. Berkeley: University of California Press.

———. 1997. What do we mean by "narrative ethics?" *Medical Humanities Review* 11, no. 2:44–57.

Nagel, T. 1986. *The View from Nowhere*. New York: Oxford University Press.

National Bioethics Advisory Commission. 1997. *Cloning Human Beings: Report and Recommendations of the National Bioethics Advisory Commission*. Washington, D.C. [Some parts of this are reproduced in Nussbaum and Sunstein (1998).]

Nelson, H. L. 2000. Stories within the moral life. *New Zealand Bioethics Journal* 1, no. 2:10–20.

Newton-Smith, W. 1981. *The Rationality of Science*. London: Routledge.

Nie, J. B. 2001. So bitter that no words can describe it: Mainland Chinese women's moral experiences and narratives of induced abortion. In *Globalizing Feminist Bioethics*, ed. R. Tong. Oxford: Westview.

Nietzsche, F. [1886] 1975. *Beyond Good and Evil.* Trans. R. J. Hollingdale. London: Penguin.

Nussbaum, M. 1990. *Love's Knowledge.* Oxford: Oxford University Press.

Nussbaum, M., and C. Sunstein. 1998. *Clones and Clones.* New York: Norton & Co.

O'Connor, T. 1991. Human immunodeficiency virus and the surgeon. *RACS Bulletin* July, 30–31.

Ofosu-Amaah, S. 1982. Ethical aspects of externally sponsored research in developing countries: An African viewpoint. In *Human Experimentation and Medical Ethics,* ed. Z. Bankowski and N. Howard-Jones. Geneva: CIOMS.

Orbach, S. 1993. *Hunger Strike.* London: Penguin.

Papps, E., and M. Olssen. 1997. *Doctoring Childbirth and Regulating Midwifery in New Zealand.* Palmerston North: Dunmore.

Parfit, D. 1976. Lewis, Perry, and what matters. In *The Identities of Persons,* ed. A. Rorty. Berkeley: University of California Press.

———. 1986. *Reasons and Persons.* Oxford: Clarendon.

Parker, M. 1990. Moral intuition, good deaths and ordinary medical practitioners. *Journal of Medical Ethics* 16, no. 1:23–29.

Paul, C. 1988. The New Zealand cervical cancer study: Could it happen again? *British Medical Journal* 316:1740–42.

———. 2000. Internal and external morality of medicine: Lessons from New Zealand. *British Medical Journal* 320:499–502.

Pellegrino, E. 1982. *The Healing Relationship: The architectonics of clinical medicine.* Houston: University of Texas Press.

———. 1994. The four principles and the doctor-patient relationship. In *Principles of Health Care Ethics,* ed. R. Gillon and A. Lloyd. Chichester: John Wiley & Sons.

———. 1997. Praxis as a keystone for the philosophy and professional ethics of medicine. In *Philosophy of Medicine and Bioethics,* ed. R. Carson and C. Burns. Dordrecht: Kluwer.

Pellegrino, E., and D. Thomasma. 1988. *For the Patient's Good.* New York: Oxford University Press.

Pietroni, P. 1992. Beyond the boundaries: Relationships between general practice and complementary therapy. *British Medical Journal* 305:564–66.

Pinching, A. 1994. AIDS: Health care ethics and society. In *Principles of Health Care Ethics,* ed. R. Gillon and A Lloyd. Chichester: John Wiley & Sons.

———. 1996. AIDS clinical and scientific background. In *AIDS: A Moral Issue,* 2d ed., ed. B. Almond. London: Macmillan.

Pinching, A., R. Higgs, and K. Boyd. 2000. The impact of AIDS on medical ethics. *Journal of Medical Ethics* 26:3–8.

Poplawski, N., and G. Gillett. 1991. Ethics and embryos. *Journal of Medical Ethics* 17:62–69.

Popper, K. R. 1959. *The Logic of Scientific Discovery.* London: Hutchinson.

Putnam, H. 1973. Meaning and reference. *Journal of Philosophy* 70:699–711.

Rabinow, Paul. 1991. *The Foucault Reader.* London: Penguin Books.

Rawls, J. 1951. Outline of a decision procedure for ethics. *Philosophical Review* 60:177–97.

———. 1955. Two concepts of rules. *Philosophical Review* 64:3–32.

Reilly, D. 2001. Enhancing human healing. *British Medical Journal* 322:120–21.

Resnick, D. 1998. The ethics of HIV research in developing nations. *Bioethics* 12, no. 4: 286–306.

Roach, J. 2000. Management blamed over consultant's malpractice. *British Medical Journal* 320:1557.

Rorty, R. 1986. Foucault and Epistemology. In *Foucault: A Critical Reader*, ed. D. Couzens Hoy. Oxford: Blackwell.

Rouse, J. 1994. Power/Knowledge. In *The Cambridge Companion to Foucault*, ed. G. Gutting. Cambridge: Cambridge University Press.

Ruskin, J. 1989. The cardiac arrhythmia suppression trial. *New England Journal of Medicine* 321, no. 6:386–88.

Sackett, D. L., et al. Evidence based medicine: What it is and what it isn't. *British Medical Journal* 312:71–72.

Sartre, J. P. 1958. *Being and Nothingness*. Trans. H. Barnes. London: Methuen & Co.

Saunders, C. 1994. The dying patient. In *Principles of Health Care Ethics*, ed. R. Gillon and A. Lloyd. Chichester: John Wiley & Sons.

Saunders, J. 1996. Alternative complementary, holistic . . . In *Philosophical Problems in Medicine*, ed. D. Greaves and H. Upton. Aldershot: Avebury.

Scally, G., and L. Donaldson. 1998. Clinical governance and the drive for quality improvement in the new NHS in England. *British Medical Journal* 317:61–65.

Schrode, K. 1995. Life in limbo: Revising policies for permanently unconscious patients. *Houston Law Review* 81, no. 5:1609–68.

Seedhouse, D., and L. Lovett. 1992. *Practical Medical Ethics*. Chichester: John Wiley & Sons.

Sharpe, R. 2001. Complementary medicine: A less than complimentary viewpoint. *New Zealand Medical Journal* 114:410–12.

Singer, P. 1979. *Practical Ethics*. Cambridge: Cambridge University Press.

———. 1992. Embryo experimentation and the moral status of the embryo. In *Philosophy and Health Care*, ed. E. Matthews and M. Menlowe. Aldershot: Avebury.

Skegg, P. 1988. *Law Ethics and Medicine*. Oxford: Clarendon.

Smith, T. 1983. Alternative medicine. *British Medical Journal* 287:307.

Stent, R. 1998. *Canterbury Health Ltd*. Auckland: Health and Disability Commission.

Strawson, P. 1974. *Freedom and Resentment*. London: Methuen.

Studdert, D., et al. 2000. Negligent care and malpractice claiming behavior in Utah and Colorado. *Medical Care* 38, no. 3:250–60.

Taylor, C. 1991. *The Ethics of Authenticity*. Cambridge, Mass.: Harvard University Press.

———. 1992. *Sources of the Self*. Cambridge: Cambridge University Press.

Temkin, O. 1991. *Hippocrates in a World of Pagans and Christians*. Baltimore: Johns Hopkins University Press.

Thielicke, H. 1970. *The Doctor as Judge of Who Shall Live and Who Shall Die*. Philadelphia: Fortress.

Thomson, J. 1971. A defense of abortion. *Philosophy and Public Affairs* 1, no. 1:47–66.

———. 2000. Legal and ethical problems of human cloning. *Journal of Law and Medicine* 8, no. 1:31–43

Tobin, T. 1993. How to implement Rogers v. Whitaker. In *What Should Patients Be Told?* ed. B. Tobin. Sydney: John Plunkett Centre.

Tong, R. 1997. *Feminist Approaches to Bioethics*. Oxford: Westview.

Tooley, M. 1972. Abortion and infanticide. *Philosophy and Public Affairs* 2:37–65.

Toulmin, S. 1997. The primacy of practice: Medicine and post-modernism. In *Philosophy of Medicine and Bioethics*, ed. R. Carson and C. Burns. Dordrecht: Kluwer.

Van Delden, J., L. Pijnenborg, and P. van der Maas. 1993. The Remmelink Study: Two years later. *Hastings Center Report* 25, no. 6:24–27.

Van der Maas, P., J. van Delden, and L. Pijnenborg. 1992. *Medical Decisions Concerning the End of Life*. Amsterdam: Elsevier.

Veatch, R. 2001. The impossibility of a morality internal to medicine. *Journal of Medicine and Philosophy* 26, no. 6:620–42.

Veatch, R., and F. Miller. 2001. The internal morality of medicine: An introduction. *Journal of Medicine and Philosophy* 26, no. 6:555–57.

Verrier, N. N. 1991. The primal wound: Legacy of the adopted child. *Proceedings of the American Adoption Congress*. Garden Grove, Calif.: American Adoption Conference.

Vincent, C., G. Neale, and M. Woloshynowych. 2001. Adverse events in British hospitals: Preliminary retrospective clinical review. *British Medical Journal* 322:517–19.

Walker, R. 1989. *The Coherence Theory of Truth*. London: Routledge.

Warren, D. 1980. Medical malpractice in the United States of America. In *Medical Malpractice*, ed. J. Leahy Taylor. Bristol: John Wright and Sons.

Warren, M. 1992. The moral significance of birth. In *Feminist Perspectives in Bioethics*, ed. H. Bequaert Holmes and L. Purdy. Bloomington: Indiana University Press.

Wartofsky, M. 1997. What can epistemologists learn from the endocrinologists? Or is the philosophy of medicine based on a mistake. In *Philosophy of Medicine and Bioethics*, ed. R. Carson and C. Burns. Dordrecht: Kluwer.

Wettstein, H. 1988. Cognitive significance without cognitive content. *Mind* 385:1–28.

Whelan, C. 1988. Litigation and complaints procedures: Objectives, effectiveness, and alternatives. *Journal of Medical Ethics* 14, no. 2:70–76.

Williams, B. 1985. *Ethics and the Limits of Philosophy*. London: Fontana.

Winch, P. 1972. *Ethics and Action*. London: Routledge.

Wittgenstein, L. 1953. *Philosophical Investigations*. Trans. G. Anscombe. Oxford: Blackwell.

———. 1967. *Zettel*. Trans. G. Anscombe. Oxford: Blackwell.

———. 1969. *Notebooks, 1914–1916*. Trans. G. Anscombe. Oxford: Blackwell.

———. 1974. Lecture on ethics. *Philosophical Review* 74:3–26.

Youngner, S., R. Arnold, and R. Schapiro. 1999. *The Definition of Death*. Baltimore: Johns Hopkins University Press.

Zuger, A., and S. Miles. 1987. Physicians, AIDS, and occupational risk. *Journal of the American Medical Association* 258, no. 14:1924–28.

Index

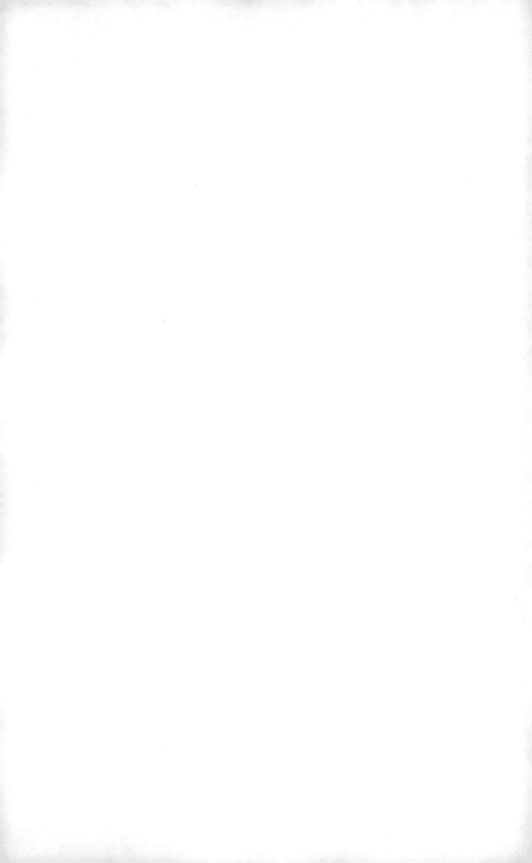

About the Author

Grant Gillett is a professor of medical ethics at the University of Otago and a practicing neurosurgeon. He qualified in medicine at the Auckland Medical School in New Zealand. While at Auckland University he also completed a master's degree in psychology and was, for some years while completing his own studies, a lecturer in physiological psychology. He qualified as a neurosurgeon and took up a post as overseas fellow in neurosurgery at the Radcliffe Infirmary in Oxford. He then enrolled for a D Phil. in philosophy at Oxford University and was appointed to a fellowship at Magdalen College in 1985. From there, he moved to the University of Otago and Dunedin Hospital.

Dr. Gillett is the author of *Representation Meaning and Thought* and *Reasonable Care* and co-author of *The Discursive Mind* and *Medical Ethics*. His latest book is *The Mind and Its Discontents*. He has edited several books and published widely in the areas of philosophy and medical ethics.

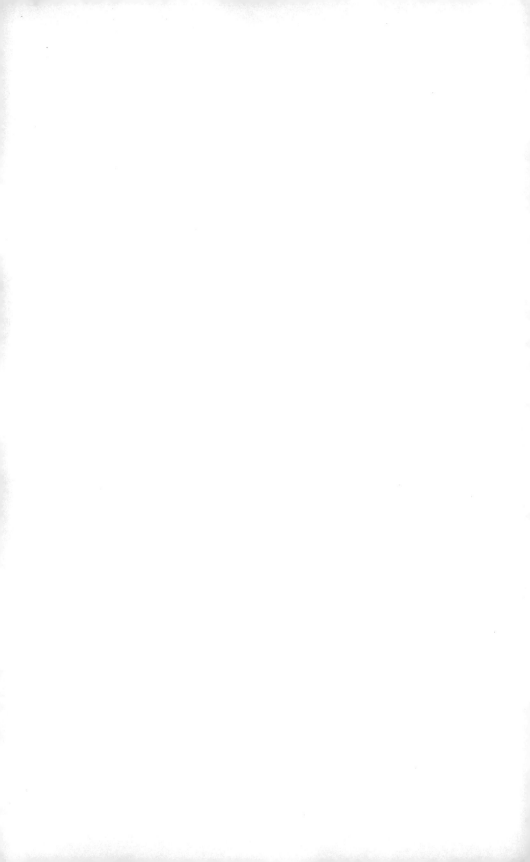